Healthcare-Driven Intelligent Computing Paradigms to Secure Futuristic Smart Cities

Healthcare-Driven Intelligent Computing Paradigms to Secure Futuristic Smart Cities presents the applications of the healthcare sector in the context of futuristic smart cities. It explores various applications like the advancements in computational and network models along with the innovative paradigms for an able healthcare model. The book discusses the state-of-the-art intelligent network and computing paradigms and machine learning models for robust healthcare. It includes several aspects of the challenges faced by a futuristic smart city in healthcare, including challenges emanating from the immense data generated by the wearable sensors, data analysis, and security concerns owing to the patient-related data. It works as a pertinent resource on how cutting-edge technologies can be integrated to aptly provide solutions for the numerous challenges faced by the healthcare industry. It includes several use-cases, practical challenges, and solutions for executing smart healthcare.

Features

- Covers a multitude of computing paradigms, namely, Cloud Computing, Fog Computing, and Mist Computing.
- Healthcare is discussed leveraging smart city, so it can potentially identify the gaps and present some newer use-cases to handle future pandemics.
- The network aspect is also covered with an inclusion of the next-generation paradigm which is software-defined networking (SDN).
- Security and privacy issues are considered, which is crucial to handle security-related aspects.
- Machine learning models are also discussed to assist any entrepreneur in developing a business model involving cutting-edge technologies.

This book is for academicians, researchers, and entrepreneurs working on healthcare-driven intelligent computing paradigms to secure futuristic smart cities.

High-Performance Computing for Smart Healthcare: New Developments and Advances

Series Editors

Rishabha Malviya
Galgotias University, India

Balamurugan Balusamy
Shiv Nadar University, India

Sonali Sundram
Galgotias University, India

Forthcoming and Published Titles:

Healthcare-Driven Intelligent Computing Paradigms to Secure Futuristic Smart Cities
Diptendu Sinha Roy, Mir Wajahat Hussain, K. Hemant Kumar Reddy, Deepak Gupta

Healthcare-Driven Intelligent Computing Paradigms to Secure Futuristic Smart Cities

Edited by
Diptendu Sinha Roy, Mir Wajahat Hussain,
K. Hemant Kumar Reddy, and Deepak Gupta

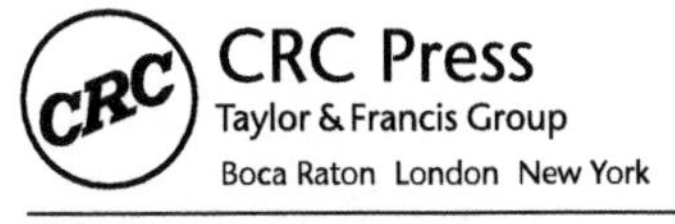

CRC Press is an imprint of the
Taylor & Francis Group, an informa business
A CHAPMAN & HALL BOOK

Designed cover image: ShutterStock Images

First edition published 2025
by CRC Press
2385 NW Executive Center Drive, Suite 320, Boca Raton FL 33431

and by CRC Press
4 Park Square, Milton Park, Abingdon, Oxon, OX14 4RN

CRC Press is an imprint of Taylor & Francis Group, LLC

Library of Congress Cataloging-in-Publication Data
Names: Roy, Diptendu Sinha, editor. | Hussain, Mir Wajahat, editor. | Reddy, K. Hemant Kumar, 1977- editor. | Gupta, Deepak (Ph.D. in physics), editor.
Title: Healthcare-driven intelligent computing paradigms to secure futuristic smart cities / edited by Diptendu Sinha Roy, Mir Wajahat Hussain, K. Hemant Kumar Reddy, Deepak Gupta.
Other titles: High-performance computing for smart healthcare: new developments and advances.
Description: Boca Raton : C&H/CRC Press, 2025. | Series: High-performance computing for smart healthcare: new developments and advances | Includes bibliographical references and index.
Identifiers: LCCN 2024024388 (print) | LCCN 2024024389 (ebook) | ISBN 9781032626895 (hardback) | ISBN 9781032631714 (paperback) | ISBN 9781032631738 (ebook).
Subjects: MESH: Delivery of Health Care | Medical Informatics Applications | Artificial Intelligence | Computing Methodologies | Cities
Classification: LCC R859 (print) | LCC R859 (ebook) | NLM W 26.5 | DDC 362.10285--dc23/eng/20240627
LC record available at https://lccn.loc.gov/2024024388
LC ebook record available at https://lccn.loc.gov/2024024389

ISBN: 978-1-032-62689-5 (hbk)
ISBN: 978-1-032-63171-4 (pbk)
ISBN: 978-1-032-63173-8 (ebk)

DOI: 10.1201/9781032631738

Typeset in Times
by SPi Technologies India Pvt Ltd (Straive)

Contents

Foreword

Healthcare has seen tremendous advancements over the past decade owing to immense technological advancements in the field of Information and Communication Technologies. This continuum of advancements has played a pivotal role in enabling a focus on smart healthcare in a smart city whose primary aim is to improve living conditions. The book *Healthcare-Driven Intelligent Computing Paradigms to Secure Futuristic Smart Cities* is a comprehensive guide to the former field and provides an inevitable resource for understanding the latest developments in the areas of smart healthcare and smart cities.

The entire book has been segregated into 20 chapters, with each chapter capturing the state-of-the-art technologies along with the healthcare-based novel use-cases, covering a wide array of key technologies such as artificial intelligence, machine learning, cloud computing, fog computing, mist computing, blockchain, Internet of Things, software-defined networking, and machine learning among others. Each chapter includes specific topics like COVID-19, pneumonia, heart diseases, and the study of various cancers, apart from the novel healthcare applications.

The book's strengths include its wide coverage of the topics and the integration of key enabling technologies with healthcare. The authors have done a handsome job of providing novel methodologies and insights into future avenues and opportunities for researchers to explore. This book will provide further impetus to undergraduates, graduates, and other experts to kickstart and explore the area in detail.

I am strongly of the opinion that this book will meet the expectations of the scientific community and, particularly, will bridge the gap between technocrats and medical professionals. I would like to applaud both the editors and authors for producing such an asset and capturing the entire essence of the area. I strongly recommend this book to those who are interested in the healthcare field, and it will be a boon to explore the cohesiveness of technologies.

Dr Xiaochun Cheng
Department of Computer Science,
Swansea University,
Bay Campus,
Fabian Way,
Swansea, SA1 8EN
Wales, UK
Email: xiaochun.cheng@swansea.ac.uk
ORCID iD: https://orcid.org/0000-0003-0371-9646
DBLP: https://dblp.uni-trier.de/pers/hd/c/Cheng:Xiaochun
Google-Scholar: https://scholar.google.com/citations?hl=en&user=0i9Ga8QAAAAJ

Preface

The concept of smart cities has gained significant traction in recent years, with advancements in Information and Communication Technologies paving the way for a more connected and efficient urban environment and healthcare being its primary focus. One crucial aspect of smart cities is the integration of healthcare-driven intelligent computing paradigms to ensure the security of futuristic healthcare services. This book *Healthcare-Driven Intelligent Computing Paradigms to Secure Futuristic Smart Cities* discusses the state-of-the-art intelligent network, computing paradigms, and machine learning models for robust healthcare.

The first chapter highlights the introduction to healthcare in a detailed manner, with a focus on smart cities. The second chapter emphasizes body transfer systems to assist the elderly and disabled. The next two chapters address artificial intelligence (AI), machine learning, and the Internet of Things (IoT) in integration with the healthcare system in a smart city. In addition to the former key technologies, AI is intertwined with the IoT to optimize the multi-hop healthcare system. As healthcare requires a stringent Quality of Service (QoS), a framework is proposed in the sixth chapter that includes the cohesion of software-defined wireless networking (SDWN) and double deep reinforcement learning (DDRL). It is followed by two chapters highlighting the issue of outlier removal for cluster identification and proposing a novel cluster weighting method. Chapter 9 discusses the pertinent issue of the security and privacy of healthcare data and identifies several novel use-cases highlighting the issue in a smart city environment. The next chapter delves into how to detect pneumonia using a mix of techniques for improving accuracy and COVID-19 detection, as well as identifying false negatives and addressing the improvement of testing efficacy.

The subsequent chapters deal with disease detection and prediction. Chapters 10 and 11 focus on depression, its symptoms, and prediction. Chapters 14–16 discuss in detail the detection and prediction of cancers using multiple techniques, including breast, ovarian, and brain cancer. Another crucial aspect of the issue addressed is heart disease detection and prediction. Chapter 17 provides a detailed survey of heart disease detection employing federated learning models. Chapter 18 proposes a novel methodology for early and correct disease prediction for diagnosis and treatment recommendations utilizing the grey wolf transfer learning model based on multi-perceptron neural networks. Chapter 19 highlights the Mist-Fog model employing federated learning integrated with an ensemble model to improve accuracy and lower the execution time for heart disease prediction. Finally, the last chapter utilizes Mist Computing, the IoT, and deep reinforcement learning for predicting cardiac disease with better-lowering energy and latency values.

This book is tailored to meet the requirements of undergraduates, postgraduates, academicians, researchers, and entrepreneurs to transform the healthcare industry. It includes several use-cases, practical challenges, and solutions for executing smarter healthcare. Healthcare-driven intelligent computing paradigms are integral to the success of secure and futuristic smart cities. In a nutshell, *Healthcare-Driven Intelligent Computing Paradigms to Secure Futuristic Smart Cities* is a pertinent resource on how cutting-edge technologies will be integrated to aptly provide solutions for the numerous challenges faced by the healthcare industry and will serve as an invaluable resource for the intended community.

Editors

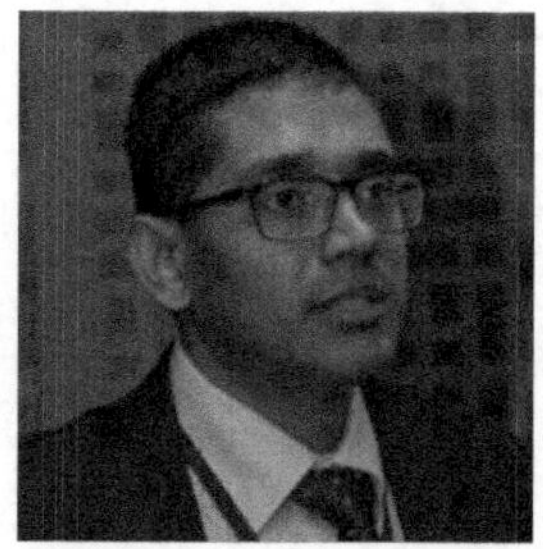

Diptendu Sinha Roy was born in Hooghly, India. He received his B.Tech. degree from Kalyani University, Kalyani, India, in 2003, and the M.Tech. and Ph.D. from the Birla Institute of Technology, Mesra, Ranchi, India, in 2005 and 2010, respectively. He is currently with the National Institute of Technology, Meghalaya, where he is the Head of the Department of Computer Science and Engineering. His current research interests include distributed, grid computing, cloud computing, fog computing, software reliability, and optimization in engineering. He also performs research on design and analysis of distributed infrastructure of power systems.

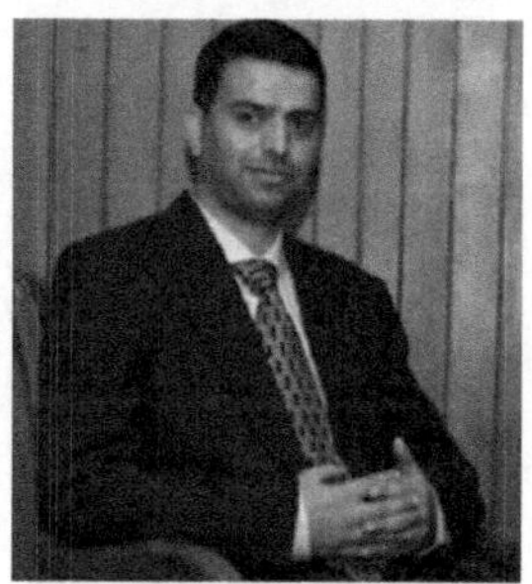

Mir Wajahat Hussain was born in Jammu & Kashmir, India. He received his B.Tech. degree from the University of Kashmir, India, in 2014, and his master's degree and Ph.D. from the National Institute of Technology, Arunachal Pradesh, and National Institute of Technology, Meghalaya, India, in 2017 and 2021, respectively. He is currently with Alliance University, India, as an Assistant Professor. His research interests include software-defined networks and big data.

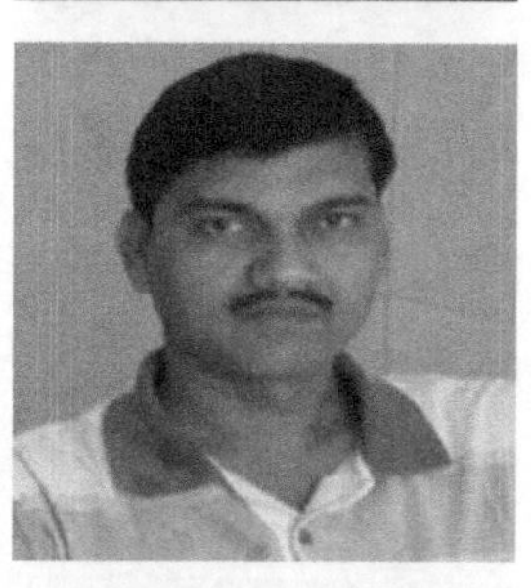

K. Hemant Kumar Reddy was born in Berhampur, India. He received the M.Tech. and Ph.D. degrees from Berhampur University, Bhanja Vihar, India, in 2008 and 2014, respectively. He is currently with the VIT-AP University, India, as an Associate Professor. He is also serving as an associate editor of *Journal of Intelligent and Fuzzy Systems* (JIFS). His research interests include distributed and grid computing, cloud computing, fog computing, and service-oriented architectures.

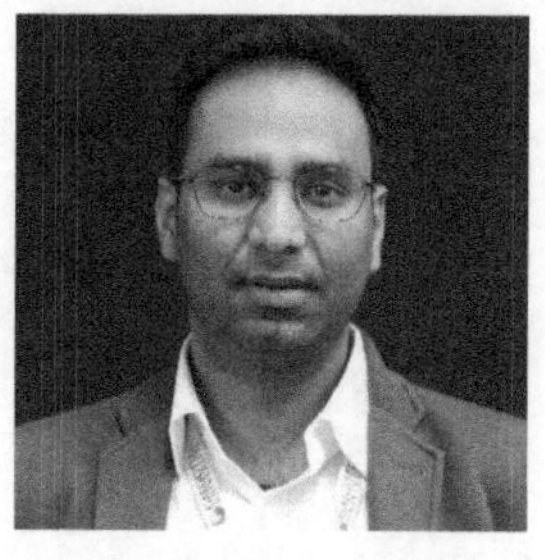

Deepak Gupta was born in Delhi, India. He has completed B.Sc. Honors in Physics from Delhi University, Delhi, and M.Sc. in Physics from Kumaun University, Nainital. He obtained his doctorate in Physics from the National Institute of Technology Meghalaya, Shillong. He also worked as a research associate at NIT Meghalaya, Shillong. He is currently working at Galgotias University, Greater Noida. His areas of interest include molecular electronics and soft matter computation.

Contributors

Inioluwa Adewuyi
Department of Computer Science
Federal University of Agriculture, Abeokuta
Nigeria

V. Aishwharya
Mepco Schlenk Engineering College
Sivakasi, India

R. Akiladevi
Department of Computer Science and Engineering
Rajalakshmi Engineering College
Chennai, India

Isuru Ariyarathne
Department of Computer Science and Engineering
Faculty of Engineering
University of Moratuwa
Moratuwa, Sri Lanka

D. Aswini
Department of Computer Science and Engineering
Kumaraguru College of Technology
India

Bahrudin
Department of Mechanical Engineering
National Taiwan University of Science and Technology
Taipei, Taiwan

Meelan Bandara
Department of Computer Science and Engineering
Faculty of Engineering
University of Moratuwa
Moratuwa, Sri Lanka

Sujit Bebortta
Department of Computer Science
Ravenshaw University
Cuttack, India

J. Jerold John Britto
Department of Mechanical Engineering
Ramco Institute of Technology
Rajapalayam, India

Giovanni Cicceri
Department of Engineering
University of Messina, Italy

Shom Prasad Das
Department of Computer Science Engineering
Birla Global University
Bhubaneswar, Odisha, India

Sima Das
Department of Computer Science and Engineering
Bengal College of Engineering and Technology
West Bengal, India

G. Gokila Deepa
Department of Artificial Intelligence and Data Science
PPG Institute of Technology
India

B. Dhiyanesh
Department of Computer Science and Engineering
Dr. N.G.P. Institute of Technology
India

A. Shahina Fathima
Mepco Schlenk Engineering College
Sivakasi, India

Idris Gbolade
Department of Computer Science
Federal University of Agriculture, Abeokuta
Nigeria

Mehdi Gheisari
Department of Computer Science
Islamic Azad University
Tehran, Iran

A. Beena Godbin
School of Computer Science and Engineering
Vellore Institute of Technology, Chennai
Chennai, India

Vaibhav Guru
Department of Computer Science and Engineering
Amity School of Engineering and Technology
Amity University Maharashtra
Maharashtra, India

R. Sree Harini
Mepco Schlenk Engineering College
Sivakasi, India

Mir Wajahat Hussain
Department of Computer Science and Engineering
Alliance University
Karnataka, India

G. Indumathi
Department of ECE
Mepco Schlenk Engineering College
Sivakasi, India

I. Janani
Department of Information Technology
Sona college of Technology
India

S. Graceline Jasmine
School of Computer Science and Engineering
Vellore Institute of Technology, Chennai
Chennai, India

Roshinie Jayasundara
Department of Computer Science and Engineering
Faculty of Engineering
University of Moratuwa
Moratuwa, Sri Lanka

Thirumoorthy Karpagalingam
Department of Computer Science and Engineering
Mepco Schlenk Engineering College
Sivakasi, India

Naufil Arif Kazi
Department of Computer Science and Engineering
Amity School of Engineering and Technology
Amity University Maharashtra
Maharashtra, India

Aadi Koshal
Amador Valley High School
Pleasanton, California

Rath Suneel Kumar
Deparment of Computer Science Engineering
C.V. Raman Global University
Bhubaneswar, Odisha, India

Vikash Kumar
Department of Mechanical Engineering
National Institute of Technology Rourkela
Odisha, India

C. B. Selva Lakshmi
Department of Computer Science and Engineering
Velammal College of Engineering and Technology
India

J. M. Sheela Lavanya
School of Computer Science and Engineering
Vellore Institute of Technology, Chennai
Chennai, India

Chyi-Yeu Lin
Department of Mechanical Engineering
National Taiwan University of Science and Technology
Taipei, Taiwan

S. K. Manasa
Department of Computer Science and Engineering
Mepco Schlenk Engineering College
Sivakasi, India

N. Malathy
Mepco Schlenk Engineering College
Sivakasi, India

Jyoteesh Malhotra
Department of Electronics and Communication Engineering
National Institute of Technology, Delhi
India

Salman Masroor
Department of Mechanical Engineering
National Taiwan University of Science and Technology
Taipei, Taiwan

Dulani Meedeniya
Department of Computer Science and Engineering
Faculty of Engineering
University of Moratuwa
Moratuwa, Sri Lanka

Umar Muhammad Modibbo
Department of Operations Research
Modibbo Adama University
Yola, Nigeria

P. Nancy
School of Computing
SRM Institute of Science and Technology
India

Abayomi Ojo
Department of Anaesthesia
Obafemi Awolowo University Teaching Hospital
Ile-Ife, Nigeria

Oluwafolake Ojo
Department of Computer Science
Federal University of Agriculture
Abeokuta, Nigeria

Oluwadolapo Oni
Department of Computer Science
Federal University of Agriculture, Abeokuta
Nigeria

Olufunke Oyinloye
Department of Computing
University of Ilesa
Ilesa, Nigeria

Deepa Parasar
Department of Computer Science and Engineering
Amity School of Engineering and Technology
Amity University Maharashtra
Maharashtra, India

M. Blessa Binolin Pepsi
Mepco Schlenk Engineering College
Sivakasi, India

Bhanu Priya
School of Electronics and Electrical Engineering
Lovely Professional University
Phagwara, India

M. Ramya
Mepco Schlenk Engineering College
Sivakasi, India

Soumya Sidhartha Ray
Department of Electrical and Computer Engineering
Ajay Binay Institute of Technology
Cuttack, India

Madhusmita Sahu
Dept of Computer Science Engineering
C.V. Raman Global University
Bhubaneswar, Odisha, India

Wasswa Shafik
School of Digital Science
University Brunei Darussalam
Brunei Darussalam

Abhishek Sharma
Department of Electronics and Communication Engineering
National Institute of Technology
Hamirpur, India

Butta Singh
Department of Engineering and Technology
Guru Nanak Dev University Regional Centre
Jalandhar, India

Kuldeep Singh
Department of Electronics Technology
Guru Nanak Dev University
Amritsar, India

Manjit Singh
Department of Engineering and Technology
Guru Nanak Dev University Regional Centre
Jalandhar, India

P. Subbulakshmi
School of Computer Science and Engineering
Vellore Institute of Technology, Chennai
Chennai, India

K. Vijaya Subasri
Mepco Schlenk Engineering College
Sivakasi, India

V. Sudha
Department of Computer Engineering
Government Polytechnic College
India

G. Sujitha
Department of ECE
Mepco Schlenk Engineering College
Sivakasi, India

J. Grace Sophia
Mepco Schlenk Engineering College
Sivakasi, India

Biswajit Tripathy
Department of Computer Science
Ravenshaw University
Cuttack, India

Niva Tripathy
Department of Computer Science and Engineering
Dhaneswar Rath Institute of Engineering and Management Studies
Cuttack, India

Subhranshu Sekhar Tripathy
School of Computer Engineering
Kalinga Institute of Industrial Technology
Bhubaneshwar, India

K. Vishveswari
Department of ECE
Mepco Schlenk Engineering College
Sivakasi, India

Lachiket Narendra Warule
Department of Computer Science and Engineering
Amity School of Engineering and Technology
Amity University Maharashtra
Maharashtra, India

T. Yawanikha
Department of Information Technology
Karpagam Institute of Technology
India

1

Healthcare and Its Applications in a Smart City

Wasswa Shafik
School of Digital Science University, Brunei, Darussalam

1.1 Introduction

The smart city is a concept that concentrates on leveraging innovation and data-driven remedies to boost the way-of-life of homeowners and enhance cosmopolitan living, ensuring good health in sustainable cities and areas with answerable consumption and manufacturing (Aldhyani et al., 2023). Smart cities stand for a vision of a connected and sustainable urban atmosphere where countless systems and solutions collaborate perfectly to enhance resources, increase efficiency, and boost the general wellness of its residents to improve user experiences (Ahmed et al., 2023; Reddy et al., 2023). These cities demonstrate an advanced innovation containing the Internet of Things (IoT), detailed artificial intelligence (AI) analytics, and connection frameworks. These aspects enable companies to gather and evaluate substantial quantities of data from numerous resources, allowing real-time insights and educated decision-making for city administrators, citizens, and companies (AlZu'bi et al., 2023).

The emphasis of sustainable cities is to attend to the problems and requirements of city living by releasing lasting alternatives across various domain names. This includes areas such as transport, power, medical care, public safety and security, waste tracking, and administration. By utilizing modern-day technology in these areas, sustainable cities aim to increase their homeowners' sustainability, general quality of life, and performance (Dutta et al., 2023). In medical care, a clever city leverages modern-day technology to reinvent treatment circulation and availability. It entails the integration of digital health and wellness treatments, telemedicine, remote person monitoring, and wearable gadgets to give tailored and favorable medical care remedies. This integration yields increased continuous interaction between customers (technology users) and physicians, remote diagnosis and therapy, early problem exploration, and trusted source allocation (Aldhyani et al., 2023).

The idea of a smart and sustainable city stands for a prediction of data-driven operations. This interconnected city environment utilizes modern technology to fix the complicated problems of urbanization. By leveraging modern technology for improved metropolitan living, smart cities aim to produce long-term, effective, and

DOI: 10.1201/9781032631738-1

comprehensive atmospheres that boost their lifestyle, entailing health (Aldossary, 2023). In addition, these cities market personal involvement and engagement by leveraging innovation systems that allow locals to contribute to decision-making treatments and supply discuss services proactively. With electronic interfaces, homeowners can access details regarding different city services, experience considerable problems, and partner with community authorities to co-create choices for everyday problems (Chakraborty et al., 2023).

By utilizing modern innovation to optimize source use, reduce eco-friendly impact, and advertise renewable energy sources, sustainable cities aim to create eco-friendly city areas. This includes efficient waste tracking, sustainable energy consumption, an environment-friendly framework, administration systems, and intelligent transportation networks, among others (Ahmed et al., 2023). In public safety, smart cities use sophisticated tracking systems, anticipating analytics, and emergency feedback systems to improve security and secure their locals. These contemporary technologies enable extremely early detection of possible risks, efficient occasion reactions, and enhanced control among different participants (AlZu'bi et al., 2023).

Moreover, the term "smart city" extends beyond the physical framework and technological innovations. It entails smart policy structures, policies, and partnerships between federal government entities, economic sector companies, the academic community, and the city residents. Partnership and collaboration are vital in realizing the vision of a smart city, as they require the experience and input of multiple stakeholders. As the international population continues to concentrate in urban locations, the smart city principle becomes progressively appropriate (Dutta et al., 2023). By leveraging technology for enhanced city living, smart cities have the potential to take on pushing difficulties such as traffic jams, environmental pollution, inadequate healthcare access, and resource shortage (Hussain, 2024; Hussain & Roy, 2021, 2022a, 2022b, 2023b).

In the context of a smart city, medical care holds tremendous significance as a result of its potential to reinvent residents' wellness and quality of life. Incorporating medical care solutions within a smart city structure addresses crucial challenges and boosts healthcare delivery access and efficiency (Ahmed et al., 2023; AlZu'bi et al., 2023). Healthcare in a sustainable city context concentrates on boosting the availability of medical solutions. By leveraging innovation, smart cities can get over geographical barriers and supply healthcare services to remote or underserved areas (AlZu'bi et al., 2023). Telemedicine platforms make online appointments possible, allowing locals to get in touch with healthcare experts without requiring physical traveling. Smart cities extend from healthcare to other areas like technology, transportation, power, atmosphere, and economic situations with AI and IoT, as exhibited in Figure 1.1.

This conserves time, decreases transport expenses, and ensures that individuals in remote areas receive prompt medical guidance and treatment. A smart city medical care system emphasizes preventive treatment and early discovery of conditions. With the assimilation of wearable gadgets and wellness monitoring technologies, individuals can track their crucial indicators, activity degrees, and other wellness indications in real time (Dutta et al., 2023). By empowering people to take aggressive actions, sustainable city healthcare advertises a shift from responsive treatments to preventive measures, eventually reducing the concern about medical care systems.

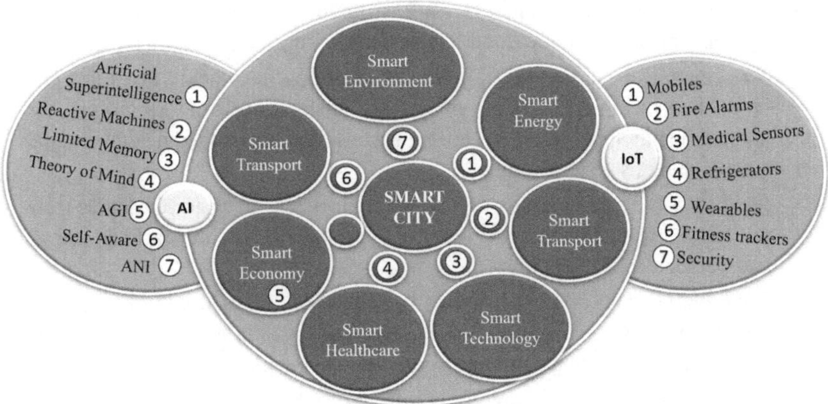

FIGURE 1.1 Application of artificial intelligence and Internet of Things in smart cities.

A sustainable city's focus on data analytics and AI applications in medical care enables more exact diagnoses, therapy optimization, and resource allowance. By assessing big volumes of medical information, including clinical imaging and electronic health records (EHRs), AI algorithms can aid healthcare experts in making accurate diagnoses and suggesting customized treatment strategies. This improves individual outcomes, decreases clinical errors, and enhances sources such as medical facility beds, medical devices, and medical care workers (Ahmed et al., 2023). Additionally, incorporating healthcare options within such a developed high-tech city framework enhances overall practical performance. Smart healthcare centers and healthcare centers utilize modern-day innovation to automate monitoring tasks, boost procedures, and improve customer management systems.

This reputable use of sources triggers far better medical care delivery and improved personal experiences and management of EHRs. Because of this, medical care in a lasting city context is vital in managing the troubles of city living and boosting people's wellness (Dutta et al., 2023). By leveraging modern-day innovation, details analytics, and AI applications, clever cities can increase the convenience of gaining access to market preventative treatment, make it feasible to get specific medical diagnoses and treatments, and enhance overall practical efficiency in healthcare circulation. Incorporating medical care options within a sustainable city framework establishes lasting and comprehensive city settings that concentrate on the health and wellness of citizens, as this phase shows (Aldhyani et al., 2023).

1.1.1 Contribution of the Chapter

This study avails the following contributions as summarized below:

- This chapter explores healthcare integration within a smart city framework, highlighting the utilization of high-tech and data-driven explanations to increase sustainable metropolitan healthcare services.

- It examines the role of smart city infrastructure elements such as connectivity, sensors, data analytics, and IoT devices in improving healthcare delivery.
- The chapter discusses the significance of remote healthcare and telemedicine, showcasing the benefits of virtual consultations, remote monitoring, and telehealth applications regarding accessibility, enhanced healthcare outcomes, and cost-effectiveness.
- It explores the incorporation of health monitoring with wearable device technologies, emphasizing their role in enabling preventive care, early detection, and personalized medicine.
- Data analytics and AI applications in healthcare are explored, focusing on disease prediction, diagnosis, treatment optimization, and resource allocation while considering challenges and ethical considerations.
- The concept of smart hospitals is introduced, highlighting their ability to enhance healthcare delivery through technology integration, automation, EHRs, and patient tracking.
- The chapter concludes by discussing the challenges, future directions, lessons learned, and policy considerations for healthcare in smart cities, providing recommendations for stakeholders to maximize the benefits of integrating healthcare within a smart city framework.

1.1.2 The Chapter Organization

Section 1.2 discovers smart city infrastructure and medical care, going over the important elements of smart city facilities, such as connectivity, sensors, information analytics, and IoT tools. It additionally clarifies exactly how these aspects can be used to improve healthcare services in a smart city by highlighting the benefits of incorporating health care right into the total smart city structure. Section 1.3 demonstrates telemedicine and remote health care, discussing the concept of telemedicine and its relevance in a smart city, reviewing how telemedicine makes it possible for remote healthcare solutions, consisting of digital consultations, remote tracking and telehealth applications, and discovering the advantages of telemedicine in terms of accessibility, cost-effectiveness, and boosting medical care results. Section 1.4 provides health and wellness surveillance and wearable gadgets and discusses the duty of wearable gadgets, such as, smartwatches, health and fitness trackers, and wellness sensing units, in a smart city healthcare community. Explain exactly how these devices can collect and transmit real-time health and wellness information to healthcare providers and people, highlighting the prospective advantages of health and wellness monitoring and wearable devices in preventive care, early detection, and individualized medicine. Section 1.5 portrays data analytics and AI in medical care, describing how data analytics and AI innovations can be leveraged in a smart city healthcare system. Go over the applications of AI in health care, such as disease forecast, diagnosis, treatment optimization, and resource allowance, and highlight the possible challenges and ethical factors to consider related to utilizing information analytics and AI in health care. Section 1.6 presents the concept of smart hospitals and medical care facilities and goes over how they incorporate technology to boost healthcare shipment. Check out the functions of a smart hospital, consisting of EHRs, smart beds, automated systems, and individual tracking. Explain just how smart hospitals boost personal results, functional effectiveness, and source monitoring. Section 1.7 shows this research's standard recognized challenges and future directions, providing the obstacles and barriers to applying medical care in a smart city context, such as information privacy, safety, and security, interoperability, and framework requirements. Discover future advancements and developments in smart city medical care, consisting of arising innovations and plan factors to consider. Finally, Section 1.8 offers the lessons gained and the chapter conclusion.

1.2 Smart City Infrastructure in Healthcare Perspective

These infrastructures are pivotal in transforming and improving health outcomes and healthcare delivery in urban environments. The integration of advanced technologies, connectivity, and data-driven solutions enables the development of innovative healthcare systems that are more accessible, efficient, and patient-centric.

1.2.1 Smart City Infrastructure

This develops the foundation of city facilities, enabling smooth interaction and information exchange between healthcare stakeholders. Dependable and high-speed web connections assist in telemedicine solutions, remote individual tracking, and real-time transmission of individual information, making it possible for healthcare specialists to offer prompt and educated treatment (Ahmed et al., 2023). Sensing units and IoT tools are indispensable to clever city frameworks that boost healthcare solutions. These gadgets can be released in healthcare centers, homes, and public areas to keep track of ecological elements, discover health-related occasions, and accumulate real-time wellness information. For example, IoT-enabled wearables can track important indicators and task degrees, equipping people to take control of their wellness and making it possible for doctors to keep track of patients from another location (AlZu'bi et al., 2023). Information analytics and AI are critical in leveraging the riches of information produced within a sustainable city medical care environment. Information analytics likewise promotes populace wellness monitoring, making it possible for policymakers to determine health and wellness fads, assign sources properly, and establish targeted treatments.

This structure further permits the development of telemedicine and remote medical care solutions. Online examinations, remote monitoring, and telehealth applications bridge the gap between medical care people and providers, especially in areas with restricted accessibility to treatment centers (Dutta et al., 2023). Clients acquire clinical assistance, prescriptions, and succeeding treatment without leaving their homes, thus decreasing the stress on physical medical care centers and improving medical care accessibility. Integration of EHRs within smart city infrastructure streamlines healthcare processes and enhances care coordination. EHRs enable secure and centralized storage of patient information, accessible to authorized healthcare providers across different healthcare settings (Aldhyani et al., 2023). This seamless exchange of medical data ensures continuity of care, reduces duplication of tests, and facilitates informed decision-making by healthcare professionals.

Smart city facilities additionally support the idea of smart healthcare facilities, where technology and automation boost performance and client care. Automated appointment scheduling, person enrollment, and prescription administration systems lessen administrative concerns, allowing healthcare specialists to concentrate extra on client treatment (Aldossary, 2023). Smart hospitals also employ IoT devices, robotics, and AI-powered systems for patient monitoring, asset management, and infection control, improving patient safety and operational efficiency. The following are the key elements of a smart city infrastructure: connectivity, sensors, data analytics, and IoT devices, as illustrated below.

1.2.1.1 Connectivity

Connection is an essential and essential element of smart city infrastructure, allowing smooth interaction and information exchange between numerous stakeholders and systems within the city setting (Aldossary, 2023). Reputable and high-speed connectivity develops the backbone that promotes the integration of advanced innovations and makes it possible for the growth of cutting-edge services in healthcare and various other industries. In healthcare, connection plays an important function in allowing telemedicine services. With robust net connections, doctors can offer digital assessments, enabling individuals to access medical recommendations and treatment from another location (Alwakeel et al., 2023). This is especially helpful for individuals living in remote or underserved locations, as they can receive medical care services without requiring carnal transportation. Telemedicine also assists in the sharing of medical information, such as examination outcomes and imaging research studies, between medical care experts, making certain reliable collaboration, and timely decision-making (Reddy Yeruva, 2023).

Moreover, connectivity enables remote client tracking, where wearable gadgets and IoT-enabled sensors collect real-time wellness data and send it to healthcare providers (Hussain et al., 2022). As an example, individuals with persistent problems can make use of connected gadgets to check their important indications, such as heart price, blood pressure, or glucose degrees (Ahmed et al., 2023). The collected information can be transferred to medical care specialists who can remotely keep track of the client's health and interfere if any irregularities or worries arise. This remote monitoring method advertises hostile treatment management and extremely early treatment, enhancing wellness outcomes and reducing medical care costs. In addition, it aids in the exchange of wellness information via EHRs (AlZu'bi et al., 2023). With joined systems, physicians can access and share personal records securely and perfectly, no matter their physical location.

This makes it feasible to link treatment, eliminates the requirement for recurring exams or treatments, and ensures that medical care specialists can access existing customer info. In addition to healthcare, connection sustains clever city initiatives, such as smart transportation systems, power tracking, and public safety and security (Aldhyani et al., 2023). For instance, attached picking-up devices and gizmos in transportation centers can supply real-time website traffic info, make the best use of internet website traffic circulation, and permit intelligent vehicle auto parking solutions (Hussain et al., 2022). In public safety and security, the connection makes it feasible for the launch of safety webcams, emergency activity systems, and communication networks that aid in prompt and collaborative activities throughout emergencies (Chakraborty et al., 2023).

1.2.1.2 Sensors

Sensing units are a crucial component of smart city infrastructure, playing a crucial duty in collecting real-time information and offering important understandings for numerous applications within metropolitan environments, including healthcare. Sensors are deployed across the city to monitor parameters, collect information, and enable data-driven decision-making (Tripathi et al., 2023). In healthcare, sensors track and monitor environmental factors, health-related events, and individual health indicators. For instance, air quality sensors measure pollutants and particulate matter, providing valuable data on air pollution levels to help identify areas with poor air quality and guide interventions to improve respiratory health (Sharma et al., 2023). Similarly, noise sensors can detect excessive noise levels in urban areas, aiding in noise pollution management and significantly impacting public health and well-being.

In specific health and wellness tracking, wearable devices equipped with various sensing units, such as heart price monitors, accelerometers, and temperature sensors, enable people to track their important indicators and task levels in real time. These sensors provide data on heart rate variability, steps taken, sleep patterns, and other health-related metrics (El-Fouly et al., 2023). This information can encourage physical activity, detect early signs of health issues, and promote overall well-being. Sensors are also employed in healthcare facilities to enhance patient care. For example, smart beds equipped with pressure sensors can detect patient movement and adjust mattress firmness to prevent pressure ulcers (Samy El menchawy et al., 2023). Motion sensors in hospitals can track the movement of healthcare staff and equipment, facilitating workflow optimization and ensuring efficient resource allocation.

Furthermore, occupancy sensors can monitor the availability of hospital beds, helping to manage patient flow and improve bed utilization. Furthermore, sensors integrated into infrastructure elements like streetlights and waste management systems contribute to the overall efficiency and sustainability of the city (Sharma et al., 2023). Smart streetlights equipped with occupancy sensors can adjust lighting levels based on the presence of pedestrians or vehicles, optimizing energy consumption. Waste management systems with fill-level sensors can monitor garbage bins' capacity, optimizing waste collection routes and reducing unnecessary truck movements, leading to cost savings and minimizing environmental impact (El-Fouly et al., 2023).

1.2.1.3 Data Analytics

Info analytics is a crucial element of the smart city framework, permitting the elimination of advantageous understandings and workable info from the large number of details generated within city setups. By leveraging ingenious analytics techniques, cities can make data-driven selections and enhance the effectiveness of numerous services, including healthcare (Hussain et al., 2023a). Information analytics are exceptionally essential in populace health surveillance (Kushwaha et al., 2023). By checking out aggregated and anonymized health details, cities can acknowledge patterns and health risks within the people. For instance, evaluating info on health problem regularity, group elements, and eco-friendly troubles can assist in figuring out locations with greater event rates of detail problems or wellness and health variations (Zakzouk et al., 2023). This information can route the development of targeted therapies, public health projects, and source slices to take care of comprehensive health issues and advertise much healthier locations.

Info analytics additionally promotes anticipating modeling and the very early discovery of wellness issues. By evaluating historical and real-time wellness information, cities can develop solutions and designs to prepare for problem breakouts, determine at-risk populations, and identify health-related abnormalities (Cabrera et al., 2023). This allows hostile therapies, timely actions, and safeguards to minimize the spread of conditions, lower healthcare costs, and enhance overall public health outcomes. Moreover, information analytics enhance treatment shipment and resource optimization (Joe et al., 2023). By assessing specific information, therapy results, and healthcare application patterns, cities can determine locations for improvement in service distribution, boost therapy paths, and appoint resources appropriately.

As an example, evaluating emergency clinic information can help in figuring out traffic jams and making the best use of procedures, decreasing delay times and boosting client fulfillment. Data analytics also supports source planning, such as designating medical care employees, medical equipment, and health center beds based on demand patterns and utilization rates (Fan et al., 2023). Moreover, data analytics allow personalized and precision medication. By incorporating numerous information resources, such as digital health records, hereditary info, and way-of-life data, cities can develop formulas and models that supply tailored recommendations for illness avoidance, treatment optimization, and medication monitoring (Fan et al., 2023). This tailored method of health care boosts personal outcomes, reduces medical errors, and improves patient experiences, as demonstrated in Figure 1.2.

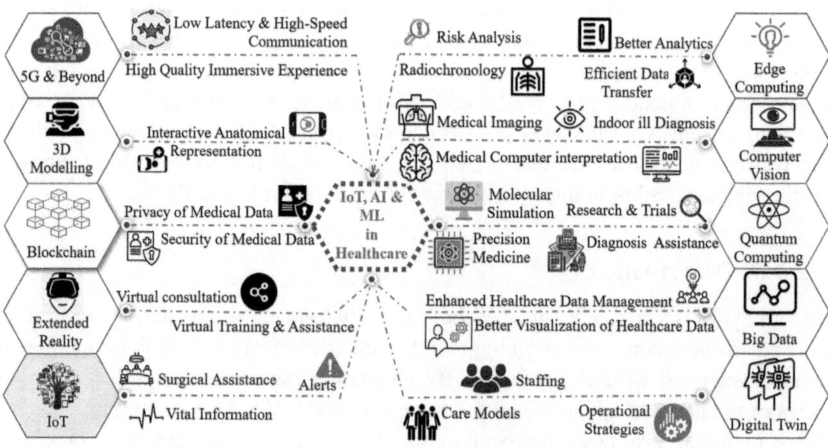

FIGURE 1.2 Application of machine learning, artificial intelligence, and Internet of Things in healthcare.

1.2.1.4 Internet of Things Devices

IoT tools enhance the efficiency, sustainability, and top quality of city services, including medical care. These gadgets can send information to doctors, help with remote individual monitoring, early discovery of health and wellness problems, and personalized medical care interventions (Ahmed et al., 2023). Also, IoT sensing units released in healthcare facilities can monitor ecological problems, occupancy prices, and equipment use, maximize source allowance, boost individual safety and security, and improve operational efficiency (AlZu'bi et al., 2023). IoT devices are indispensable to creating a connected and intelligent smart city community, driving advancements in health care, and facilitating the delivery of positive, tailored, and effective healthcare services.

1.2.2 Integration Benefits Healthcare

The integration of connectivity, sensors, data analytics, and IoT devices within a smart city framework offers significant opportunities to enhance healthcare services and bring about numerous benefits, as demonstrated in the following ways.

1.2.2.1 Improved Access to Healthcare, Proactive, and Preventive Care

By leveraging connectivity and telemedicine services, smart cities can offer enhanced access to medical care services, especially for individuals living in remote or underserved areas. Virtual consultations, remote surveillance, and telehealth applications enable individuals to obtain clinical guidance and diagnoses (Ahmed et al., 2023). Information analytics and IoT gadgets promote positive and precautionary care campaigns. By examining populace health and wellness data, cities can determine health patterns, danger aspects, and disease patterns (AlZu'bi et al., 2023). This info allows the development of targeted interventions and wellness promotion projects to avoid diseases, promote healthy actions, and boost total wellness within the neighborhood.

1.2.2.2 Enhanced Resource Efficiency

Smart city framework optimizes the usage of medical care resources through data-driven understandings. By examining patient information, resource allocation patterns, and healthcare use, cities can recognize locations for renovation, reduce ineffectiveness, and improve resource allowance (Aldhyani et al., 2023). This leads to enhanced operational efficiency, minimized wait times, and far better usage of healthcare facilities, resulting in set-back savings and enhanced individual experiences.

1.2.2.3 Personalized and Precision Medicine

Integrating information analytics and IoT gadgets permits personalized and precision medication strategies. By evaluating different medical datasets and patient acceptance, including digital wellness and health documents, hereditary information, and lifestyle details, clinical experts can develop tailored therapy methods and referrals customized to a person's unique demands and functions (Aldossary, 2023). This enhances treatment results, decreases damaging celebrations, and boosts specific satisfaction.

1.2.2.4 Early Detection and Disease Surveillance

IoT devices and sensors enable early detection of health issues and enhance disease surveillance. For instance, wearable devices can monitor vital signs and detect abnormalities, allowing for early intervention and timely medical assistance (Chakraborty et al., 2023). Sensor networks can monitor environmental factors, detect disease outbreaks, and provide real-time public health surveillance and response data, leading to more effective disease control and management.

1.2.2.5 Data-Driven Decision-Making

Incorporating information analytics within sustainable city infrastructures equips policymakers and healthcare experts with important understandings for evidence-based decision-making (Hussain et al., 2021). By evaluating health and wellness information, demographics, and ecological aspects, cities can determine top-priority locations, designate sources properly, and carry out targeted healthcare treatments (Alwakeel et al., 2023). This leads to even more enlightened decision-making, boosted source allowance, and much better health and wellness results for the populace.

1.2.2.6 Collaboration and Care Coordination

Smart city facilities help with smooth wellness information sharing and advertise treatment synchronization among doctors. With interoperable digital wellness documents and protected information exchange, healthcare experts can access thorough person info, decreasing replication of examinations, guaranteeing connection of treatment, and assisting in working with and incorporating healthcare solutions (Reddy Yeruva, 2023; Sharma et al., 2023). In compliance with the area, we should get more information on telemedicine and remote health care.

1.3 Remote Healthcare and Telemedicine

Telemedicine describes utilizing innovative interactions, modern technologies, and electronic frameworks to provide medical care solutions from another location. It leverages a sustainable city's connection and data-driven abilities to change just how medical care is accessed and offered (Chakraborty et al., 2023). Telemedicine incorporates different online medical care experiences, consisting of video clip assessments, remote tracking, digital wellness documents, and safe and secure messaging systems, as described next.

1.3.1 Improved Access to Healthcare

Telemedicine removes geographical obstacles and improves the ease of access to treatment solutions for homeowners of lasting cities. Individuals staying in remote or underserved locations can conveniently get in touch with doctors, overcoming variety and transportation problems (Sharma et al., 2023). This is specifically valuable for those who handle restricted mobility devices, do not have transportation alternatives, or stay in locations with an absence of healthcare facilities.

1.3.2 Time and Cost Savings, Remote Monitoring, and Management

Telemedicine decreases the need for individuals to travel to medical care centers, conserving time and costs related to transport and waiting locations. Individuals can get scientific referrals, examinations, and follow-up therapy from the convenience of the comfort of their own homes, allowing much better comfort and flexibility in handling their healthcare needs (El-Fouly et al., 2023). It makes remote individual surveillance possible by utilizing linked devices and sensing units. Clients can place on wearable gadgets or use home monitoring tools that transfer health and wellness details to physicians in real time (Samy El Menchawy et al., 2023). This makes it possible for healthcare specialists from another location to track important signs, medication adherence, and disease monitoring, making it feasible for prompt therapies, individualized treatment strategies, and boosted total therapy results.

1.3.3 Continuity of Care, Urgent, and Emergency Care

Smart cities with bundled telemedicine systems make sure links in therapy, specifically for individuals with relentless problems or detailed medical history. With telemedicine, people maintain routine contact with their doctor, obtain recurring assistance, and handle their healthcare requirements successfully (Kushwaha et al., 2023). This decreases the danger of spaces in treatment, boosts treatment synchronization, and boosts a person's complete satisfaction. Telemedicine is essential in providing emergency and immediate treatment solutions within a smart city. Telemedicine makes it possible for medical care specialists to analyze and triage clients from another location, offer first clinical guidance, and overview emergency-responders on suitable activities (Zakzouk et al., 2023). This in-log run helps optimize resource allocation and ensures timely access to critical care, potentially saving lives when immediate in-person medical attention is not feasible.

1.3.4 Collaborative Healthcare

Telemedicine facilitates collaboration among healthcare providers within a smart city ecosystem. Through secure communication platforms, healthcare professionals can quickly consult with specialists, share medical records, and seek second opinions, fostering a multidisciplinary approach to patient care (Joe et al., 2023). This collaborative environment enhances healthcare outcomes, promotes knowledge sharing, and enables faster decision-making. To attain a detailed analysis of healthcare in a smart city, Figure 1.3 illustrates the current possible computation as far as a smart city is concerned from the sensor or terminal level, edge computing, fog computing, and cloud computing.

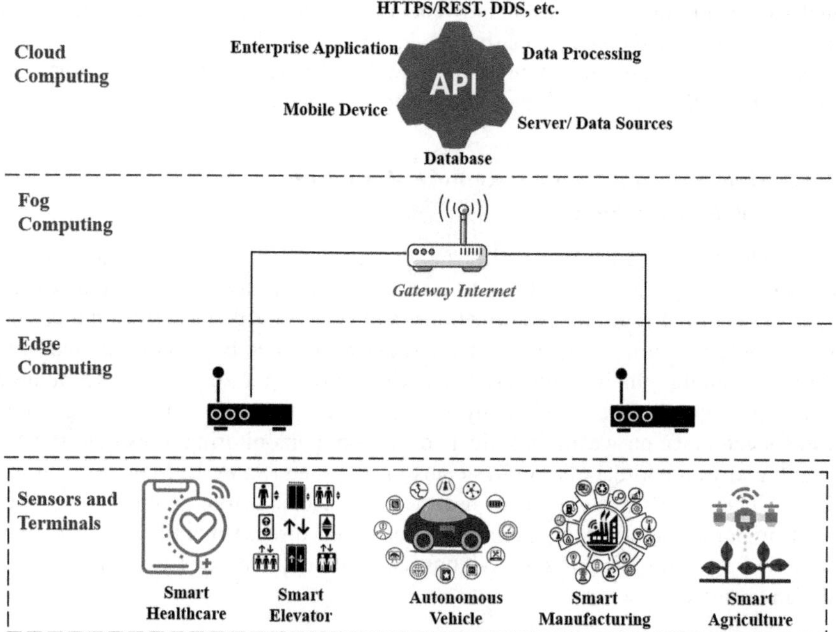

FIGURE 1.3 The current state of computation entailing smart healthcare.

1.3.5 Accessibility and Connectivity

Telemedicine removes geographical obstacles and boosts healthcare accessibility for locals of smart cities. With online assessments, patients can connect with doctors no matter their physical location, ensuring that healthcare solutions come to people in remote or underserved locations (Fan et al., 2023). This is especially helpful for people with minimal mobility, transportation challenges, or those living far away from medical care centers. The sophisticated connection infrastructure of a smart city enables seamless and trusted interaction between healthcare providers and patients. High-speed internet, cordless networks, and broadband connection help with real-time video appointments, secure messaging, and remote monitoring (Mohammed & Hasan, 2023). This ensures that healthcare encounters are conducted efficiently, permitting efficient interaction and information exchange.

1.3.6 Remote Monitoring and Care

Telemedicine enables remote patient monitoring through the use of connected devices and sensors. Smart city infrastructure supports integrating wearable devices, home monitoring equipment, and IoT sensors, which can collect and transmit health data to healthcare providers (Fong et al., 2023). This enables continuous monitoring of vital signs, medication adherence, and disease management, allowing for proactive interventions and personalized treatment plans.

1.3.7 Health Data Integration, Collaboration, and Care Coordination

From a smart city point of view, telemedicine includes incorporating and sharing health data throughout different medical care setups. EHRs can be firmly accessed and shared between doctors, guaranteeing a smooth connection of care (Berawi, 2023). This provides healthcare experts with a detailed view of a client's medical history, helping with accurate diagnoses, treatment planning, and collaborative care. More still, Telemedicine supports collaborative healthcare within a sustainable city ecosystem. Doctors can quickly connect and talk to experts, share medical records, and look for second opinions via electronic platforms (Ahmed et al., 2023; Berawi, 2023). This joint setting promotes interdisciplinary treatment, improves clinical decision-making, and makes certain coordinated and effective personal healthcare services.

1.3.8 Patient Empowerment

Telemedicine empowers patients by giving them greater control over their healthcare. Via digital examinations, clients have a lot more adaptability in organizing visits and accessing medical care solutions. They can proactively join their treatment, get medically educated, increase their learning, and take part in common decision-making with doctors (AlZu'bi et al., 2023). Telemedicine boosts ease of access by getting over geographical and wheelchair obstacles, provides price financial savings via decreased traveling expenditures, and boosts medical care results by providing prompt accessibility to care and allowing remote tracking and professional examinations. These benefits add to a much more patient-centric and effective healthcare system, profiting people who would certainly or else deal with difficulties accessing healthcare solutions (Dutta et al., 2023).

1.4 Health Monitoring and Wearable Devices

Health and wellness surveillance from a sustainable smart city point of view involves making use of innovative innovations, information analytics, and interconnected systems to keep an eye on and handle the health and wellness and health of people within a city. It entails the combination of different sensing units, wearable tools, and data-driven systems to gather, evaluate, and analyze health-related information in real time.

1.4.1 Wearable Devices and Sensors

Medical wearable gadgets like smart heart monitoring, stress watches, health and fitness trackers, and clinical sensing units play an essential function in health and wellness tracking. These tools can gather a wide variety of information, consisting of heart price, high blood pressure, rest patterns, and task degrees. The information is transferred to a central system or doctor for evaluation and surveillance (Aldhyani et al., 2023; Dutta et al., 2023). Sensing units released in public rooms, homes, and healthcare centers can additionally catch ecological information, such as high air quality, temperature level, and sound degrees, affecting people's health and wellness.

1.4.1.1 Real-Time Data Collection and Analytics

Wellness surveillance in a sustainable city entails constantly gathering health-related information from different resources. This information is refined, examined, and changed right into purposeful understandings with progressed information analytics strategies. Real-time analytics permit healthcare specialists to recognize patterns, spot abnormalities, and track health and wellness indications to make enlightened choices immediately (Tareen et al., 2023). This positive method allows very early discovery of health and wellness problems and prompt treatments.

1.4.1.2 Remote Patient Monitoring

Smart city framework sustains remote individual tracking, where people can be checked in real time from their homes or various other areas. A doctor can, from another location, track clients' important indicators, medicine adherence, and illness administration with wearable tools and linked sensing units (El-Shafai et al., 2023). This makes prompt treatments and individualized therapy strategies possible and lowers the demand for regular medical facility check-outs.

1.4.1.3 Predictive and Preventive Healthcare

Wellness tracking from a clever city viewpoint stresses preventative and anticipating health care. By constantly checking wellness information, medical doctors can determine patterns and fads that might suggest prospective wellness dangers (Ahmed et al., 2023). This aggressive technique makes it possible for the advancement of tailored treatments, health and wellness education and learning programs, and safety nets to enhance total health and wellness results.

1.4.1.4 Data Integration and Interoperability

Health and wellness surveillance in a sustainable city calls for smooth health and wellness information combination and interoperability throughout various medical care systems and systems. It offers doctors a thorough sight of a person's health and wellness info, consisting of case history, diagnostics, and real-time surveillance information (AlZu'bi et al., 2023). This combination promotes extra exact medical diagnoses, tailored therapy strategies, and reliable treatment synchronization.

1.4.1.5 Public Health Surveillance

Health and wellness tracking from a high-tech city point of view expands past private wellness checking to population-level security. By assessing aggregated and anonymized health and wellness information, public health authorities can spot illness breakouts, keep track of public health fads, and execute targeted treatments to safeguard the area's health (Dutta et al., 2023). This data-driven method enhances public health preparation, source appropriation, and feedback to public health emergencies. Health and wellness tracking from a sustainable city point of view improves healthcare distribution by leveraging sophisticated modern technologies, information analytics, and interconnected systems (Aldhyani et al., 2023). It allows real-time tracking, very early discovery of health and wellness concerns, customized treatments, and positive healthcare monitoring. This strategy advertises precautionary and anticipated medical care, encourages people to organize their health and wellness, and sustains public health efforts for the health of the whole sustainable city area (Aldossary, 2023).

1.4.1.6 Health Monitoring and Fitness

Wearable gadgets such as smartwatches, health and fitness trackers, and health and wellness brands allow people to track their exercises and check heart prices, rest patterns, calorie usage, and various other health-related metrics. These medical tools offer real-time comments and motivate sick individuals to preserve an energetic, healthy, and balanced way of living (Chakraborty et al., 2023). In a smart city, wearable gadgets advertise public wellness by encouraging people to check their wellness and take safety nets, as depicted in Figure 1.4.

1.4.1.7 Chronic Disease Management

Using wearable innovation has been revealed to be useful in the monitoring of lasting health and wellness problems like diabetic issues, hypertension, and breathing diseases. As an example, gadgets that constantly keep track of sugar degrees can give

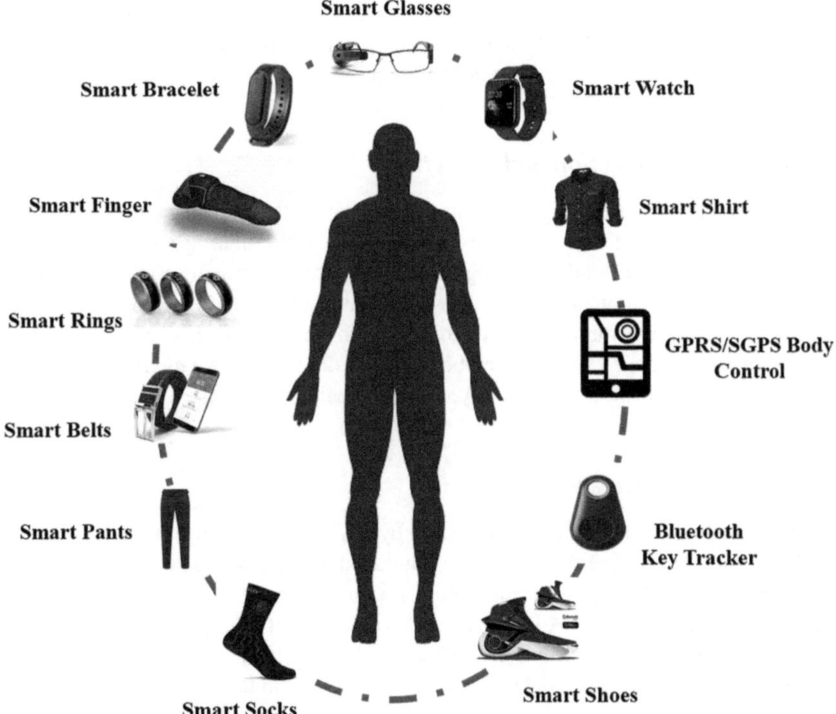

FIGURE 1.4 Wearable medical electronics.

prompt analyses for people with diabetic issues, allowing them to make necessary modifications to their therapy or day-to-day regimens (Alwakeel et al., 2023). Wearable gadgets with integrated sensing units can additionally track important indicators, determine abnormalities, and inform medical care specialists or caretakers in emergency circumstances, leading to far better condition control and reduced healthcare facility admissions.

1.4.1.8 Safety and Security

Medical wearable devices have demonstrated improved patient security and safety in a smart city atmosphere. For example, smartwatches or sustainable fashion jewelry with integrated panic buttons or general practitioners' capacities can be used to demand instant aid throughout emergencies (Reddy Yeruva, 2023). These gadgets can send area information to emergency responders or loved ones, allowing quicker action times and ensuring the safety and security of troubled people.

1.4.1.9 Environmental Monitoring

Wearable gadgets can additionally be added to environmental monitoring in a sustainable city. For instance, wearable air pollution sensing units can gauge air top quality, ultraviolet radiation, or sound degrees. This information can be gathered and examined to examine the effect of ecological elements on people's health and wellness and health (Sharma et al., 2023). It can sustain city planning initiatives even more to boost ecological problems and reduce wellness threats.

1.4.1.10 Data Collection and Analytics

Wearable devices produce large amounts of information that can be gathered, assessed, and incorporated right into smart city systems. By accumulating and assessing this information, beneficial understandings can be acquired relating to populace wellness patterns, urban planning, and source allowance (El-Fouly et al., 2023). As an example, information from wearable gadgets can offer info on patterns of exercise, rest high quality, or tension degrees, which can be made use of to maximize metropolitan facilities, advertise energetic living, and layout much healthier settings.

1.4.1.11 Citizen Engagement

Wearable gadgets foster resident interaction by advertising empowerment and responsibility for individual health and wellness and health. They motivate people to proactively join their health and wellness administration and make educated choices (Samy El menchawy et al., 2023). Additionally, wearable gadgets can promote communications with sustainable city solutions and applications, enabling people to access customized health and wellness details, get notices, and get in touch with doctors.

1.5 Data Analytics and Artificial Intelligence (AI) in Healthcare

Information analytics checks out and translates huge quantities of information to discover purposeful patterns and understandings (Hussain et al., 2021; 2022). It includes utilizing different analytical and computational methods to draw out important info and make notified choices. Information analytics includes information cleansing, improvement, modeling, and visualization (Kushwaha et al., 2023). It makes it possible for companies to get workable understandings, boost decision-making, maximize procedures, and drive service development.

1.5.1 Data Analytics in Healthcare

Information analytics can assess individual documents and recognize relationships between particular therapies and results, enabling medical persons to make evidence-based choices and enhance client treatment, as illustrated next.

1.5.1.1 Predictive Analytics

Information analytics strategies can be related to historical and real-time medical care information to determine patterns, fads, and relationships. By assessing information from numerous resources, consisting of wearable tools, digital health and wellness documents, and public health data sources, anticipating analytics can assist in anticipating condition episodes, preparing for medical care source requirements, and recognizing risky populaces (Zakzouk et al., 2023). This allows aggressive treatments, source appropriation, and safety nets to boost public health results.

1.5.1.2 Personalized Medicine

Modern technologies can assess private health and wellness information, consisting of hereditary info, case history, and way of life elements, to produce individualized therapy strategies. By taking into consideration a person's special attributes, AI formulas can advise customized treatments, medicine, and safety nets (Cabrera et al., 2023). This technique improves the efficiency of healthcare treatments, decreases damaging occasions, and boosts client results.

1.5.1.3 Alert Systems and Real-time Monitoring

Information analytics and AI formulas can allow real-time surveillance and sharp systems within a sustainable city healthcare system. Constant information evaluation from wearable tools, sensing units, and healthcare tracking systems can identify unusual patterns or vital occasions and cause notifications to doctors or emergency reaction groups (Joe et al., 2023). This assists in very early treatment, prompts clinical interest, and boosts individual security.

1.5.1.4 Healthcare Resource Optimization

Information analytics can be related to medical care source administration in a clever city. By evaluating client circulation, tenancy prices, and source applications, AI formulas can enhance the appropriation of medical care centers, personnel, and devices (Mohammed & Hasan, 2023). This helps reduce waiting times, boosts performance, and ensures the accessibility of sources where they are most required.

1.5.1.5 Telemedicine and Remote Monitoring

Information analytics can be put into medical care source monitoring in a smart city. By examining client circulation, tenancy prices, and source use, AI formulas can enhance the allotment of medical care centers, personnel, and devices (Mohammed & Hasan, 2023). This helps reduce waiting times, improve effectiveness, and make sure the accessibility of sources is where they are most required.

1.5.1.6 Risk Assessment and Fraud Detection

Intelligence analytics can be utilized to find deceptive tasks and examine medical care threats within a sustainable city system. AI formulas can assess invoicing documents, insurance coverage cases, and doctor action patterns to determine abnormalities and prospective scams. In addition, anticipating analytics can analyze populace health and wellness dangers, such as determining locations susceptible to condition breakouts or people at high threat of persistent problems (Tripathy et al., 2023). This info sustains targeted treatments, source allowance, and public health preparation.

1.5.2 Applications of AI in Healthcare

Modern AI technologies use smart formulas and systems that resemble human cognitive procedures such as finding out, thinking, and analyzing. AI includes different subfields, consisting of AI, natural language processing, computer system vision, and robotics. AI, a part of AI, concentrates on formulas that allow computer systems to gain information and make forecasts or choices without specific programs. For example, in self-governing automobiles, modern AI technologies examine real-time sensing unit information to spot and react to website traffic problems, allowing cars to browse securely. In health care, AI can be utilized to evaluate clinical pictures, for example, MRIs or X-rays, to detect or forecast illness development.

1.5.2.1 Medical Imaging Analysis, Remote monitoring, and telemedicine

AI formulas can evaluate clinical pictures, for example, X-rays, CT scans, and MRIs, to aid in medical diagnosis. For instance, a deep understanding of formulas can discover problems or help radiologists determine malignant growths (Badr, 2023). This modern technology boosts the precision and performance of clinical imaging analysis, bringing about much faster medical diagnoses and even more reliable therapy strategies. AI allows remote tracking of clients' essential indicators, enabling doctors to track wellness problems in real time. As an example, wearable tools outfitted with AI formulas can continually keep an eye on heart price, high blood pressure, and various other physical specifications (Pandya et al., 2023). The gathered information can be transferred to healthcare experts that can from another location to evaluate people's health and wellness conditions and give prompt treatments, lowering the demand for healthcare facilities. Figure 1.5 demonstrates the real-time application of the net of clinical points in the ecological community.

Interconnected clinical tools, wearables, sensing units, and information analytics systems work together flawlessly to collect, transfer, and evaluate important health and wellness info in real time. As an example, in a health center setup, wearable tools can continually check clients' essential indicators, such as heart price, high blood pressure, and oxygen degrees, sending this information to a central system. This real-time surveillance permits medical care caregivers to spot any abnormalities or degeneration immediately, making prompt treatments possible and lowering the danger of difficulties. In remote client surveillance circumstances, IoMT tools make it possible for doctors to track individuals' problems beyond standard medical care setups, permitting aggressive treatment administration and lowering medical facility readmissions. Additionally, IoMT's real-time applications prolong past client-like medical care procedures. Smart supply administration systems can keep track of clinical materials and tools, instantly activating orders when supply degrees are reduced, hence guaranteeing smooth accessibility of important sources.

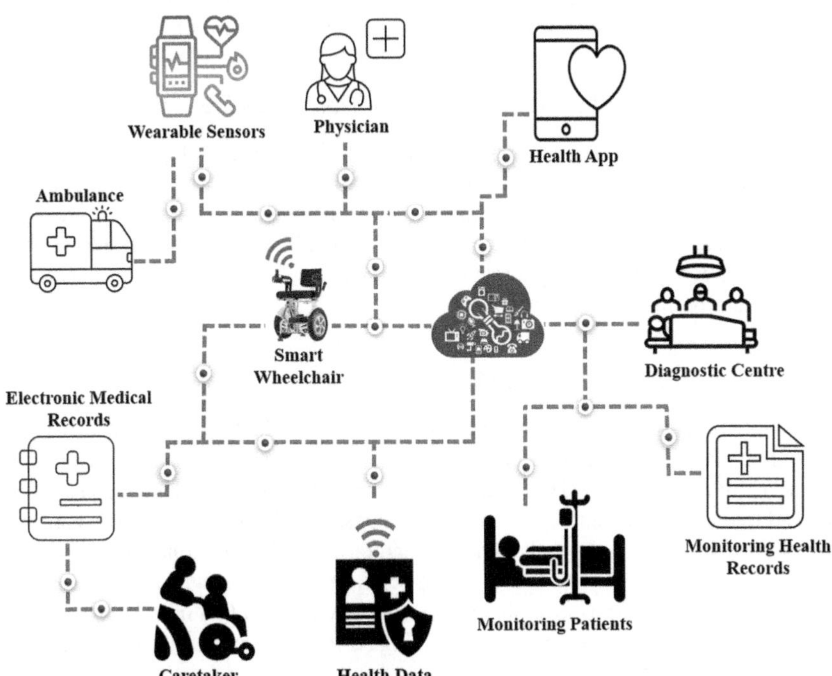

FIGURE 1.5 Real-time artificial intelligence of the Internet of Medical Things ecosystem implementation.

The suggested safe Artificial Intelligence of the Internet of Medical Things that can be executed in Figure 1.5 has the potential to change medical care by offering customized and reliable treatment while ensuring the safety, security, and personal privacy of personal information. Nonetheless, it is necessary to attend to honest and regulative problems and make certain that the advantages of AI in health care are stabilized with ideal safeguards and honest factors to consider.

1.5.2.2 Predictive Analytics for Disease Outbreaks

AI formulas can evaluate numerous information resources, consisting of client documents, ecological information, and social media site feeds, to anticipate and find condition episodes. By determining very early indications and patterns, healthcare authorities can take positive actions to avoid the spread of illness within a smart city (Mengash et al., 2023). As an example, AI versions can assess signs and symptoms reported by people in real time to determine prospective condition collections and promote targeted treatments.

1.5.2.3 Healthcare Resource Management

AI formulas can maximize the allowance of healthcare sources in a clever city. AI can forecast person circulation by assessing client information, tenancy prices, and source usage, making it possible to make much better staffing choices and source allotment (Gagliardi & Albergo, 2023). This makes certain reliable usage of healthcare centers, decreases waiting times, and boosts total medical care solution shipment.

1.5.2.4 Personalized Treatment and Precision Medicine

AI modern technologies can assess massive datasets, consisting of genomics, medical documents, and way of living information, to establish customized therapy strategies. AI formulas can determine patterns and relationships that aid dressmaker therapies to specific clients' qualities and choices (Tareen et al., 2023). This method allows accurate medication, guaranteeing that clients get targeted treatments most efficiently for their certain problems.

1.5.2.5 Smart Health Assistants

AI-enabled digital aides and chatbots can supply individualized health and wellness recommendations, respond to clinical questions, and overview people in handling their health and wellness. These online aides can utilize natural language processing and AI to comprehend and reply to customer questions. For instance, people can communicate with a clever city's healthcare chatbot to obtain info concerning signs and symptoms, locate nearby medical care centers, or make routine visits (El-Shafai et al., 2023). These applications show the transformative capacity of AI in medical care from a sustainable city point of view. By leveraging AI innovations, healthcare systems can improve medical diagnosis precision, allow remote surveillance and telemedicine, forecast condition episodes, maximize source appropriation, individualize therapies, and offer available medical care info to people.

1.5.3 Potential Challenges and Ethical Considerations

This combination of AI in medical care solutions adds to enhancing populace wellness, boosting personal experiences, and maximizing healthcare distribution in clever cities. Nevertheless, some prospective obstacles and honest factors to consider are related to making use of information analytics and AI in health care.

1.5.3.1 Data Privacy and Security

Accumulating and examining delicate health and wellness information elevates problems regarding personal privacy, safety, and security. Person details need to be protected to avoid unapproved gain access to or information violations. As an example, when sharing personal information between doctors and AI systems for evaluation, there is a threat of information leak or abuse if correct protection procedures are not in a position (Gagliardi & Albergo, 2023). Guaranteeing durable information file encryption, gaining access to controls, and anonymization methods are vital to shielding clients' privacy.

1.5.3.2 Bias and Fairness

AI systems depend on historical information, which might consist of prejudices and differences, resulting in discriminatory decision-making. As an example, if an anticipating design is educated utilizing information that primarily stands for a details market team, it might result in unreliable medical diagnoses or therapy referrals for underrepresented populations (Mengash et al., 2023). Resolving predispositions in information collection and formula style is critical to ensuring justness and equity in healthcare results.

1.5.3.3 Explainability and Transparency

Several AI versions run as "black boxes," making it challenging to comprehend the thinking behind their choices. This absence of openness can weaken trust funds and prevent the fostering of AI in medical care. As an example, when an AI system advises a certain therapy strategy, medical care experts and clients might intend to recognize the elements that affect that referral (Pandya et al., 2023). Creating explainable AI versions and offering clear decision-making procedures are necessary to acquire individual depend on and approval.

1.5.3.4 Legal and Regulatory Compliance

Information analytics and AI in medical care need to follow lawful and regulative structures, such as information security laws (for instance, the General Information Security Policy), which information needs to be refined per personal privacy regulations (Badr, 2023). Guaranteeing conformity with these laws and developing moral standards for AI in health care are needed to safeguard clients' civil liberties and guarantee the accountable use of modern technology.

1.5.3.5 Liability and Accountability

As AI systems play an even more considerable function in healthcare decision-making, inquiries of responsibility and liability emerge. That is accountable if an AI formula offers a defective medical diagnosis or therapy suggestion. For instance, establishing responsibility can be intricate if an independent medical robotics technician makes a mistake throughout a treatment (Ahmed et al., 2023). Developing clear structures for liability, consisting of recognizing medical care experts' and innovation programmers' duties, is important to attend to these difficulties.

1.5.3.6 Human–AI Collaboration

Stabilizing the duties of healthcare experts and AI systems is a vital moral factor to consider. While AI can give beneficial understandings and boost decision-making, it does not change human judgment and compassion (AlZu'bi et al., 2023). Guaranteeing suitable human–AI partnership, where medical care specialists continue to be in control and preserve honest obligation, is vital. For instance, when making use of AI in radiology, radiologists must utilize AI formulas as choice assistance devices instead of completely relying upon automated analyses.

Dealing with these difficulties and honest factors requires interdisciplinary cooperation among healthcare specialists, information researchers, policymakers, and ethicists. It includes creating clear and responsible AI systems, advertising information administration methods, developing clear standards for liable AI usage, and constantly assessing and checking the effect of AI on healthcare results and personal wellness (Dutta et al., 2023). By proactively attending to these difficulties, medical care systems can harness the possibility of information analytics and AI while guaranteeing client's personal privacy, justice, openness, and honesty in medical care.

1.6 Smart Hospitals and Healthcare Facilities

Smart medical facilities are medical care centers that utilize progressed modern technologies and data-driven methods to boost individual treatment, enhance functional effectiveness, and maximize source use. These health centers incorporate numerous interconnected systems and tools to develop a smart and interconnected medical care atmosphere (Aldhyani et al., 2023). The principle of clever healthcare facilities focuses on making use of innovation to enhance healthcare shipment, improve client results, and improve medical facility procedures. In clever medical facilities, an essential part is the assimilation of IoT gadgets and sensing units throughout the center. These gadgets can consist of wearable wellness trackers, intelligent beds, clinical devices, and ecological sensing units. They gather real-time information on clients' essential indications, device use, and ecological problems (Aldossary, 2023). This information is evaluated to make positive and customized healthcare treatments possible.

An additional facet of intelligent health centers is the execution of EHRs and electronic systems. These systems allow healthcare experts to safely access and exchange personal info, enhancing treatment synchronization and decreasing the threat of mistakes related to paper-based documents (Chakraborty et al., 2023). Additionally, digital systems automate management jobs such as organizing visits and taking care of stock, allowing doctors to concentrate a lot more on personal treatment (Alwakeel et al., 2023). Smart healthcare facilities likewise use real-time place systems (RTLS) to track the area of devices, materials, and employees within the center. This aids in maximizing source allowance, simplifying processes, and enhancing individual security by making sure essential sources are readily available when and where they are required.

AI plays a considerable duty in clever healthcare facilities by supplying choice assistance to healthcare specialists. AI formulas can examine huge quantities of client information and medical records and study literary works to help in medical diagnosis, therapy preparation, and anticipating client results. AI-powered chatbots and online aides likewise boost individual communications and offer tailored healthcare details. Additionally, smart healthcare facilities stress clever person surveillance (Yang et al., 2021). This includes making use of innovative tracking systems that constantly track people's crucial indications and health and wellness criteria.

Wearable gadgets, biosensors, and remote tracking innovations transfer real-time information to doctors, making it possible for prompt treatments and remote individual surveillance. This technique helps in reducing medical facility readmissions and enhances personal results. Smart medical facilities are medical care centers that utilize progressed innovations and data-driven strategies to boost client treatment, enhance functional effectiveness, and maximize source application (Shafik et al., 2020a). These health centers incorporate numerous interconnected systems and tools to produce a smart and interconnected medical care atmosphere, as shown below.

1.6.1 Internet of Things Integration

Smart healthcare facilities utilize IoT tools and sensing units throughout the center to collect real-time information and keep an eye on different specifications. These gadgets can consist of wearable wellness trackers, clever beds, clinical tools, and ecological sensing units (Shafik et al., 2020b). The accumulated information is, after that, evaluated and used to improve client surveillance, maximize operations, and enhance total medical facility procedures.

1.6.2 Electronic Health Records (EHR) and Digital Systems

Smart medical facilities take on digital health and wellness documents and electronic systems for smooth personal info storage space and exchange. EHR systems allow medical care specialists to access client information firmly, helping with exact and prompt medical diagnosis, therapy, and treatment control (Ahmed et al., 2023). Digital systems additionally allow the automation of management jobs, minimizing documentation and simplifying processes.

1.6.3 Real-Time Location Systems (RTLS)

RTLS innovations, like RFID tags and Bluetooth signs, are used to track the area of tools, products, and employees (AlZu'bi et al., 2023). This aids in simplifying supply administration, possession monitoring, and team appropriation, boosting performance, decreasing waiting times, and boosting individual security (Dutta et al., 2023).

1.6.4 Artificial Intelligence (AI) for Decision Support

Smart health centers utilize AI formulas and AI methods to aid medical care specialists in decision-making. AI can evaluate individual information and medical records and study literary works to give scientific choice assistance, help in medical diagnosis, and suggest therapy strategies (Aldhyani et al., 2023). AI-powered chatbots and digital aides likewise assist in individual communication and offer customized medical care details.

1.6.5 Smart Patient Monitoring

Smart healthcare facilities execute innovative tracking systems that constantly track individuals' essential indicators and health and wellness specifications. These systems make use of wearable gadgets, biosensors, and remote surveillance innovations to transfer real-time information to doctors (Aldossary, 2023). This makes it possible for very early discovery of modifications in client problems, punctual treatments, and remote individual surveillance, lowering health center readmissions and enhancing individual results.

1.6.6 Data Analytics and Predictive Analytics

Smart health centers utilize information analytics and anticipating analytics to evaluate large quantities of medical care information and create important understandings. By extracting personal documents, clinical imaging information, and various other resources, healthcare facilities can determine patterns, anticipate condition development, enhance therapy strategies, and expect healthcare source demands (Chakraborty et al., 2023). This data-driven strategy aids in boosting individual results, source allowance, and functional effectiveness. Smart medical facilities stand for a transformative technique to healthcare shipment, incorporating innovation, information, and automation to improve client treatment, improve procedures, and enhance total healthcare results (Reddy Yeruva, 2023). Smart medical facilities aim to produce an interconnected healthcare ecological community that makes individualized, effective, and patient-centric treatment possible by incorporating IoT, electronic systems, AI, and progressed analytics.

1.7 Challenges and Future Research Directions

This section discusses the challenges and barriers to implementing healthcare in a smart city context, followed by future developments and advancements in smart city healthcare.

1.7.1 Challenges and Limitations

Carrying out medical care in a sustainable city context features numerous difficulties and obstacles that need to be resolved for effective combination, as discussed next.

1.7.1.1 Interoperability and Data Integration

Incorporating numerous medical care systems, tools, and information resources can be tested because of interoperability concerns. Various systems might utilize various information layouts and procedures, making it challenging to trade details effortlessly (Sharma et al., 2023). For instance, incorporating EHRs from numerous doctors right into a unified system might call for getting over compatibility problems and ensuring safe and secure information sharing.

1.7.1.2 Privacy and Data Security

Smart city healthcare systems entail gathering and assessing delicate personal information, elevating problems concerning personal privacy and information protection. Safeguarding personal info from the unapproved gain access to information violations and abuse is important (Aldhyani et al., 2023; Aldossary, 2023; Dutta et al., 2023). For example, when executing remote person tracking systems that transfer health and wellness information online, durable safety steps have to remain in a location to protect a person's privacy.

1.7.1.3 Infrastructure and Connectivity

A reputable and durable framework is vital for a clever city healthcare system. Nonetheless, making certain ample connections and facilities can be difficult, particularly in underdeveloped or remote locations (Alwakeel et al., 2023). For instance, releasing high-speed net gain access to and cordless networks might be hard in specific areas, restricting the performance of telemedicine or remote surveillance campaigns.

1.7.1.4 Cost and Financial Considerations

Applying clever city healthcare options usually needs a substantial framework, innovation, and training financial investment. The monetary problem can be an obstacle, especially for resource-constrained medical care companies (Reddy Yeruva, 2023). For instance, releasing sophisticated clinical gadgets, executing information analytics systems, and preserving the required framework can stress the spending plans of doctors, specifically in financially deprived locations.

1.7.1.5 Digital Divide and Access Disparities

The electronic divide describes the void inaccessibility to modern technology and electronic sources among various populations. This divide can impede the application of clever city healthcare campaigns, as not all people might have access to essential gadgets or web connections (El-Fouly et al., 2023). For example, deprived neighborhoods or senior populations might face obstacles to taking on telemedicine because of restricted access to smart devices or net solutions.

1.7.1.6 Regulatory and Legal Frameworks

Carrying out medical care in a sustainable city context calls for browsing complicated governing and lawful structures. Conformity with information defense policies, client authorization needs, and clinical principles standards are vital (Samy El menchawy et al., 2023). As an example, guaranteeing conformity with personal privacy policies, such as the GDPR, when gathering and refining individual information is vital. Still, it can be tested as a result of the complicated nature of information cooperating in a sustainable city environment (Kushwaha et al., 2023).

1.7.1.7 Stakeholder Collaboration and Adoption

Successful implementation of smart city healthcare initiatives requires collaboration among various stakeholders, including healthcare providers, technology vendors, policymakers, and the community (Kushwaha et al., 2023). Achieving buy-in and adoption from these stakeholders can be a challenge, especially if there is resistance to change or skepticism regarding the effectiveness and benefits of smart city healthcare solutions (Zakzouk et al., 2023).

1.7.1.8 Ethical and Social Considerations

Effective execution of clever city medical care efforts calls for partnership among different stakeholders, consisting of doctors, innovation suppliers, policymakers, and the area (Kushwaha et al., 2023). Accomplishing buy-in and fostering from these stakeholders can be a difficulty, specifically if there is resistance to alteration or uncertainty relating to the efficiency and advantages of smart city healthcare remedies (Zakzouk et al., 2023).

1.7.1.9 User Acceptance and Trust

Carrying out health care in a clever city context increases moral and social factors to consider that require to be thoroughly attended to. For example, making sure fair accessibility to medical care solutions is vital to stop aggravating existing wellness variations (Joe et al., 2023). It is essential to think about the demands of prone populations, such as low-income areas or people with restricted technical proficiency, and make sure that they are not left to embrace intelligent city healthcare options (Reddy Yeruva, 2023).

1.7.1.10 Regulatory Alignment and Standardization

Getting individual approval and counting on it is crucial for the effective execution of medical care in an intelligent city. Individuals are required to feel great about the dependability, precision, and safety of the modern technologies and systems being made use of (Mohammed & Hasan, 2023). For instance, people might be reluctant to share their health and wellness information or rely upon automated medical diagnosis without human participation. Structure counts on clear interaction, durable information safety steps, and showing the performance of intelligent city healthcare campaigns, which are important (Berawi, 2023).

1.7.1.11 Education and Training

Carrying out medical care in a smart city context commonly calls for straightening with existing laws and developing information exchange, personal privacy, and safety requirements. Balancing laws and requirements throughout various territories can be difficult (Tripathy et al., 2023). For instance, wellness information interoperability between various doctors might call for standardization of information layouts, terms, and procedures to ensure smooth exchange and compatibility (Badr, 2023).

1.7.1.12 Scalability and Sustainability

Healthcare specialists and teams require appropriate education, learning, and training to efficiently use and browse clever city medical care innovations (Mengash et al., 2023). They have to be geared up with the needed abilities to analyze and make use of information analytics, AI formulas, and IoT tools. Making sure thorough training programs and continual education and learning for medical care experts is vital to taking full advantage of the advantages of intelligent city healthcare systems (Gagliardi & Albergo, 2023).

1.7.2 Future Research Directions

As smart city medical care efforts expand and broaden, making sure scalability and sustainability end up being critical. Preparation for future development, suiting raising information quantities, and preparing for technical developments are essential (El-Shafai et al., 2023). Likewise, taking into consideration the ecological effect of clever city medical care systems and embracing lasting techniques is important for long-lasting practicality (Tareen et al., 2023).

1.7.2.1 Advanced Artificial Intelligence (AI) Applications

Additional research studies can concentrate on creating innovative AI formulas and designs for health care in clever cities. This consists of enhancing the precision and performance of AI-based medical diagnosis and therapy referrals, enhancing anticipating analytics for condition avoidance and very early treatment, and discovering the capacity of AI in individualized medication and accurate medical care (Ahmed et al., 2023).

1.7.2.2 Block Chain Technology for Data Security

Block chain modern technology guarantees the improvement of information safety and personal privacy in clever city medical care systems. Future research studies can discover the application of block chain to take care of wellness documents firmly, allow protected information sharing and authorization monitoring, and guarantee openness and stability in healthcare information exchange (Dutta et al., 2023).

1.7.2.3 Internet of Medical Things (IoMT)

The IoMT includes interconnected clinical tools, wearables, and sensing units that gather and send real-time client information. Future studies can concentrate on creating brand-new IoMT gadgets, enhancing their interoperability, and incorporating them right into intelligent city healthcare systems (Aldossary, 2023). This can allow a lot more exact and extensive wellness tracking, remote person administration, and individualized healthcare treatments.

1.7.2.4 Human-Centered Design and User Experience

Future studies can highlight human-centered style concepts to make certain that intelligent city medical care modern technologies are straightforward, available, and satisfy varied customer requirements. This consists of developing user-friendly user interfaces, thinking about the requirements of senior or handicapped populations, and enticing customers to establish and examine medical care innovations (Chakraborty et al., 2023).

1.7.2.5 Ethical and Legal Implications

As medical care in clever cities becomes even more common, there is a demand to resolve the honest and lawful ramifications related to information collection, authorization, and usage. Future studies can check out structures for honest information administration, educated approval versions, and standards for the liable use of AI and information analytics in medical care (Alwakeel et al., 2023).

1.7.2.6 Health Equity and Social Determinants of Health

Research studies can concentrate on leveraging sustainable city modern technologies to attend to wellness variations and social components of wellness. This consists of researching the effect of clever city treatments on at-risk populations, establishing methods to make sure fair accessibility to medical care solutions, and incorporating social and ecological information to educate healthcare decision-making (Reddy Yeruva, 2023).

1.7.2.7 Sustainability and Environmental Impact

Future research studies can discover means to make clever city healthcare systems extra lasting and eco-friendly. This can include maximizing power use, minimizing waste, and using renewable resource resources in the medical care framework (Sharma et al., 2023). In addition, researching the ecological effects of electronic healthcare technologies and creating environment-friendly medical care methods can add to an extra-lasting future.

1.7.2.8 Real-Time Analytics for Decision Support

Future research studies can concentrate on establishing real-time analytics devices and formulas that supply medical care experts with prompt understanding and choice assistance. This can make it possible for doctors to make educated choices on client treatment, source allotment, and medical care treatments (El-Fouly et al., 2023). Real-time analytics can aid in finding patterns, recognizing abnormalities, and anticipating prospective health and wellness threats, permitting aggressive and tailored medical care shipment.

1.7.2.9 Integration of Social and Behavioral Data

Incorporating social and behavioral information right into clever city medical care systems can supply a much more extensive understanding of people's wellness and health. Future studies can discover approaches to incorporate information from social networks, wearable tools, and various other resources to get an understanding right into a way of living aspects, social components of health and wellness, and populace health and wellness fads (Kushwaha et al., 2023; Samy El menchawy et al., 2023). This combination can educate targeted treatments, public health projects, and individualized medical care techniques.

1.7.2.10 Data-Driven Preventive Healthcare

Future research studies can utilize information analytics and AI to establish reliable precautionary medical care techniques. This consists of making use of anticipating analytics to determine people in danger of creating persistent illness, making customized health care, and executing aggressive treatments to advertise healthy and balanced actions and protect against condition development (Zakzouk et al., 2023; Alnssyan et al., 2023). By taking advantage of the power of information, clever city medical care systems can move the emphasis from responsive therapy to aggressive avoidance.

1.7.2.11 Privacy-Preserving Data Sharing and Collaboration

Making sure of personal privacy and safety while making it possible for information sharing and cooperation is a continuous obstacle in clever city health care. Future studies can check out methods, for instance, federated knowing, homomorphic security, and differential personal privacy, to make it possible for privacy-preserving information sharing and joint research studies (Cabrera et al., 2023). These strategies enable several stakeholders to assess aggregated information without endangering specific personal privacy, promoting large healthcare studies, and understanding exploration.

1.7.2.12 Smart City Healthcare Infrastructure Resilience

Strength is vital for the sustainability and connection of clever city medical care systems. Future studies can concentrate on establishing a durable and resistant framework that can endure all-natural catastrophes, cyberattacks, and various other interruptions. This consists of applying backup systems, catastrophe healing strategies, and protected information storage space remedies to guarantee undisturbed healthcare solutions in tough scenarios (Joe et al., 2023). By attending to these research study instructions, intelligent city health care can continue to progress and boost, offering ingenious services that boost personal treatment, boost health and wellness results, and maximize medical care distribution in metropolitan settings.

1.8 Lessons Learned and Conclusion

The partnership between scientists, doctors, policymakers, and innovation specialists will certainly play a vital duty in driving innovations in clever city medical care and resolving the advancing requirements of city populaces.

1.8.1 Lessons Learned from the Chapter

As we conclude the chapter, some lessons can be learned, as presented next.

1.8.1.1 Collaboration and User-Centric Design

Effective application of medical care in an intelligent city needs partnership among different stakeholders, consisting of doctors, modern technology suppliers, policymakers, and the area. Cooperation assists in making sure that varied points of view are thought about, obstacles are attended to jointly, and remedies are customized to satisfy the populace's detailed requirements. Likewise, user-centric layout concepts need to go to the leading edge of intelligent city healthcare campaigns. Taking into consideration the requirements, choices, and capacities of end-users, consisting of clients, medical care experts, and caretakers, is critical for fostering functionality. Including individuals in the layout and analysis procedure aids in producing options that are instinctive, available, and reliable.

1.8.1.2 Privacy and Security must be Prioritized

Provided the delicate nature of medical care information, making sure personal privacy and safety is vital. Durable information defense procedures, protected communication channels, and adherence to personal privacy laws are necessary. Lessons from previous information violations and safety events highlight the demand for solid safeguards to keep individuals dependent on and protect delicate details.

1.8.1.3 Infrastructure and Connectivity Are Foundational

A trusted and durable facility consisting of high-speed web connection and durable networks develops the structure for reliable, intelligent city medical care. Financial investment in the framework and guaranteeing global accessibility to connection are important for allowing telemedicine, remote surveillance, and information exchange, particularly in underserved locations.

1.8.1.4 Regulatory Frameworks Need to Evolve

The quick innovation of innovation in health care requires nimble and versatile regulative structures. Rules and plans need to equal technical advancements to attend to honest factors to consider, such as information administration, approval, and responsibility. Cooperation between policymakers, healthcare experts, and modern technology specialists is necessary to establish receptive and future-proof guidelines.

1.8.1.5 Data Integration and Interoperability Are Challenges

Incorporating information from several resources and systems continues to be a difficulty. Creating standard information layouts, interoperability criteria, and smooth information exchange procedures is vital. Lessons discovered highlight the significance of buying information assimilation facilities and advertising interoperability to help with the smooth circulation of info throughout healthcare systems.

1.8.1.6 Continuous Evaluation and Improvement Are Necessary

Smart city medical care campaigns need to go through a constant assessment to examine their efficiency, influence, and complete customer satisfaction. Routine responses from individuals, doctors, and various other stakeholders can determine locations for enhancement and overview future advancements. Examination metrics must exceed technical facets and take into consideration healthcare results, personal experiences, and cost-effectiveness.

1.8.1.7 Equity and Inclusivity Should be Prioritized

Attending to wellness differences and making sure fair accessibility to healthcare solutions must be main too clever city healthcare campaigns. Lessons found emphasize the demand to think about the requirements of underserved populations, bridge the electronic divide, and include social components of health and wellness in the layout and execution of healthcare options.

1.8.1.8 Upskilling and Training Are Vibrant

Developing the required abilities and capabilities among healthcare specialists, innovation experts, and end-users is vital. Education, learning and training programs must be developed to outfit people with the expertise and abilities required to use and browse clever city healthcare modern technologies successfully. Constant knowledge and expert advancement are important to equaling progressing innovations.

1.8.1.9 Flexibility and Adaptability Are Vital

Smart city medical care campaigns must be versatile and versatile to fit rising modern technologies, transforming medical care requirements and progressing customer assumptions. Welcoming a society of technology, cultivating nimble growth methods, and preparing for future patterns can assist in making certain that healthcare systems stay receptive and lasting. These lessons discovered can indicate future growth and lead to the application of health care in smart city contexts, cultivating enhancements in healthcare access, top quality, and results for city populations. By using these lessons, cities can develop durable and comprehensive healthcare systems that harness the power of innovation and information to profit all.

1.8.2 Conclusions

The chapter discovered the idea of health care in a smart city, highlighting the combination of innovation to boost metropolitan living. It reviews the crucial elements of a sustainable city framework, consisting of connection, sensing units, information analytics, and IoT gadgets, and their applications in boosting medical care solutions. The benefits of incorporating health care right into the intelligent city structure consist of boosted availability, cost-effectiveness, and enhanced healthcare results. The idea of telemedicine is described thoroughly, highlighting its importance in a smart city context and its perspective on conquering geographical obstacles and enhancing medical care access. Furthermore, health and wellness tracking and wearable gadgets are checked out, showcasing their function in encouraging people to take control of their health and wellness and allowing real-time information collection. The chapter further looked into making use of information analytics and AI innovations in intelligent city health care, reviewing their possibility of driving individualized medication, maximizing source allowance, and allowing very early condition discovery. Honest factors to consider and difficulties related to making use of information analytics and AI in medical care are likewise talked about. The principle of intelligent healthcare facilities is presented, highlighting their assimilation of sophisticated modern technologies and patient-centered treatment. The phase ends by dealing with obstacles to applying health care in a sustainable city context, like facility restrictions, personal privacy problems, and stakeholder partnerships. Future study instructions are recommended, highlighting sophisticated AI applications, modern block chain technology, and wellness equity.

REFERENCES

Ahmed, S. T., Basha, S. M., Ramachandran, M., Daneshmand, M., & Gandomi, A. H. (2023). An Edge-AI enabled Autonomous Connected Ambulance Route Resource Recommendation Protocol (ACA-R3) for eHealth in Smart Cities. *IEEE Internet of Things Journal*. https://doi.org/10.1109/JIOT.2023.3243235

Aldhyani, T. H. H., Khan, M. A., Almaiah, M. A., Alnazzawi, N., Hwaitat, A. K. A., Elhag, A., Shehab, R. T., & Alshebami, A. S. (2023). A Secure Internet of Medical Things Framework for Breast Cancer Detection in Sustainable Smart Cities. *Electronics (Switzerland), 12*(4). https://doi.org/10.3390/electronics12040858

Aldossary, M. (2023). Multi-Layer Fog-Cloud Architecture for Optimizing the Placement of IoT Applications in Smart Cities. *Computers, Materials and Continua, 75*(1). https://doi.org/10.32604/cmc.2023.035414

Alnssyan, B., Ahmad, Z., Malela-Majika, J. C., Seong, J. T., & Shafik, W. (2023). On the Identifiability and Statistical Features of a New Distributional Approach with Reliability Applications. *AIP Advances, 13*(12). https://doi.org/10.1063/5.0178555

Alwakeel, A., Alwakeel, M., Zahra, S. R., Saleem, T. J., Hijji, M., Alwakeel, S. S., Alwakeel, A. M., & Alzorgi, S. (2023). Common Mental Disorders in Smart City Settings and Use of Multimodal Medical Sensor Fusion to Detect Them. *Diagnostics, 13*(6). https://doi.org/10.3390/diagnostics13061082

AlZu'bi, S., Elbes, M., Mughaid, A., Bdair, N., Abualigah, L., Forestiero, A., & Zitar, R. A. (2023). Diabetes Monitoring System in Smart Health Cities Based on Big Data Intelligence. *Future Internet, 15*(2). https://doi.org/10.3390/fi15020085

Badr, N. G. (2023). Smart Cities for People with IDD - Foundations for Digitally Inclusive Healthcare Ecosystems. *ITM Web of Conferences, 51.* https://doi.org/10.1051/itmconf/20235104002

Berawi, M. A. (2023). Smart Cities: Accelerating Sustainable Development Agendas. *International Journal of Technology, 14*(1). https://doi.org/10.14716/ijtech.v14i1.6323

Cabrera, C., Svorobej, S., Palade, A., Kazmi, A., & Clarke, S. (2023). MAACO: A Dynamic Service Placement Model for Smart Cities. *IEEE Transactions on Services Computing, 16*(1). https://doi.org/10.1109/TSC.2022.3143029

Chakraborty, A., Banerjee, J. S., Bhadra, R., Dutta, A., Ganguly, S., Das, D., Kundu, S., Mahmud, M., & Saha, G. (2023). A Framework of Intelligent Mental Health Monitoring in Smart Cities and Societies. *IETE Journal of Research.* https://doi.org/10.1080/03772063.2023.2171918

Dutta, A., Kovid, R. K., Thatha, M., & Gupta, J. (2023). Adoption of IoT-Based Healthcare Devices: An Empirical Study of End Consumers in an Emerging Economy. *Paladyn, 14*(1). https://doi.org/10.1515/pjbr-2022-0106

El-Fouly, F. H., Kachout, M., Alharbi, Y., Alshudukhi, J. S., Alanazi, A., & Ramadan, R. A. (2023). Environment-Aware Energy Efficient and Reliable Routing in Real-Time Multi-Sink Wireless Sensor Networks for Smart Cities Applications. *Applied Sciences (Switzerland), 13*(1). https://doi.org/10.3390/app13010605

El-Shafai, W., Ali, R., Sedik, A., Taha, T. E. S., Abd-Elnaby, M., & Abd El-Samie, F. E. (2023). Analysis of Brain MRI: AI-Assisted Healthcare Framework for the Smart Cities. *Intelligent Automation and Soft Computing, 35*(2). https://doi.org/10.32604/iasc.2023.019198

Fan, J., Yang, W., Liu, Z., Kang, J., Niyato, D., Lam, K. Y., & Du, H. (2023). Understanding Security in Smart City Domains from the ANT-centric Perspective. *IEEE Internet of Things Journal.* https://doi.org/10.1109/JIOT.2023.3252040

Fong, B., Kim, H., & Sai, V. (2023). Special Section: Consumer Healthcare Technologies in Smart Cities. *IEEE Consumer Electronics Magazine.* https://doi.org/10.1109/MCE.2023.3245303

Gagliardi, A. R., & Albergo, F. (2023). The Rise of Smart Healthcare in Smart Cities: A Bibliometric Literature Review and Avenue for a Research Agenda. *ITM Web of Conferences, 51.* https://doi.org/10.1051/itmconf/20235103002

Joe, S. S. A., Mary, S. J. J., Cordova, R. S., Kalash, H. S., & Al-Badi, A. (2023). IoT-based Smart Campus Monitoring Based on an Improved Chimp Optimization-Based Deep Belief Neural Network. *Indonesian Journal of Electrical Engineering and Informatics (IJEEI), 11*(1). https://doi.org/10.52549/ijeei.v11i1.4410

Hussain, M. W., Moulik, S., & Roy, D. S. (2021, December). A broadcast based link discovery scheme for minimizing messages in software defined networks. In *2021 IEEE Globecom Workshops (GC Wkshps)* (pp. 1–6). IEEE.

Hussain, M. W., & Roy, D. S. (2021). Enabling indirect link discovery between SDN switches. In *Proceedings of the International Conference on Computing and Communication Systems: I3CS 2020*, NEHU, Shillong, India (pp. 471–481). Springer Singapore.

Hussain, M. W., & Roy, D. S. (2022a). Intelligent node placement for improving traffic engineering in hybrid SDN. In *Advances in Communication, Devices and Networking: Proceedings of ICCDN 2020* (pp. 287–296). Springer Singapore.

Hussain, M. W., & Roy, D. S. (2022b). A Counter-Based Profiling Scheme for Improving Locality Through Data and Reducer Placement. In *Advances in Machine Learning for Big Data Analysis* (pp. 101–118). Singapore: Springer Nature Singapore.

Hussain, M. W., & Roy, D. S. (2023a). Performance Optimization Strategies for Big Data Applications in Distributed Framework. In *Intelligent Technologies: Concepts, Applications, and Future Directions*, Volume *2* (pp. 221–252). Singapore: Springer Nature Singapore.

Hussain, M. W., Khan, M. S., Reddy, K. H. K., & Roy, D. S. (2022). Extended indirect controller-legacy switch forwarding for link discovery in hybrid multi-controller SDN. *Computer Communications*, *189*, 148–157.

Hussain, M. W., & Roy, D. S. (2023b). Performance Optimization Strategies for Big Data Applications in Distributed Framework. In *Intelligent Technologies: Concepts, Applications, and Future Directions*, Volume *2* (pp. 221–252). Singapore: Springer Nature Singapore.

Kushwaha, R., Shambharkar, R., Gupta, S., & Malik, M. (2023). Integration of Block Chain Model for Energy Efficient WSN for IOT Application. *International Journal for Research in Applied Science and Engineering Technology*, *11*(2). https://doi.org/10.22214/ijraset.2023.48942

Mengash, H. A., Alharbi, L. A., Alotaibi, S. S., AlMuhaideb, S., Nemri, N., Alnfiai, M. M., Marzouk, R., Salama, A. S., & Duhayyim, M. A. (2023). Deep Learning Enabled Intelligent Healthcare Management System in Smart Cities Environment. *Computers, Materials and Continua*, *74*(2). https://doi.org/10.32604/cmc.2023.032588

Mohammed, B. G., & Hasan, D. S. (2023). Smart Healthcare Monitoring System Using IoT. *International Journal of Interactive Mobile Technologies*, *17*(1). https://doi.org/10.3991/ijim.v17i01.34675

Pandya, S., Srivastava, G., Jhaveri, R., Babu, M. R., Bhattacharya, S., Maddikunta, P. K. R., Mastorakis, S., Piran, M. J., & Gadekallu, T. R. (2023). Federated Learning for Smart Cities: A Comprehensive Survey. *Sustainable Energy Technologies and Assessments*, *55*. https://doi.org/10.1016/j.seta.2022.102987

Reddy Yeruva, A. (2023). Providing A Personalized Healthcare Service To Patients Using AIOPs Monitoring. *Eduvest - Journal of Universal Studies*, *3*(2). https://doi.org/10.36418/eduvest.v3i2.742

Reddy, K. H. K., Roy, D. S., Mishra, T. K., & Hussain, M. W. (Eds.). (2023). *Handbook of Research on Network-Enabled IoT Applications for Smart City Services*. IGI Global.

Samy El Menchawy, A., Hassan Moustafa, H., & Ibrahim Abdel-Hamid, N. (2023). Smart Capital Cities: Towards a Smart New Administrative Capital (NAC). *F1000Research*, *12*. https://doi.org/10.12688/f1000research.130322.1

Shafik, W., Matinkhah, S. M., & Ghasemzadeh, M. (2020a). Theoretical Understanding of Deep Learning in UAV Biomedical Engineering Technologies Analysis. *SN Computer Science*, *1*(6). https://doi.org/10.1007/s42979-020-00323-8

Shafik, W., Mojtaba Matinkhah, S., & Ghasemzadeh, M. (2020b). *Internet of Things-Based Energy Management, Challenges, and Solutions in Smart Cities*. https://doi.org/10.22385/jctecs.v27i0.302

Sharma, O., Rathee, G., Kerrache, C. A., & Herrera-Tapia, J. (2023). Two-Stage Optimal Task Scheduling for Smart Home Environment Using Fog Computing Infrastructures. *Applied Sciences (Switzerland)*, *13*(5). https://doi.org/10.3390/app13052939

Tareen, F. N., Alvi, A. N., Malik, A. A., Javed, M. A., Khan, M. B., Saudagar, A. K. J., Alkhathami, M., & Abul Hasanat, M. H. (2023). Efficient Load Balancing for Blockchain-Based Healthcare System in Smart Cities. *Applied Sciences (Switzerland)*, *13*(4). https://doi.org/10.3390/app13042411

Tripathi, A. K., Akul Krishnan, K., & Pandey, A. C. (2023). A Novel Blockchain and Internet of Things-Based Food Traceability System for Smart Cities. *Wireless Personal Communications*. https://doi.org/10.1007/s11277-023-10230-9

Tripathy, S. S., Imoize, A. L., Rath, M., Tripathy, N., Bebortta, S., Lee, C. C., Chen, T. Y., Ojo, S., Isabona, J., & Pani, S. K. (2023). A Novel Edge-Computing-Based Framework for an Intelligent Smart Healthcare System in Smart Cities. *Sustainability (Switzerland), 15*(1). https://doi.org/10.3390/su15010735

Yang, Z., Jianjun, L., Faqiri, H., Shafik, W., Talal Abdulrahman, A., Yusuf, M., & Sharawy, A. M. (2021). Green Internet of Things and Big Data Application in Smart Cities Development. *Complexity, 2021*. https://doi.org/10.1155/2021/4922697

Hussain, M. W. (2024). Centralized Traffic Engineering. In *Towards Wireless Heterogeneity in 6G Networks* (pp. 180–193). CRC Press https://doi.org/10.1201/9781003369028

Zakzouk, A., El-Sayed, A., & Hemdan, E. E. D. (2023). A Blockchain-Based Electronic Medical Records Management Framework in Smart Healthcare Infrastructure. *Multimedia Tools and Applications*. https://doi.org/10.1007/s11042-023-15152-z

2

Role of Body-Transfer System in Active Assistive Living for Effective Healthcare

Chyi-Yeu Lin, Bahrudin, and Salman Masroor
National Taiwan University of Science and Technology, Taipei, Taiwan

2.1 Introduction

2.1.1 Aiming Towards an Active Assistive Living Environment

This chapter discusses a variety of health, sociological, and economic issues that arise globally because of changes in the demographic structure. The long-term effects felt by various nations of the world due to the demographic changes are elaborated. Furthermore, the healthcare burden and their financial estimates for various nations and regions are discussed later. Furthermore, the concept of active assistive living (AAL) is presented as a possible solution for maintaining individuals' independence in a community that is aging.

2.1.2 Demographic Structural Change

2.1.2.1 Drastic Increase in the Life Expectancy

The repercussions of a demographic shift are being felt in countries all across the world, and it is frequently cited as one of the most enduring problems facing future generations. The average age of an individual in Europe has reached almost 78 years. This is because individual life expectancies have significantly increased during the modern era (Commissi, 2006; Nehmer, Becker, Karshmer, & Lamm, 2006). By 2025, around 1.2 billion people will reach the age of 60, based on projections presented by the World Health Organization (WHO). Moreover, forecasts also state that by 2050, 2 billion people, or 22% of the worldwide population, are going to be 60 years of age or older (Laleci et al., 2008). Over the same time span, it is anticipated that the population of people over the age of 85 will increase by more than six times (Vergados, Alevizos, Mariolis, & Caragiozidis, 2008).

Recent shifts occurring in Europe are not an anomaly to this widespread trend. The population of Europe is aging because of longer life spans and persistently low birth rates. Senior citizens now outnumber children in Europe by 2050, that ratio is expected

DOI: 10.1201/9781032631738-2

to be more than double (Coughlin, D'Ambrosio, Reimer, & Pratt, 2007). By 2025, about one-third of Europeans will be 60 years of age or older, as per WHO projections (WHO, 2022).

The more developed Asian countries can also be viewed to be in a similar situation. The case of Japan has almost negligible population growth because the population is aging at an exponential rate. Almost 25 million Japanese individuals are over the age of 65, and 20,000 are over the age of 100 (Stadlmayer, 2009). Right now, the population structure of Japan has converted from a pyramid-shaped structure into a cone-shaped structure. Additionally, the WHO estimates that the original structure of Japan's population will be inverted into an upside-down pyramid by 2035 (WHO, 2022). With the continuation of such a trend, there will be a deficiency of younger caregivers who can care for their elderly relatives by 2050 (Nehmer et al., 2006). Similar traits can be seen in other Asian nations. In Singapore, for instance, 20% of the population is expected to be 65 or older within the next 30 years (Chen, Zhang, Kam, & Shue, 2005). Figure 2.1 shows the factors that cause the aging population to rise and the consequences these elderly people face due to aging. To accommodate these people, the family members play the role of caregiver, or they hire a professional caregiver.

However, the population upheaval is affecting more than just the Western world. Dependency ratios are predicted to sharply increase in emerging economies like China

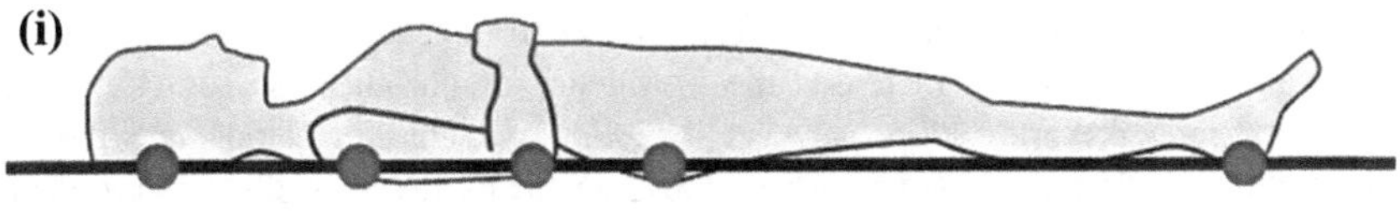

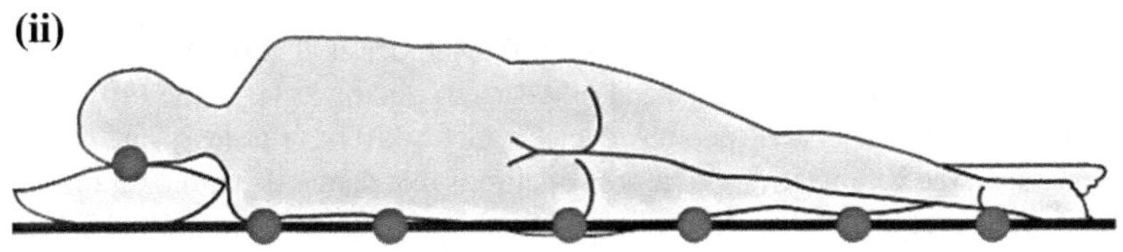

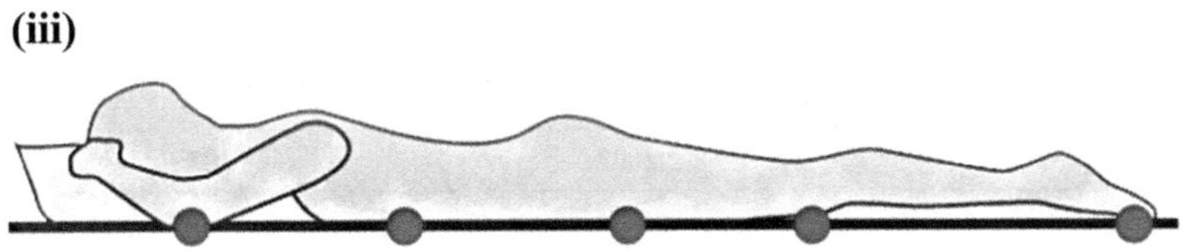

FIGURE 2.1 Various lying positions of elderly and physically challenged persons.

and India until 2050 (Commissi, 2006). China has also seen a sharp increase in the number of senior citizens, with almost 140 million individuals in the country having 60 years of age or older (Coughlin et al., 2007). According to the WHO projections, the amount of adults 60 and over will rise from 400 million to almost 840 million until 2025, making up 70% of the world's elderly population (WHO, 2022).

2.1.2.2 Reduced Birth Rate

Given the dramatic drop in birth rates and an increasing lifespan of the elderly, there is very little likelihood that demographic patterns will reverse in the ensuing decades. In the absence of immigration, the fertility rate in Europe should be 2.1 for maintaining the population pyramid. However, currently, it has reduced to 1.5 children per woman (Commissi, 2006).

The estimates presented by WHO (2022) show a rapid rise in old-age dependency ratios across the globe. According to Table 2.1, by 2025, there will be 66 elderly persons in Japan for every 100 citizens between the ages of 15 and 60, an increase from 0.39 in 2002 to 0.66. According to the United Nations, by 2045, more people will be over 60 than under 15 (Coughlin et al., 2007).

2.1.2.3 Drastic Rise in Chronic Conditions and Disabilities

Individuals are living longer and recovering faster from acute illnesses as a result of medical advances, which increases the prevalence of chronic diseases (Campana, Moreno, Riano, & Varga, 2008; Laleci et al., 2008; Podtschaske, Glende, & Friesdorf, 2009; Villar, Federici, & Annicchiarico, 2007). Diabetes and heart disease, for example, are growing more common as people age, according to current study (Braun, Nelles, & Rumm, 2009). Morbidity data show that over 75% of older citizens in all sociological, economic, and cultural situations suffer a chronic condition (Rasmus Hoffmann, 2008). Cardiovascular illnesses, hypertension, stroke, cancer, diabetes, dementia, and musculoskeletal problems are only a few of the frequent high-age diseases that impact seniors worldwide (Jones, 1998; Nehmer et al., 2006).

While more than 60% of persons aged 60 years are facing at least one or multiple chronic illnesses. Over 95% of persons over the age of 70 have at least one chronic condition, and over 30% have five or more conditions that demand continuing medical treatment (Kruse et al., 2002). According to Wichert, Gaugisch, Norgall, & Becker (2009), about 40% of the people suffering from such chronic illnesses cause individuals to have long-term activity limits. In addition, new research indicates individuals over 65 report one serious health event on average per year (Atchley, 1985).

TABLE 2.1

Old-Age Dependency Ratios for Selected Countries and Regions Based on UN (2001)

Country	2002	2025
Japan	0.39	0.66
North America	0.26	0.44
European Union	0.36	0.56

Age is also a significant factor that raises the risk of impairment, in addition to chronic conditions (Schäper, Schüller, Dieckmann, & Greving, 2010). According to the Living Britain Survey (Office for National Statistics (ONS), 1995), mobility, visual, and hearing impairments are the most prevalent issues for the majority of disabled people aged 65 or older. As people get older, the likelihood of having a disability, particularly a sensory disability, increases. As per the study presented by the British Department of Health study, approximately 80% of those persons who are over the age of 60 have a vision impairment, and similarly, 75% of those persons who are over the age of 60 have a hearing impairment, and 22% of the individuals have both (Office for National Statistics (ONS), 1995).

A higher likelihood of falling is another major danger associated with deteriorating physical capabilities. As per WHO estimates, every year, roughly 30% of individuals beyond the age of 65 and 50% of those over the age of 80 pass away. According to Nehmer et al. (2006), one-quarter of persons aged 65–74 had at least one autumn year. While the majority of mishaps are minor, 20–30% of such incidents result in long-term functional impairments for the patients (De Ruyter and Pelgrim, 2007). According to Lohman, Sonnega, Nicklett, Estenson, and Leggett (2019), falls are a major source of impairment in those over the age of 75, as well as a significant cause of injury-related mortality. Hip fractures are the most common major injury caused by falls in the elderly, costing England alone about 2 billion euros per year (Dolan & Torgerson, 1998).

2.1.2.4 Requirement for Continuous Care

In the upcoming years, it has been estimated that there will be drastic rise in the number of elderly individuals who require care and assistance in performing activities of daily living. As per the estimates presented in (Campana et al., 2008), the population of severely impaired persons who require time care is equivalent to the population of elderly people. According to estimates, 5% of adults aged 65–69 require care, 10% of those aged 70–79 require care, and 80% of those over the age of 80 require care (Walker, 2011).

Recent numbers from Germany illustrate the gravity of the situation. Approximately 8 million people are currently incapacitated, and in 85% of these situations, previous diseases are to blame (Wegge, 2009). While just 10% of individuals 65 and older require care, the number climbs to 50% for those 85 and beyond (Wilkes, 2009). Furthermore, the general population in need of care has increased considerably during the last ten years. In Germany, the proportion of persons in need of care increased by 48.8% from 2.9% in 2007 to 4.3% in 2017 (Schwinger & Tsiasioti, 2018). The population requiring stationary care, in particular, is constantly growing. According to Wichert et al. (2009), the number of people living in care institutions increased by 6 years, from 573,200 in 1999 to 676,600 in 2005. And the population of people in need of care is expected to expand significantly over the next ten years. Presently, the study in Germany shows that there are 2.15 million people who require care and assistance through institutional services and estimated to reach 3 million by 2025 (Heinze, Hilbert, & Paulus, 2009). In addition to the prevalence of chronic medical diseases, the deterioration of physical capacities in older individuals contributes to the need for assistance. As a result of diminished mobility, performing daily tasks at home and elsewhere becomes increasingly difficult, if not impossible (Horter et al., 2009; Lee, Chen, Lin, Chang, & Chen, 2000; Rialle, Lamy, Noury, & Bajolle, 2003; Vergados et al., 2008).

2.1.2.5 Shortage of Caregiving People Force

In almost every Western country, the shrinking working-age population (15–64 years old) is inextricably related to increased life expectancy. Additionally, research indicates that throughout the same span of time, the dependency ratio will nearly increase by 51%, and by 2050, 48 million fewer individuals in Europe are likely to be employed (Commissi, 2006). This means that the ratio of elderly persons over 65 to the working population will fall from 4:1 to 2:1 in the next 40 years. Many writers and organizations, such as Britton (2003) and Wilkes (2009), forecast that throughout the next few decades, there will be a severe shortage of healthcare workers for providing care to functionally dependent individuals.

A primary concern in this context is the increasing number of people afflicted with chronic conditions such as diabetes. According to Reinhart Hoffmann (2009), the annual cost of diabetes (including comorbidities and indirect expenditures) in Germany is around 60 billion euros. According to Bernnat et al. (2017), the ambulant industry bears a sizable amount of these costs. Diabetes patients, who account for less than 10% of insurance holders in Germany, are expected to bear over 29% of the country's overall health insurance (Heuzeroth, 2009).

2.1.2.6 Long-Term Elder People Care

The number of older individuals in danger of institutionalization has increased as a result of longer life expectancies, lower birth rates, and a rise in single-person homes (Vergados et al., 2008). The figures from Germany and the United States in Nehmer et al. (2006) show that only 3–4% of Americans are today institutionalized in aged care institutions, about 1.5 million people in Germany live out their entire lives in such facilities. They estimate that the old-age population in both nations will get doubled, as the young generation starts to get older based on the current developments. This desire is frequently connected to a sense of improved quality of life in a comfortable setting. Generali (2017) surveyed $N = 4133$ participants between the ages of 65 and 85 to learn more about the living conditions of older adults in Germany. According to the study, the majority of seniors are content with their existing living arrangements, particularly those who own their homes or apartments.

The current changes in family arrangements occurring in most developed countries are another driving force behind the need for new care paradigms. While internal support mechanisms for senior family members were traditionally given through extended family structures, in recent years the approach of keeping large families is now becoming obsolete (Dewsbury & Edge, 2000). The severity of the issue is also exacerbated by two other developments: (1) the rise in single-family homes and (2) the growing percentage of elderly individuals who reject care provided by the family members.

It is frequently stated that changes to the social structures in many Western societies are to blame for the sharp rise in single-person families over the past several years. The fact that elderly individuals frequently reject family support because they see fulfilling family responsibilities as an attack on their moral values and dignity goes largely undetected (Lindley, Harper, & Sellen, 2008). According to poll findings, almost 95% of older individuals surveyed did not want to live with relatives (Dewsbury & Edge, 2000).

2.2 Active Assistive Living

2.2.1 Concept and Definition

AAL is a concept that blends active aging, assistive technology, and supportive surroundings to improve the quality of life and independence of seniors and people with disabilities. This method attempts to improve physical, cognitive, and social well-being while allowing people to live more freely in their homes or communities (Dobre, Bajenaru, Marinescu, & Tomescu, 2019).

Recent advancements in information and communication technology are laying the framework for new patient-centered homecare solutions. Previously, most of the computer-assistive healthcare equipment that has emerged in the past few decades has primarily been intended to help caregivers and medical personnel (Reddy et al., 2023). However, this trend has recently been reversed by the emergence of assistive technology that provides help and flexible support to caregivers and medical personnel in addition to sick or disabled individuals (Cortés et al., 2008). Several authors, including De Ruyter and Pelgrim (2007) and Vergados et al. (2008), anticipate that in the future, healthcare systems will be primarily focused on providing assistance at home. This approach will shift the paradigm from providing care and assistance in the traditional hospital environment to the patient's home. According to Villar et al. (2007), the focus of this relatively new sector of research is to safeguard the autonomy of the care-requiring individuals. This not only increases the quality of life for elderly and disabled people but also caregivers by allowing them to stay at their homes for as long as practical. This method of providing care to disabled and elderly individuals is also known as AAL.

AAL systems play a significant role in enhancing the quality of life and independence of elderly individuals or people with disabilities. These systems combine technology, healthcare, and various forms of assistance to create an environment that supports individuals in their daily activities and promotes their well-being. Here are some key significances of utilizing AAL systems:

2.2.2 Enhanced Quality of Life, Independence, and Autonomy

Initially and most notably, AAL environments represent a significant advancement in improving the overall quality of life for elderly and disabled individuals within their homes (Heinze et al., 2009; Meyer, 2009; Nehmer et al., 2006). Through the reduction of dependence on caregivers, personal nursing services, and the necessity to relocate to nursing homes, AAL environments have the potential to enhance the everyday lives of elderly individuals, enabling them to age in place (Adam, Mukasa, Breiner, & Trapp, 2008; Britton, 2003; Glende, Podtschaske, & Friesdorf, 2009; Palen & Aaløkke, 2006). Preserving one's independence for as long as feasible and avoiding becoming reliant on one's children is broadly acknowledged as a pivotal factor contributing to a high quality of life in later years (Forlizzi et al., 2004; Hirsch et al., 2000; Lindley et al., 2008). Thus, AAL systems enable individuals to remain in their own homes and maintain a higher level of independence and autonomy. By providing assistance in tasks such as medication management, meal preparation, and personal care, these systems help individuals retain control over their lives.

Research conducted by Kane and Kane (1987) further demonstrates that, in comparison to patients who receive traditional treatment compared to those who receive home care, typically exhibit more positive sentiments when it comes to assessing the satisfaction in life and perceived health. Likewise, another study contends that there is substantial evidence indicating that individuals residing in nursing homes are more prone to increased hospitalizations, doctor visits, and a higher likelihood of experiencing depression due to their diminished sense of independence (Helal et al., 2003). Furthermore, delivering medical services in patients' own homes enhances their privacy and dignity (Finkelstein et al., 1998; Vergados et al., 2008). Assistive technologies can also play a positive role in enhancing the quality of life for individuals with disabilities. According to Schalock (1996), the quality of life for disabled individuals is impacted by eight key dimensions, including self-determination and social inclusion. Many authors, such as Klauß (1999), emphasize the significance of self-determination as a pivotal factor in improving the quality of life for individuals with disabilities. Contemporary research underscores the significance of personal independence, as evidenced by findings that establish a link between decreased mobility and lower self-esteem (Motl et al., 2005; Saizmaa & Kim, 2008). AAL technologies can assume a critical role in empowering individuals with disabilities to engage in daily activities by catering to individual limitations and facilitating novel forms of computer-mediated communication (Garrels & Arvidsson, 2019).

The term "active aging" was formally introduced by the WHO in 2002, defining it as "the process of optimizing opportunities for health, participation, and security, in order to enhance the quality of life and well-being as people age" (WHO, 2022). However, the concept itself is not new. Walker (2002) offers a comprehensive historical perspective on the term's evolution and its relationships and distinctions from earlier terms like "successful aging" and "productive aging" (Morrow-Howell, Hinterlong, & Sherraden, 2001). Drawing on his previous work (Fernández-Ballesteros, 2008), Fernández-Ballesteros et al. (2012) succinctly summarize the fundamental attributes of active aging as encompassing "low probability of illness and disability, high physical fitness, high cognitive functioning, positive mood and coping with stress, and being engaged with life" (Fernández-Ballesteros, Robine, Walker, & Kalache, 2013). In this context, Walker (2002) emphasizes that "active aging must encompass all older people, even those who are, to some extent, frail and dependent." Consequently, AAL systems can be regarded as technology that empowers independence and inclusion, particularly for individuals who may not enjoy the same level of health and autonomy (Walker, 2002).

2.2.3 Medical Benefits

AAL systems have enormous potential, especially when taken into account in relation to illness prevention and early detection (Orwat et al., 2008). Effective therapeutic support and early recognition of aberrant circumstances are made possible by the remote patient monitoring, but it has also demonstrated its capacity to significantly reduce hospitalizations and enhance the success of long-term therapies (Biley, 2002; Braun et al., 2009).

2.2.4 Cost-Efficiency

AAL goes beyond merely enhancing service quality. It also holds the potential to substantially decrease the expenses associated with long-term care (Braun et al., 2009; Britton, 2003; Kühne, Behner, Henke, & Nelles, 2009; Mynatt, Melenhorst, Fisk, & Rogers, 2004). As an illustration, Heinze et al. (2009) believe that implementing remote healthcare for patients with cardiovascular problems could result in up to 30% in cost reductions. Comparable research conducted by Gothe, Storz, Daroszewska, and Freytag (2009) and Johnston, Weeler, Deuser, & Sousa (2000) also yielded similarly positive outcomes. Thus, it comes as no surprise that technology-supported home care will emerge as one of the most rapidly expanding sectors within the healthcare industry in the coming decades (Demiris & Tan, 2005). Recent research conducted in Europe, for instance, projects a potential value of around 39 billion Euros for electronic healthcare solutions. This amounts to over 12% of the overall healthcare expenses in Europe (Bernnat et al., 2017).

Nowadays, the technical considerations of system providers and medical professionals largely influence the design of contemporary homecare systems (Ballegaard, Hansen, & Kyng, 2008). Even though the value of interdisciplinary collaboration is well recognized, discipline-spanning research is uncommon, particularly in the field of healthcare technologies and aging (Hennessy & Walker, 2011). Consequently, advances in this field are frequent demonstrations of technological possibilities instead of responses to the actual demands of the potential users. It is frequently cited as one of the main causes of poor adoption behavior (Leonard & Rayport, 1997). One cause of this difficulty is a developer's lack of knowledge. Engineers and system designers usually know a great deal about their technological capabilities but not as much about the societal setting within which their solutions will be used (Haines, Mitchell, Cooper, & Maguire, 2007; Lindley et al., 2008; Venkatesh, 1996; Venkatesh & Vitalari, 1992). According to Quigley & Tweed (2000), "Thoughts about what modern technology may accomplish for the elderly are often grounded in a thorough grasp of requirements and, occasionally, are just overt attempts to promote technology."

2.3 Problems Identified Based on Previous Research Studies

2.3.1 Lack of User Integration

Even though modern assistive systems have addressed certain glaring flaws in their design, many systems are still missing user integration (Bias & Mayhew, 2005; Cooper, 2004). Time and money restraints are among the most often mentioned justifications for not including users in the creation of new technologies (Glende et al., 2009). Therefore, numerous products are inaccessible to huge segments of the population since designers' design focus is on the users who are able-bodied. Or they are either unaware of or unable to consider the demands of users with varied capacities during the design process (Keates, Clarkson, Harrison, & Robinson, 2000).

2.3.2 Lack of Adopting User-Centered Approach

Numerous research studies have proved the relevance of user-centered design approaches. For example, in Ziefle (2008) and Ziefle and Bay (2005), it has been demonstrated that age-specific design approaches could dramatically minimize age-related handicaps, allowing older persons to operate modern technology more efficiently. Furthermore, user-centered design additionally benefits end users by making medical products more usable, but it is additionally likely to have a significant positive financial impact on suppliers and manufacturers since it is significantly less expensive to adapt technical concepts and aid features early in the design process (Vahs & Burmester, 2005). Thus, potential users should be involved in exploratory studies frequently for the development of new systems. During this process, it is critical to give special consideration to two areas, i.e., the participation of potential users and their homes, which are major areas of application. This is especially important because elderly consumers will certainly be the first to adopt electronically improved healthcare solutions (Coughlin et al., 2007).

2.3.3 Poor Adoption of AAL Systems Due to Lack of Workspace Considerations

Previous design techniques are founded on actual knowledge gathered in the workplace, and these studies have frequently ignored the core rationalities of stakeholder's desires, demands, and comfort (Crabtree, Hemmings, & Rodden, 2002). It is sometimes overlooked when building home technology that the same design considerations that are used in offices cannot be translated to a domestic context (Hindus, 1999). Since various resources and factors considered by home users differ completely compared to those found within workplaces. The poor adaptation of new assistive technology is the result of this misalignment in approach. Since AAL systems can give personalized medical help and allow older people to live independently, many present products are not well accepted by potential users. According to Fichten, Barile, Asuncion, and Fossey (2000), nearly 50% of people who require assistive technologies do not utilize them.

Usage that is insufficient or inconsistent indicates that providers have not yet satisfied end customers' true needs and preferences (Abowd, Edwards, & Grinter, 2003). When tackling this issue, keep in mind that technological approval is a highly situational phenomenon. Various studies have been conducted to show the improvement in the quality of life of physically challenged individuals at home. However, the usage of assistive technology in a social context is not known broadly (Haines et al., 2007). As a result, rather than attempting to transfer current knowledge from other application areas, it is critical to carefully examine the application of future healthcare technology in home scenarios. To fully grasp the context of later usage, the design of successful AAL systems for home use necessitates strong communication with possible end users (Ballegaard et al., 2008). Understanding the impact of caregiving on persons who provide care to older adults or people with disabilities requires assessing the load and stress on caregivers in the context of AAL. AAL strives to improve care recipients' independence and well-being while simultaneously taking caregivers' needs and well-being into account. The Zarit-Burden Interview and the caregiver Strain Index are used to assess the caregiver's load (Hagell, Alvariza, Westergren, & Årestedt, 2017).

Typically, these tools include questions about the physical, emotional, economic, and social elements of caregiving.

2.4 Body-Transfer System

This section describes the design methodology of the body-transfer system (BTS) in detail. The BTS comprises three modules, namely, a body-transfer bed (BTB), a body-transfer wheelchair (BTW), and a body-transfer toilet wheelchair (BTTW). Lin, Masroor, Bahrudin, and Bulut (2023) depicts the schematic diagram of BTS. Since the BTS has to be used in the AAL facility, the user can provide commands through various sources like vision or audio sensors. The health monitoring system is used to continuously monitor health, and it can also provide data to health professionals in case of emergency. All BTS modules, input modules, and health-management systems are connected by a local network.

2.4.1 Design of Body-Transfer Bed

The standard proposed by the International Organization for Standardization (ISO) and the International Electrotechnical Commission (IEC) is IEC/EN 60601-2-52. This is the dimensional standard set for the development of various assistive devices such as home-based healthcare systems, nursing, and hospital beds. However, there is no fixed dimension regarding the length of the bed, i.e., the length between the head and the end panel of the bed. Therefore, it can be inferred that the commercial manufacturers of this technology are allowed to keep dimensions of their own choice, but it should still comply with the other dimensions proposed in the aforementioned standard. Manufacturers frequently construct beds with distances of up to 2300 mm between head and foot panels. However, the most typical length is 2000 mm. According to the statistics in Annex A (which shows the percentile distribution of height in the Taiwanese adult population), beds with a height of 1810 mm will cover more than 99% of the population. Using this information, it is possible to determine that a device with a length of 1880 mm will cover the majority of the population. Furthermore, the anthropometric estimates for Chinese adults (see Annex A) depict that the shoulder breadth of the male population is less than 450 mm. These measurements are significant because a relatively flat space on which the shoulders are able to rest comfortably without discomfort is required. Therefore, it can be analyzed that if this portion of the body is curled in, the thorax is compressed, and if this section is arched, the patient may fall off the device.

Additionally, the mass of those individuals who will be transferred is also necessary for deciding the overall specifications of the BTS. If the system is over-designed for exaggerated loads, then it will increase the cost of the system and adversely affect its overall functionality. Thus, evaluating a mass value that can accommodate a large population is required. For this reason, in Chen, Lin, Lee, Chen, and Ho (2021), the weight distribution of Taiwanese adults has been shown to be 72.2±10.5 kg for males and 57.4 ±8.8 kg for females. Thus, to accommodate 99% of Taiwan's population, the BTS has been designed to have a payload capacity of 110 kg.

2.4.2 Assessment of Lying Positions of Elderly and Physically Challenged Persons

It has been observed that the individuals lying on the bed have three distinct positions. Figure 2.1 shows the lying positions of these individuals. They may be lying on the bed (decubitus) in a supine state (dorsal decubitus), which means that they will be lying on their back, as shown in Figure 2.1 (i). They may be lying on one side of the body (lateral decubitus), either on the left or the right, as depicted in Figure 2.1 (ii). The third possible state of lying on the bed is lying on their stomach (ventral decubitus), as shown in Figure 2.1 (iii). However, for achieving stability, safety, and comfort while transferring, a supine state is preferred.

2.4.3 Load Distribution Assessment According to Human Body Segmentation

For conducting the load distribution analysis, a previously developed system has considered a general value of the weight of the human body that is concentrated on a single point. However, when designing BTS, human body load distribution with reference to human body segments is considered. In this regard, for evaluation, the high-pressure concentration areas are assessed. This is done by considering the pressure mapping (mmHg) of a person lying on the bed in a supine state, as shown in Figure 2.2.

The pressure distribution mapping shows that most of the human body weight is concentrated on the chest, pelvis, and legs. Furthermore, the low-pressure concentration region is the head and neck, abdomen, and lastly, the upper thighs and knee part.

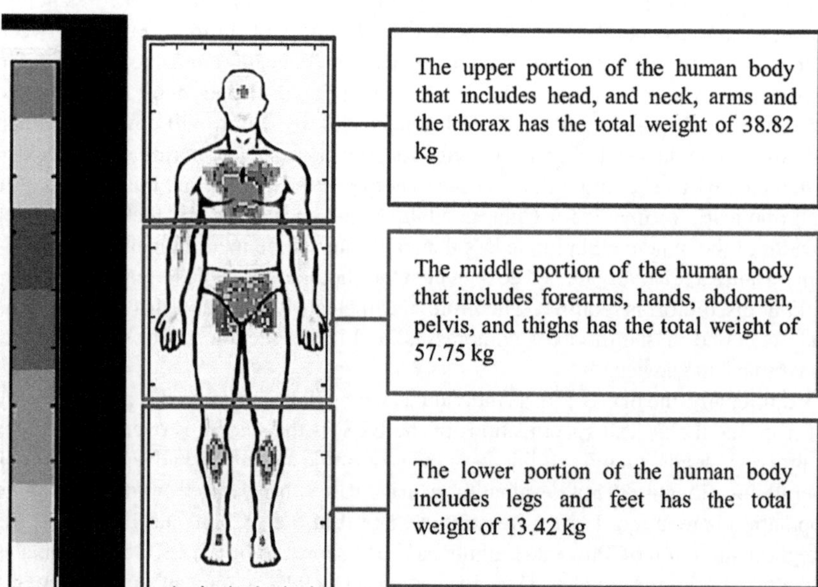

FIGURE 2.2 Concentration of pressure on the array of pressure sensors when a person lay on the bed.

Thus, it can be inferred that the weight distribution can be used for calculating the force exerted by each segment of the human body. Moreover, a conveyor belt solution for transferring the physically disabled is an optimal solution. With regard to human body segmentation, the weight distribution of each segment of the human body is studied in Kärki and Lekkala (2006), and according to the study, a human having a mass of 110 kg has the weight distribution as shown in Table 2.2. Thus, the distribution is mentioned in Table 2.2, and the distribution of mass of the human body at various portions of the body is shown in Figure 2.3.

From Figure 2.2, it can be inferred that most of the weight concentration is on the middle section of the body. So, the transfer should be designed in such a manner that it can transfer the human body properly without altering the human body angle and

TABLE 2.2
Human Body Mass Segmentation

	Relative Mass	Individual Member Mass	Combined Mass of Body Parts
Body Segment	**(%)**	**(kg)**	**(kg)**
Head and neck	8.1	8.91	8.9
Forearm	3.2	1.76	3.52
Thorax	21.6	23.76	23.76
Arm	5.6	3.08	6.2
Hand	1.2	0.66	1.32
Abdomen	13.9	15.29	15.29
Pelvis	14.2	15.62	15.62
Thigh	20.0	11	22
Leg	9.3	5.115	10.23
Foot	2.9	1.595	3.19
Total Mass			110

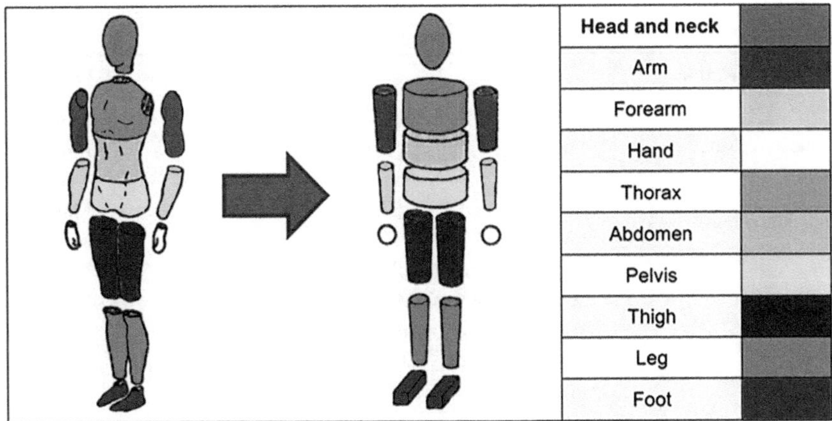

FIGURE 2.3 Body-segmentation with reference to its geometric shape.

posture in the sagittal plane, as shown in Figure 2.4. These operational requirements can be used to design, develop, and test the BTS. Table 2.3 displays the specifications of the BTB. The transfer and safety modules are the two modules that make up the BTB. These conveyor belts are placed opposite to one another and are driven by two synchronized AC servomotors. The BTB measures 1880 x 1060 x 200 mm, while the BTB frame has 2075 x 1150 x 580 mm dimensions. Two center-driven conveyor belts have been attached to the BTB to enable transfers of an individual from the bed to both wheelchairs. Upper and lower conveyor belts with dimensions of 3600 x 590 x 3 mm and 3600 x 900 x 3 mm, respectively, have been chosen.

These conveyor belts are covered with a Velcro-secured material that serves as a bedsheet to preserve proper cleanliness. The upper and lower conveyor belts are driven by two friction rollers with 606 and 910 mm lengths, respectively. Both rollers have a

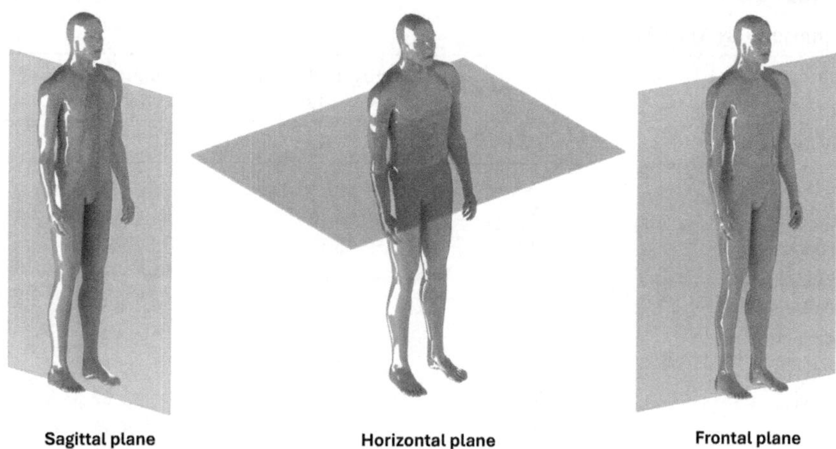

FIGURE 2.4 Planes of motion in the human body.

TABLE 2.3

Overall Specifications of Body-Transfer Bed (Lin et al., 2023)

BTB Specifications		Value	Unit
Fame dimensions	Length	2075	Mm
	Width	1150	Mm
	Height	580	Mm
Bed dimensions	Length	1880	Mm
	Width	1060	Mm
Conveyor dimensions	Upper conveyor length	3600	Mm
	Upper conveyor width	5900	Mm
	Lower conveyor length	3600	Mm
	Lower conveyor width	900	Mm
Load	Transfer load capacity	110	Kg
Safety flap dimensions	Height	250	Mm
	Width	400	Mm

diameter of 76.5 mm. Crown rollers are mounted on both sides of BTB, maintaining the belt's trajectory in a straight path. To lessen friction across the sidewalls between the belt and the bed, supplementary 500 mm idler rollers have been added on both sides of the BTB. Since the patient's body must pass over the rollers during the transfer, the rollers have been covered with 75 mm of thick foam to ensure the patient's comfort. A spring-loaded tension device has been incorporated into the transfer system to maintain tension on both conveyor belts. To keep the driving rollers vertical, roller supports have been bolted to a horizontal sliding frame. Due to the bi-directional nature of the conveyor belts, there is a risk that a patient who is physically impaired may be seriously injured as a result of an accident involving the belts. Therefore, it is necessary to include a safety module. According to this module consists of a motorized guiding rail, a double rail, and a motorized protective flap. The motorized guide rail's purpose is to move the flap out of the way so that the transfer can proceed. These guide rails are bolted below the frame. L-shaped brackets are bolted with these guides for countering the unbalanced forces on the flap while moving. The guide rail is driven by a NEMA23XL stepper motor with a 1000 mm travel stroke. Limit switches are used for safe movement of the guide rails. Safety motorized flaps are mounted on both sides of the BTB. A motorized flap panel with a flange for holding the motor, which rotates the flap frame, has been attached to the L-shaped bracket using a pipe. Two limit switches that are firmly fastened to the flange control the rotation of the DC-geared motor that drives the flap.

2.4.4 Task Scenarios of BTS

BTS has been designed to perform various tasks, i.e., transferring the person from bed to wheelchair and vice versa, moving the person around the home, and assisting the person in performing toileting and bathing. In the AAL facility, all modules are connected to a local Wi-Fi network that monitors the position of each module, and the central control unit acts according to the user's instructions. Figure 2.5 shows various task scenarios of different BTS modules as per the user's instructions.

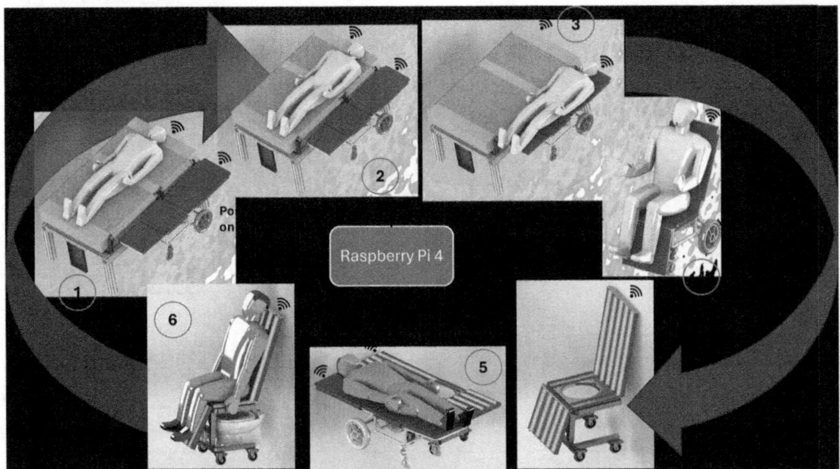

FIGURE 2.5 Smart bed and wheelchair transfer devices and communication concept.

It can be inferred that all the modules of BTS are designed according to the dimensions and standards set by the ISO. Therefore, there is no space limitation issue in operating the modules of BTS. All modules communicate with the central control unit, which helps in assisting various people in the AAL facility, and every module is connected to the WI-FI network. Figure 2.6 shows the architecture on which the BTS is working. The cloud-based service ensures the safety and well-being of each individual living in the AAL facility (Reddy et al., 2023; Hussain and Roy, 2023).

2.4.5 Advantages of Utilizing BTS in AAL Facility

Improved independence in performing ADLs: The BTS can empower physically disabled and bedridden individuals to have more control over their mobility and transfers. Additionally, it also allows them to perform the ADLs with increased independence.

Reduced caregiver burden: When helping bedridden patients be transferred and transported, caregivers frequently run into difficulties. Your app might make it possible for caregivers to complete these chores more effectively and safely, potentially lightening their physical and mental load.

Safety: Transferring a physically disabled person is a tedious and dangerous task. Most of the accidents and injuries occur during the transfers. BTS lowers the risk of accidents and falls during transfers. Contrary to the previously developed approaches, the seat of the BTW does not have any electrical parts. This ensures that the chances of electrocution should be mitigated.

Personalized assistance: The modules of BTS can be utilized individually and in integrated form. This helps the users to fulfill their specific needs and capabilities. Therefore, BTS provides a personalized approach to mobility and transfers.

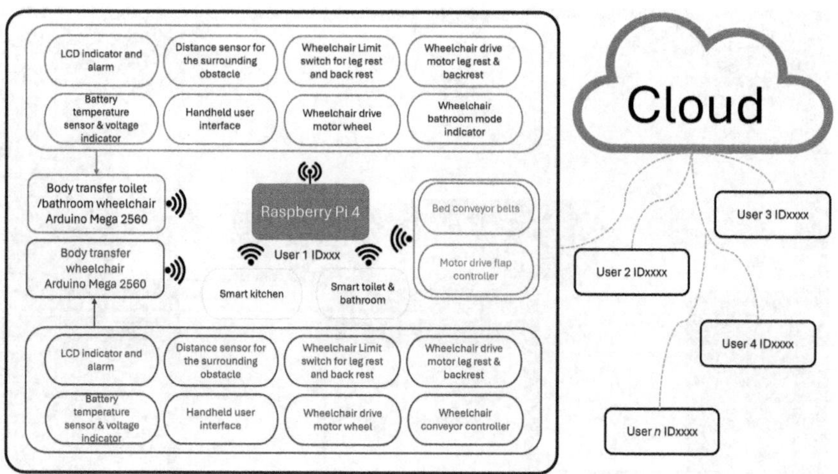

FIGURE 2.6 Data communication between smart-care devices and cloud data services.

2.4.6 Discussion

Functionally disabled and elderly people generally require assistance in transfers, bathing, and toileting because they require complex movements of limbs. Studies have shown that these individuals can be moved by a lifting system, and various commercially available systems have been developed. However, this approach has not been able to provide safe and secure outcomes since the person has to be lifted against gravity, so there are chances of accidents. In most cases, they require some infrastructural changes, which is also a drawback of these systems. Table 2.4 shows the comparative analysis of the BTS with the previously developed systems. Previous approaches have focused their emphasis on transferring physically challenged individuals via a lifting transfer approach that involved various risks. The proposed mode of transfer proved to be effective in transferring people safely and securely. Previous systems were also unable to transfer the individuals adequately. Furthermore, some lifting transfer devices require the involvement of two caregivers for the systems to work safely. However, contrary to the lifting approach, sliding transfer has proved to be more effective in transferring the person. In an AAL facility, people try to be more independent, and they want to achieve freedom and privacy, which is not achievable through lifting transfer devices. After various experimentations and user evaluations mentioned in Lin and Masroor (2023) and Lin, Masroor, Bahrudin, and Bulut (2023), it can be inferred that the BTS can transfer the person more effectively, comfortably, and securely. Additionally, the focus of the existing system was to assist the people in a single task, as mentioned in Mori (2012), using reverse transfer. This approach is dangerous and keeps the individual in an awkward position. It puts immense pressure on the spine of the individual while toileting. Furthermore, the BTS also ensures that the person who is being cared for and the caregiver should be safe while performing various tasks. For this reason, the BTTW that is being used in the toilet and bathroom does not contain any electrical appliances. Contrary to RIBA (Mukai et al., 2011), the proposed system assures that it is electrically safe for the caregivers and the dependent individual. Furthermore, BTS also takes into account the fact that the caregiver should bear the least amount of burden while assisting the dependent person, so the sliding transfer method ensures that the caregiver should not face chronic illness because of lifting continuous loads.

2.4.7 Conclusion

This chapter discusses various issues regarding the demographic changes occurring globally. Previously developed systems used various approaches to provide assistance and care to the elderly and physically disabled individuals. Furthermore, these systems have also focused on the reduction of load from the healthcare community, especially the caregivers. However, they are unable to provide smarter solutions regarding assistance in performing ADLs. Additionally, it has also been analyzed that the lifting approach in person transfer is dangerous. Because while lifting the person, the system works against gravity. The person being transferred is also uncomfortable with lifting transfer systems. Contrary to the lifting transfer approach, BTS is a novel contribution in smart healthcare system. This system uses a sliding transfer approach for person transfer, which is more suitable, comfortable, and safe. Furthermore, in the lifting approach, various dangers are also associated, like chances of falling and other

TABLE 2.4
Comparison of Various Person Transfer Assisted Systems (PTAS) with BTS

PTAS	Purpose/Provide Assistance in Performing:	Transfer Approach	Load (kg)	Transfer Mode	Sensing Technology	Issues/Limitations
Wheelchair mounted robotic-assisted transfer device (RTAD) (Grindle et al., 2015)	• Lifting • Transfer	Lifting	84	Sitting	• Three-axis load sensor	• A bed-ridden person cannot be transferred using this system • Lifting system sometimes distorts the posture of the person being transferred
Transfer system by Yoshihiko Takahashi et al (2003)	• Transferring from wheelchair to toilet and vice versa	Lifting	70	Sitting	• Nil	• Applies huge force on the chest • Upper limb disabled person is not able to use that
Intelligent sweet home (ISH) concept	• Lifting • Transfer • Locomotion	Lifting	70	Sitting	• Pressure sensor • Torque sensor • Laser range finder	• Lifting through robotic hoist is not safe for one caregiver • Dependence of disabled person on the caregiver is not resolved • Caregiver still has to bear the load of the dependent person
Robot for interactive body assistance (RIBA) (Mukai Toshiharu, 2011)	• Lifting • Transfer • Locomotion	Lifting	60	Sitting	• Tactile sensors • Vision sensors • Auditory sensors	• Risk of slippage of user from the arms of RIBA • Electrical input so it is dangerous to use it in toilets or bathrooms
Wheelchair by Mori et al. (2012)	• Lifting • Toileting	Lifting	-	Sitting	• Nil	• Approaching the toilet in the absence of a caregiver can be very difficult and dangerous • Lack of maneuverability in toilet and bathroom.

Home lift position and rehabilitation (HLPR) chair (Bostelman and Albus, 2007)	• Lifting • Transfer • Locomotion • Rehabilitation	Lifting	93	Sitting	• 3D imaging camera • Wheel encoders • RFID • LIDAR	• Bulky and complex structure • Lack of maneuverability in toilet and bathroom.
Advanced hydraulically actuated patient transfer assist device (Humphreys, Book, & Deetjen, 2018)	• Lifting • Transfer • Locomotion	Lifting	350	Sitting	• Ultrasonic sensors • Force sensors	• Lack of maneuverability in toilet and bathroom • Lifting a Multiple Sclerosis patient can be dangerous
Agile Life patient transfer system (PTS) (Kulich, Wei, Crytzer, Cooper, & Koontz, 2023)	• Transfer from wheelchair to bed and vice versa Locomotion	Sliding	159	Supine	• Nil	• Requires infrastructural modification. • It cannot assist in bathing and toileting
Mechatronic system for handling bedridden people (Da Silva, 2015)	• Transfer from stretcher to bed and vice versa	Sliding	155	Supine	• Force sensing resistor • Wheel encoders	• This system can only be used to transfer from bed to stretcher • It cannot assist in bathing and toileting
Novel person transfer (Tian et al., 2021)	• Transfer from stretcher to bed and vice versa	Sliding	120	Supine	• Pressure sensors • Optoelectronic switches • Range sensors • Torque sensor	• This system can only be used to transfer from bed to stretcher • It cannot assist in bathing and toileting
Body-transfer system (BTS) (Lin & Masroor, 2023; Lin et al., 2023)	• Transfer from bed to vice versa Locomotion Bathing • Toileting	Sliding	110	Supine	• Ultrasonic sensor • Wheel encoders	• It requires infra-structural modification of toilet • Approaching the toilet from the rear side is a tedious task for the physically challenged individual

accidents. Various caregivers who are using lifting transfer systems also report that they feel pain in the wrist and shoulder because of frequent transfers. So, BTS mitigates this issue by the use of a sliding transfer approach mechanism. Finally, the lifting transfer system is not capable of keeping the person's posture and body angle in the sagittal plane unaltered. However, BTS ensures that the posture and the person's body angle would not change while transferring BTB to other systems.

REFERENCES

Abowd, G. D., Edwards, K., & Grinter, B. (2003). Smart homes or homes that smart? *SIGCHI Bulletin*, p. 13.

Adam, S., Mukasa, K. S., Breiner, K., & Trapp, M. (2008). An apartment-based metaphor for intuitive interaction with ambient assisted living applications. *People and Computers XXII Culture, Creativity, Interaction 22*, 67–75.

Atchley, R. C. (1985). *Social forces and aging: An introduction to social gerontology*. Thomas Wadsworth, Belmont, CA, USA.

Ballegaard, S. A., Hansen, T. R., & Kyng, M. (2008). Healthcare in everyday life: designing healthcare services for daily life. Paper presented at the *Proceedings of the SIGCHI Conference on Human Factors in Computing Systems*, New York, NY, USA.

Bernnat, R., Bauer, M., Schmidt, H., Bieber, N., Heusser, N., & Schönfeld, R. (2017). Effizienzpotentiale durch eHealth: Studie im Auftrag des Bundesverbands Gesundheits-IT–bvitg e. V. und der CompuGroup Medical SE. strategy. https://www.strategyand.pwc.com/de/de/studien/effizienzpotentiale-durch-ehealth.pdf. Zugegriffen, 16.

Bias, R. G., & Mayhew, D. J. (2005). *Cost-Justifying Usability: An Update for the Internet Age*. Elsevier.

Biley, A. (2002). National service framework for older people: Promoting health. *British Journal of Nursing*, *11*(7), 469–476.

Bostelman R & Albus, J. (2007). A multipurpose robotic wheelchair and rehabilitation device for the home. In: *Proceedings of the IEEE/RSJ International Conference on Intelligent Robots and Systems*, San Diego, California, USA, 3348–3353.

Braun, G., Nelles, S., & Rumm, P. (2009). Telemonitoring von Gesundheits-und Vitaldaten–Ökonomischer und qualitativer Nutzen bei chronischen Erkrankungen. Paper presented at the *Proceedings of the Second German Congress on Ambient Assisted Living*.

Britton, B. P. (2003). *American Telemedicine Association's Home Telehealth Clinical Guidelines*. Retrieved from Washington, DC, USA:

Campana, F., Moreno, A., Riano, D., & Varga, L. Z. (2008). K4care: Knowledge-based homecare e-services for an ageing Europe. In: R. Annicchiarico, U. Cortès, C. Urdiales (Eds.): *Agent Technology and E-Health*. Birkhäuser, Basel, Switzerland, 95–115.

Chen, S.-C., Lin, C.-W., Lee, P.-F., Chen, H.-L., & Ho, C.-C. (2021). Anthropometric characteristics in Taiwanese adults: Age and gender differences. *International Journal of Environmental Research and Public Health*, *18*(14), 7712.

Chen, J., Zhang, J., Kam, A. H., & Shue, L. (2005). *An automatic acoustic bathroom monitoring system*. Paper presented at the *2005 IEEE International Symposium on Circuits and Systems (ISCAS)*.

Commissi, E. (2006). *The Demographic Future of Europe - From Challenge to Opportunity. Commission Communication, COM(2006) final, Commission of the European Communities. EUR-Lex* Brussels.

Cooper, A. (2004). *The Inmates Are Running the Asylum: Why High Tech Products Drive Us Crazy and How to Restore the Sanity*: Sams Publishing, Carmel, Indiana, USA.

Cortés, U., Annicchiarico, R., Urdiales, C., Barrué, C., Martínez, A., Villar, A., & Caltagirone, C. (2008). Supported human autonomy for recovery and enhancement of cognitive and motor abilities using agent technologies. *Agent Technology and e-health*, 117–140.

Coughlin, J. F., D'Ambrosio, L. A., Reimer, B., & Pratt, M. R. (2007). Older adult perceptions of smart home technologies: implications for research, policy & market innovations in healthcare. Paper presented at the *2007 29th Annual International Conference of the IEEE Engineering in Medicine and Biology Society*.

Crabtree, A., Hemmings, T., & Rodden, T. (2002). Pattern-based support for interactive design in domestic settings. Paper presented at the *Proceedings of the 4th Conference on Designing Interactive Systems: Processes, Practices, Methods, and Techniques*.

Da Silva, B. M. F. (2015). *Design of Mechatronic System for Handling Bedridden People*.

De Ruyter, B., & Pelgrim, E. (2007). Ambient assisted-living research in carelab. *ACM Interaction*, *14*(4), 30–33.

Demiris, G., & Tan, J. (2005). Rejuvenating home health care and tele-home care. In: J. Tan (Ed.): *E-Health Care Information Systems: An Introduction for Students and Professionals*. Jossey-Bass, San Francisco, CA, USA, 267–290.

Dewsbury, G., & Edge, M. (2000). Designing the Home to Meet the Needs of Tomorrow…. Today: Deconstructing and rebuilding the home for life. Paper presented at the *ENHR 2000 Conference*.

Dobre, C., Bajenaru, L., Marinescu, I. A., & Tomescu, M. (2019). Improving the quality of life for older people: From smart sensors to distributed platforms. Paper presented at the *2019 22nd International Conference on Control Systems and Computer Science (CSCS)*.

Dolan, P., & Torgerson, D. (1998). The cost of treating osteoporotic fractures in the United Kingdom female population. *Osteoporosis International*, *8*, 611–617.

Fernández-Ballesteros, R. (2008). *Active Aging. The Contribution of Psychology*. Hogrefe, Göttingen, Germany.

Fernández-Ballesteros, R., Robine, J. M., Walker, A., & Kalache, A. (2012). Active Aging: A Global Goal. In: *Current Gerontology and Geriatrics Research*, 2013, Article ID 298012, 4 pages.

Fernández-Ballesteros, R., Robine, J. M., Walker, A., & Kalache, A. (2013). Active aging: A global goal. In: *Current Gerontology and Geriatrics Research*. Vol. *2013*, Article ID 298012, 4

Fichten, C. S., Barile, M., Asuncion, J., & Fossey, M. (2000). What government, agencies, and organizations can do to improve access to computers for postsecondary students with disabilities: Recommendations based on Canadian empirical data. *International Journal of Rehabilitation Research*, *23*(1), 191–199.

Finkelstein, J., Hripcsak, G., & Cabrera, M. (1998). Telematic system for monitoring of Asthma severity in patients' homes. In: *Studies in Health Technology and Informatics*, *52*, 272–276.

Forlizzi, J., DiSalvo, C., & Gemperle, F. (2004). Assistive robotics and an ecology of elders living independently in their homes. In: *Human-Computer Interaction*, *19*(1), 25–59.

Garrels, V., & Arvidsson, P. (2019). Promoting self-determination for students with intellectual disability: A Vygotskian perspective. *Learning, Culture and Social Interaction*, *22*, 100241. https://doi.org/10.1016/j.lcsi.2018.05.006

Generali. (2017). *Generali Age Study 2017 - How older people in Germany think and live*. Retrieved from Heidelberg, Germany.

Glende, S., Podtschaske, B., & Friesdorf, W. (2009). Senior User Integration: Ein ganzheitliches Konzept zur Kooperation von Herstellern und älteren Nutzern während der Produktentwicklung. Paper presented at the *Proceedings of the Second German Congress on Ambient Assisted Living*.

Gothe, H., Storz, P., Daroszewska, A., & Freytag, A. (2009). Health and economic Effects of the future use of AAL technologies: telemonitoring heart failure patients. Paper presented at the *Proceedings of the Second German Congress on Ambient Assisted Living (AAL'09)*. VDE, Berlin, Germany.

Grindle, G. G., Wang, H., Jeannis, H., Teodorski, E., & Cooper, R. A. (2015). Design and user evaluation of a wheelchair mounted robotic assisted transfer device. *BioMed Research International, 2015*(1), 198476.

Hagell, P., Alvariza, A., Westergren, A., & Årestedt, K. (2017). Assessment of burden among family caregivers of people with Parkinson's disease using the zarit burden interview. *Journal of Pain and Symptom Management, 53*(2), 272–278.

Haines, V., Mitchell, V., Cooper, C., & Maguire, M. (2007). Probing user values in the home environment within a technology driven Smart Home project. *Personal and Ubiquitous Computing, 11*, 349–359.

Heinze, R., Hilbert, J., & Paulus, W. (2009). Der Haushalt: Ein zukunftssicherer Baustein für moderne Versorgungsstrukturen. *Professional Process: Zeitschrift für Modernes Prozessmanagement im Gesundheitswesen, 2*, 3–5.

Helal, S., Winkler, B., Lee, C., Kaddoura, Y., Ran, L., Giraldo, C., … Mann, W. (2003, March). Enabling location-aware pervasive computing applications for the elderly. In *Proceedings of the First IEEE International Conference on Pervasive Computing and Communications, 2003. (PerCom 2003)* (pp. 531–536). IEEE.

Hennessy, C. H., & Walker, A. (2011). Promoting multi-disciplinary and inter-disciplinary ageing research in the United Kingdom. *Ageing & Society, 31*(1), 52–69.

Heuzeroth, V. (2009). Schwerwiegende Komplikationen zu Hause behandeln [My home is my hospital]. Paper presented at the *Proceedings of the 2nd German Ambient Assisted Living Conference*.

Hindus, D. (1999). The importance of homes in technology research. Paper presented at the *Cooperative Buildings. Integrating Information, Organizations, and Architecture: Second International Workshop, CoBuild'99*, Pittsburgh, PA, USA, October 1–2, 1999. Proceedings 2.

Hirsch, T., Forlizzi, J., Hyder, E., Goetz, J., Stroback, J., & Kurtz, C. (2000). The ELDer project: Social, emotional, and environmental factors in the design of eldercare technologies. In: *Proceedings on the International Conference on Universal Usability (CUU'00)*. ACM Press, New York, NY, USA, 72–79.

Hoffmann, R. (2008). *Socioeconomic Differences in Old Age Mortality* (Vol. 25): Springer Science & Business Media. Berlin, Germany.

Hoffmann, R. (2009). Prävention vor Kuration–Gesundheit 2010 unsere chance. Paper presented at the *Proceedings of the Second German Congress on Ambient Assisted Living*.

Horter, H., Linti, C., Loy, S., Planck, H., Kotterba, B., & Günther, U. (2009). Health Wear–Sensorische Textilien zur Erfassung von Vitalparametern. Paper presented at the *Proceedings of the Second German Congress on Ambient Assisted Living (AAL'09)*.

Humphreys, H., Book, W. J., & Deetjen, G. (2018). Advanced patient transfer assist device. Paper presented at the *2018 International Symposium on Medical Robotics (ISMR)*.

Hussain, M. W., & Roy, D. S. (2023). Performance Optimization Strategies for Big Data Applications in Distributed Framework. In *Intelligent Technologies: Concepts, Applications, and Future Directions*, Volume 2 (pp. 221–252). Singapore: Springer Nature Singapore.

Johnston, B., Weeler, L., Deuser, J., & Sousa, K. H. (2000). Outcomes of the Kaiser permanente tele-home health research project. *Archives of Family Medicine*, *9*(1), 40.

Jones, J. S. (1998). Life in the 21st century, A vision for all. In *The World Health Report.*

Kane, R. A., & Kane, R. L. (1987). *Long-Term Care: Principles, Programs and Policies.* Springer, New York, USA.

Kärki, S., & Lekkala, J. (2006). Pressure mapping system for physiological measurements. Paper presented at the *Imeko World Congress–Metrology for A Sustainable Development.*

Keates, S., Clarkson, P. J., Harrison, L.-A., & Robinson, P. (2000). *Towards a practical inclusive design approach.* Paper presented at the *Proceedings on the 2000 conference on Universal Usability.*

Klauß, T. (1999). Self-determination of people with intellectual disabilities: Individual, interactive and structural conditions. *Special Education*, *29*, 123–139.

Kruse, A., Gaber, E., Heuft, G., Oster, P., Re, S., & Schulz-Nieswandt, F. (2002). Themenheft 10 "Gesundheit im Alter".

Kühne, H., Behner, U., Henke, S., & Nelles, S. (2009). Das selbstbestimmte Leben älterer chronisch Kranker und Risikopatienten im eigenen Zuhause erfordert innovative und bezahlbare Versorgungslösungen. Paper presented at the *Proceedings of the Second German Congress on Ambient Assisted Living.*

Kulich, H. R., Wei, L., Crytzer, T. M., Cooper, R. A., & Koontz, A. M. (2023). Preliminary evaluation of an automated robotic transfer assist device in the home setting. *Disability and Rehabilitation: Assistive Technology*, *18*(5), 511–518.

Laleci, G. B., Dogac, A., Olduz, M., Tasyurt, I., Yuksel, M., & Okcan, A. (2008). SAPHIRE: A multi-agent system for remote healthcare monitoring through computerized clinical guidelines. In: R. Annicchiarico, U. Cortès, C. Urdiales (Eds.): *Agent Technology and E-Health.* Birkhäuser, Basel, Switzerland, 25–44.

Lee, R.-G., Chen, H.-S., Lin, C.-C., Chang, K.-C., & Chen, J.-H. (2000). Home telecare system using cable television plants-an experimental field trial. *IEEE Transactions on Information Technology in Biomedicine*, *4*(1), 37–44.

Leonard, D., & Rayport, J. F. (1997). Spark innovation through empathic design. *Harvard Business Review*, *75*, 102–115.

Lin, C.-Y., & Masroor, S. (2023). Efficient body-transfer wheelchair for assisting functionally impaired people. *Computers, Materials & Continua*, *74*(3), 4881–4900.

Lin, C.-Y., Masroor, S., Bahrudin, B., & Bulut, H. (2023). The design and user evaluation of body-transfer system via sliding transfer approach for assisting functionally impaired people. *Machines*, *11*(5), 555.

Lindley, S. E., Harper, R., & Sellen, A. (2008). Designing for elders: Exploring the complexity of relationships in later life. *People and Computers XXII Culture, Creativity, Interaction 22*, 77–86.

Lohman, M. C., Sonnega, A. J., Nicklett, E. J., Estenson, L., & Leggett, A. N. (2019). Comparing estimates of fall-related mortality incidence among older adults in the United States. *The Journals of Gerontology: Series A*, *74*(9), 1468–1474.

Meyer, S. (2009). Der Nutzer im Zentrum. Anforderungen, Wünsche, Erfahrungen jüngerer Senioren. *BMBF/VDE Innovationspartnerschaft AAL (Hg.): Ambient Assisted Living.*

Mori, Y., Sakai, N., & Kaoru, K. (2012b). Development of a wheelchair with a lifting function. *Advanced in Mechanical Engineering 2012*, 1–9.

Mori, Y., Sakai, N., & Katsumura, K. (2012a). Development of a Wheelchair with a Lifting Function. *Advances in Mechanical Engineering*, *4*, 803014.

Morrow-Howell, N., Hinterlong, J., & Sherraden, M. (2001). *Productive Aging: Concepts and Challenges*. JHU Press, Baltimore, USA.

Motl, R. W., Konopack, J. F., McAuley, E., Elavsky, S., Jerome, G. J., & Marquez, D. X. (2005). Depressive symptoms among older adults: Long-term reduction after a physical activity intervention. *Journal of Behavioral Medicine*, *28*, 385–394.

Mukai, T., Hirano, S., Nakashima, H., Sakaida, Y., & Guo, S. (2011). Realization and safety measures of patient transfer by nursing-care assistant robot RIBA with tactile sensor. *The Journal of Mechanisms and Robotics*, *23*(3), 360–369.

Mynatt, E. D., Melenhorst, A.-S., Fisk, A.-D., & Rogers, W. A. (2004). Aware technologies for aging in place: Understanding user needs and attitudes. *IEEE Pervasive Computing*, *3*(2), 36–41.

Nations Unies, O. (2001). *World population prospects: the 2000 revision*.

Nehmer, J., Becker, M., Karshmer, A., & Lamm, R. (2006). Living assistance systems: an ambient intelligence approach. Paper presented at the *Proceedings of the 28th International Conference on Software Engineering*.

Office for National Statistics (ONS) (1995). *General Household Survey 1994: Living in Britain, Population Censuses and Surveys Office*. UK Data Service. SN: 3170. http://doi.org/10.5255/UKDA-SN-3170-1

Orwat, C., Rashid, A., Wölk, M., Holtmann, C., Scheermesser, M., & Kosow, H. (2008). Pervasive computing in medical care. In: *Technology Assessment - Theory and Practice, Institute for Technology Assessment and Systems Analysis (ITAS)*. *17*, 5–12.

Palen, L., & Aaløkke, S. (2006). Of pill boxes and piano benches: " home-made" methods for managing medication. Paper presented at the Proceedings of the *2006 20th Anniversary Conference on Computer Supported Cooperative Work*.

Podtschaske, B., Glende, S., & Friesdorf, W. (2009). Ein ganzheitliches Konzept zur Realisierung der informationellen Selbstbestimmung älterer Nutzer. Paper presented at the *Proceedings of the Second German Congress on Ambient Assisted Living*.

Quigley, G., & Tweed, C. (2000). *Added-Value Services from the Installation of Assistive Technology for the Elderly*, Research Report EPSRC GR/M05171, Queen's University of Belfast, UK.

Reddy, K., Roy, D. S., Mishra, T. K., & Hussain, M. W. (Eds.). (2023). *Handbook of Research on Network-Enabled IoT Applications for Smart City Services*. IGI Global.

Rialle, V., Lamy, J.-B., Noury, N., & Bajolle, L. (2003). Telemonitoring of patients at home: A software agent approach. *Computer Methods and Programs in Biomedicine*, *72*(3), 257–268.

Saizmaa, T., & Kim, H.-C. (2008). A holistic understanding of HCI perspectives on smart home. Paper presented at the *2008 Fourth International Conference on Networked Computing and Advanced Information Management*.

Schalock, R. L. (1996). Reconsidering the conceptualisation and measurement of quality of life. In: R. L. Schalock, G. N. Siperstein (Eds.): *Quality of Life., Volume I: Conceptualization and Measurement. American Association on Mental Retardation, Washington*, Washington DC, USA, 123–139.

Schäper, S., Schüller, S., Dieckmann, F., & Greving, H. (2010). Anforderungen an die Lebensgestaltung älter werdender Menschen mit geistiger Behinderung in unterstützten Wohnformen. *Ergebnis einer Literaturanalyse und Expertenbefragung*.

Schwinger, A., & Tsiasioti, C. (2018). Pflegebedürftigkeit in Deutschland. *Pflege-Report 2018: Qualität in der Pflege*, 173–204.

Stadlmayer, T. (2009). Weiblich, ledig, alt-und unabhängig. In: *Financial Times Deutschland, June 8, 2009, Germany*.

Takahashi Y, Manabe, G., Takahashi, K., & Hatakeyama, T. (2003). Simple self-transfer aid robotic system. In *Proceedings of the IEEE International Conference on Robotics and Automation*, Taipai, Taiwan, September, 2305–2309.

Tian, Y., Wang, H., Zhang, Y., Su, B., Wang, L., Wang, X., … & Niu, J. (2021). Design and evaluation of a novel person transfer assist system. *IEEE Access*, *9*, 14306–14318.

Vahs, D., & Burmester, R. (2005). *Innovationsmanagement: Von der Produktidee zur erfolgreichen Vermarktung (3, überarb Aufl.)*. Stuttgart: Schäffer-Poeschel (Praxisnahes Wirtschaftsstudium).

Venkatesh, A. (1996). Computers and other interactive technologies for the home. *Communications of the ACM*, *39*(12), 47–54.

Venkatesh, A., & Vitalari, N. P. (1992). An emerging distributed work arrangement: An investigation of computer-based supplemental work at home. *Management Science*, *38*(12), 1687–1706.

Vergados, D., Alevizos, A., Mariolis, A., & Caragiozidis, M. (2008). Intelligent services for assisting independent living of elderly people at home. Paper presented at the *Proceedings of the 1st international conference on PErvasive Technologies Related to Assistive Environments*.

Villar, A., Federici, A., & Annicchiarico, R. (2007). K4care: Knowledge-based homecare eservices for an ageing europe. In: R. Annicchiarico, U. Cortès, C. Urdiales (Eds.): *Agent Technology and E-Health*. Birkhäuser, Basel, Switzerland, 141–148.

Walker, A. (2002). A strategy for active ageing. *International Social Security Review*, *55*(1), 121–139.

Walker, A. (2011). *The Future of Ageing Research in Europe: A Road Map*. University of Sheffield: Sheffield, UK.

Wegge, K.-P. (2009). Barrierefreie AAL Services–Nutzer mit besonderen Anforderungen. Paper presented at the *Proceedings of the Second German Congress on Ambient Assisted Living*.

WHO. (2022). *Active Aging: A Policy Framework*. World Health Organization, Geneva, Switzerland.

Wichert, R., Gaugisch, P., Norgall, T., & Becker, M. (2009). Individuelle Gestaltung und Anpassung bestehender Wohnkonzepte. Paper presented at the *Proceedings of the Second German Congress on Ambient Assisted Living*.

Wilkes, B. (2009). Genderspezifische Produktentwicklung für AAL-Notwendigkeit oder Übertreibung. Paper presented at the *Proceedings of the Second German Congress on Ambient Assisted Living*.

Ziefle, M. (2008). Age perspectives on the usefulness on e-health applications. Paper presented at the *International Conference on Health Care Systems, Ergonomics, and Patient Safety (HEPS), Straßbourg*, France.

Ziefle, M., & Bay, S. (2005). How older adults meet complexity: aging effects on the usability of different mobile phones. *Behaviour & Information Technology*, *24*(5), 375–389.

3

An In-Depth Analysis of Machine Learning and Artificial Intelligence Advancements in Healthcare for Smart Cities

Soumya Sidhartha Ray
Ajay Binay Institute of Technology, Cuttack, India

Niva Tripathy
Dhaneswar Rath Institute of Engineering and Management Studies, Cuttack, India

Subhranshu Sekhar Tripathy
Kalinga Institute of Industrial Technology, Bhubaneshwar, India

Mehdi Gheisari
Islamic Azad University, Tehran, Iran

3.1 Introduction

The "smart cities" concept has appeared as an urbanization phenomenon solution to provide better living conditions, more efficient resource management, and also greater opportunities for civil society participation (Reddy et al., 2023). The cities are aimed at maximizing the potential of information and communications technology (ICT) to become highly functioning ecosystems that are interdependent upon one another (Hallur et al., 2022). ICT contributes primarily in the conceptualization of planning, implementation, and also management strategies for smart city initiatives as it permits a wide variety of creative responses to the inevitable challenges that accompany urbanization. The provision of healthcare services in smart cities as a way to ensure the quality of health and wellness for all their citizens is one major element (Jiwani et al., 2022).

It's a "smart city" when digital technology, data analytics, and several other forms of artificial intelligence are fused together to make living in the cities much easier. The ICT-based infrastructure in these metropolitan regions facilitates the transfer of information between different sectors, thus providing more informed decision-making

DOI: 10.1201/9781032631738-3

(Dhaya and Kanthavel, 2021). An intelligent city seeks to achieve the best percentage in utilizing the resources, improve lives of its citizens, and sustain economic viability over a long time while taming its environmental footprint.

ICTs serve as the foundation of smart development, providing real-time data collection, analysis and also communication. ICT solutions like sensors, data networks, and also cloud computing facilitate proper management of the different urban domains such as transportation, energy governance, and healthcare (Mala, 2022). In doing so, these technologies contribute to laying the requisite ground for implementing data-driven solutions that enhance the urban living standards.

Increasing the amount of access and quality of medical care available to people is one of the main goals of smart city initiatives. When healthcare services are integrated into smart city infrastructures, early sickness detection, treatment, and prevention all improve (Tejaswi and Gnana Swathika, 2023). There is more potential than ever before to improve healthcare systems in smart cities thanks to recent developments in machine learning (ML) and artificial intelligence (AI).

Notwithstanding the numerous advantages that may ensue, a lot of obstacles must be overcome before ML and AI may be effectively applied in the healthcare sector (Bhowmik, 2023). Because of the enormous volumes of healthcare data that are produced by wearable sensors and other medical equipment, there have been some concerns expressed regarding the volume of data and the capacity of storage. Protecting the privacy of patients' personal information becomes an increasingly pressing concern as interdependence between healthcare systems increases. The necessity of latency for real-time health monitoring systems adds an additional layer of complication to healthcare application development (Haque and Rahman, 2023). Figure 3.1 broadly describes the use of smart city applications. Because of these problems, inventive solutions are required in order to find a middle ground between the positive aspects of technology and the moral and legal repercussions that are associated with healthcare data.

The healthcare industry relies heavily on foundational technologies like ML and AI. This chapter provides a foundational understanding of ML and AI by exploring their various forms and their potential medical applications.

ML, a kind of AI, allows computers to gain knowledge and proficiency by analyzing data and making adjustments accordingly (Pradhan et al., 2022). It entails creating algorithms for computers to use data to form inferences and detect trends. However, AI refers to a wider range of technologies with the same overarching goal – to give robots human-level intelligence. Healthcare is only one of several fields where ML and AI have proven useful.

In this chapter, we have given the details of the role and application of AI and ML in healthcare, ML model for healthcare, comparison of different computing paradigms, integration of block chain for secure healthcare data management, and a case study to justify our approach.

The rest of the chapter is organized as follows. Section 3.2 gives the total overview of related work. Section 3.3 provides the application of ML and AL in healthcare. Section 3.4 describes software-defined networking. Section 3.5 gives the future trends in AI-powered healthcare. Section 3.6 provides a case study of smart healthcare implementation. Finally, the conclusion and future scope are discussed.

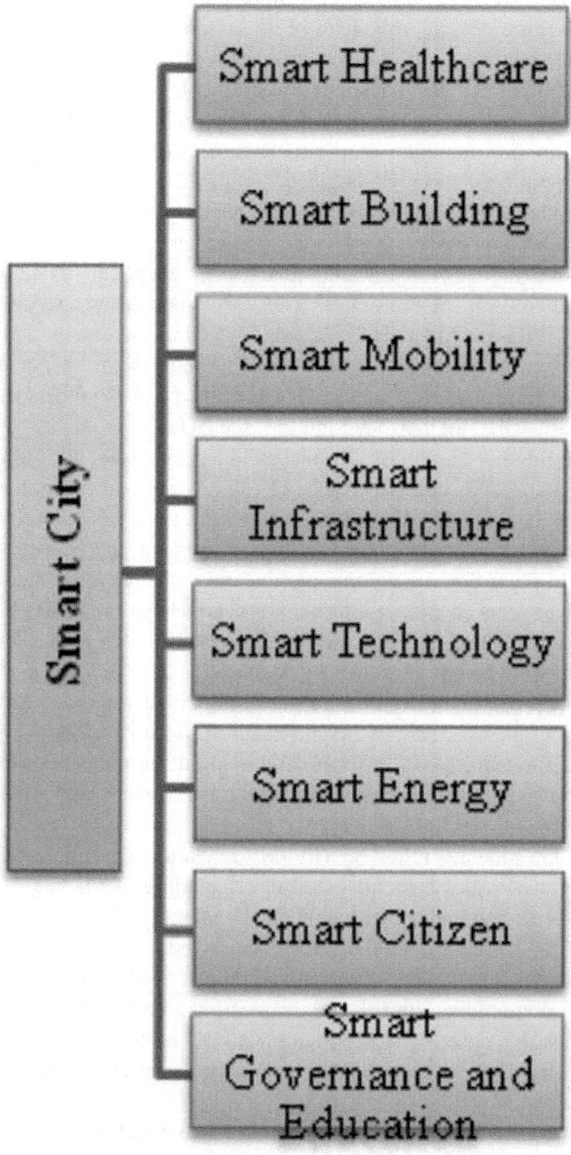

FIGURE 3.1 Key components of a smart city.

3.2 Related Work

There are many different kinds of ML algorithms, and each one is designed to handle a specific kind of application.

Supervised learning entails teaching a system to do a task by exposing it to labeled data and allowing the system to learn from its mistakes. In order to forecast or categorize unknown data, it is necessary to develop a mapping among inputs and outputs (Saxena and Chandra, 2021). We can use this to classify or forecast information that was previously unavailable. Models can be used in the field of disease diagnosis to learn to classify patients in accordance with their diseases by analyzing patient data that has been appropriately labeled. In the context of making a medical diagnosis, this is done.

Learning without labels, or unsupervised learning, is the process of combing through data in search of hidden patterns. Clustering and decreasing dimensionality are two methods frequently used in unsupervised learning. For instance, based on their medical records, unsupervised learning can be used to categorize patients into groups with shared characteristics, which can facilitate the creation of individualized treatment plans.

Algorithmic programmers learn by observing and interacting with their environment, according to the principles of reinforcement learning. The algorithm makes decisions so as to maximize the sum of all rewards it receives, and then "learns" from the outcomes of those decisions. The field of medicine can benefit from reinforcement learning. The method takes the patients' reactions and the results into account (Kumari et al., 2022).

The application of AI has the potential to drastically transform the current structure of the healthcare system, primarily through the enhancement of diagnostics, therapy, and follow-up care. The ability of AI-powered systems to quickly and effectively assess medical data paves the way for early disease identification and diagnosis (Padmavathi, 2021). ML algorithms, by examining massive amounts of data, can identify subtle patterns and relationships that a human analyst might miss, leading to more accurate diagnoses (Hussain and Roy, 2023). In addition, AI can assist with personalized medicine by enabling medical professionals to modify treatments according to the specific characteristics of each individual patient. Table 3.1 describes the types of ML algorithms used so far.

TABLE 3.1

Types of Machine Learning Algorithms

Algorithm Type	Description	Example Application	References
Supervised Learning	Algorithms learn from labelled data, mapping inputs to outputs	Predicting house prices using linear regression	(Halur et al.)
Unsupervised Learning	Algorithms identify patterns and relationships in unlabelled data	Grouping customers using K-means clustering	(Kumar et al.)
Semi-supervised Learning	A combination of labelled and unlabelled data is used for predictions	Sentiment analysis with limited labelled data	(Jiwani et al.)
Reinforcement Learning	Agents gather up behaviors that enhance the environment's cumulative rewards	Q-Learning for instructing game-playing agents	(Mohaghegh et al.)
Deep Learning	Neural networks with multiple layers are used for complex pattern recognition	Image recognition with convolution neural networks	(Chen et al.)
Ensemble Learning	Multiple models are combined to improve performance	Predicting disease outcomes using Random Forest	(Motwani et al.)

3.3 Applications of ML and AI in Healthcare

With the use of AI and ML, more recent healthcare applications have been created that perform better in terms of administration systems, diagnostics, specific treatment plans, and patient condition monitoring. Table 3.2 gives the details of application of Al and Ml in healthcare.

- **Early Disease Detection Using ML Algorithms**

  ML algorithms have significantly transformed the process of early disease detection by looking for tiny interrelations in data that point to early-stage illnesses (Chandra and Mazumdar, 2022). To find discrepancies that can point to the existence of malignant diseases like cancer, ML algorithms, for example, can be used to evaluate medical images. In order to guarantee speedier and more accurate diagnoses and better patient outcomes, these algorithms supplement the expertise of medical personnel.
- **Personalized Medicine and Treatment Planning**

  By allowing the customization of care for each patient on an individual basis, AI-based technologies are opening the door for personalized medicine. The optimal course of treatment will be determined by machine-learning algorithms by analyzing a patient's genetic information, medical history, and other pertinent data (Chen et al., 2021). Figure 3.2 describes the application of AI in the healthcare field. This technique demonstrates how AI can increase the efficacy rate and eliminate or reduce adverse effects, thereby changing the way patients are treated.
- **Remote Patient Monitoring through AI-Driven Systems**

  AI-driven technologies have made great gains in enhancing remote patient monitoring, opening the door to continuous health monitoring outside of the clinical setting. Wearables loaded with sensors have the potential to collect patient data, which can afterward be processed by AI algorithms (Mohaghegh, 2022). These algorithms are able to recognize out-of-the-ordinary health data in the event of a medical emergency and sound an alarm, which may be heard by medical professionals or careers. The patient is able to become more self-reliant, and timely interventions are no longer out of the question, thanks to remote monitoring.
- **Smart Healthcare Infrastructure Management**

  In addition to its employment in the treatment of individual patients, ML and AI are also beneficial in the overall management of healthcare systems. The use of AI-powered systems that process large amounts of data can positively impact hospital operations, resource allocation, and also patient fluidity. Figure 3.3 illustrates the application of ML in healthcare. For example, predictive models allow hospitals to better plan their allocation of resources based on estimated patient admissions (Sundaresan et al., 2021). Such plans help to reduce the total healthcare costs and also improve the service provision in general.

TABLE 3.2

Applications of ML and AI in Healthcare

Application	Description	References
Smart Healthcare Applications	Discusses various applications of AI and ML in healthcare, potentially covering diagnosis, patient monitoring, and treatment recommendations	(Hallur et al.)
Smart Healthcare Informatics	Covers ML approaches for healthcare informatics, implying the use of data analysis to enhance healthcare processes	(Jiwani et al.)
Intelligent Healthcare Assistant	Focuses on the development of an ML-based intelligent assistant for healthcare, which could aid in patient interaction, data analysis, and decision support	(Mala et al.)
AI-Assisted Security Analysis of Healthcare Systems	Explores the use of AI for enhancing the security of healthcare systems, likely addressing data privacy, fraud detection, and secure information sharing	(Haque et al.)
AI Challenges and Applications in Smart Healthcare	Discusses challenges and principles of applying AI in healthcare, potentially addressing areas like data quality, ethical considerations, and patient outcomes	(Kumari et al.)
AI and ML in Healthcare	Offers insights into the broader implications of AI and ML in healthcare, which might include patient care improvement, disease prediction, and treatment optimization	(Ahmed et al.)
Diagnosis of Brain Disorders Using AI	Focuses on using AI for diagnosing brain disorders, which could involve analyzing medical imaging data to detect conditions such as tumors or neurological diseases	(Mir et al.)
Machine Learning for Disease Assessment	Explores the use of ML for assessing diseases, potentially discussing techniques to predict disease progression, severity, or response to treatment	(Saha et al.)
Ubiquitous Healthcare Monitoring with ML	Discusses frameworks for monitoring healthcare using ML, which could include wearable devices, remote patient monitoring, and predictive health analytics	(Motwani et al.)

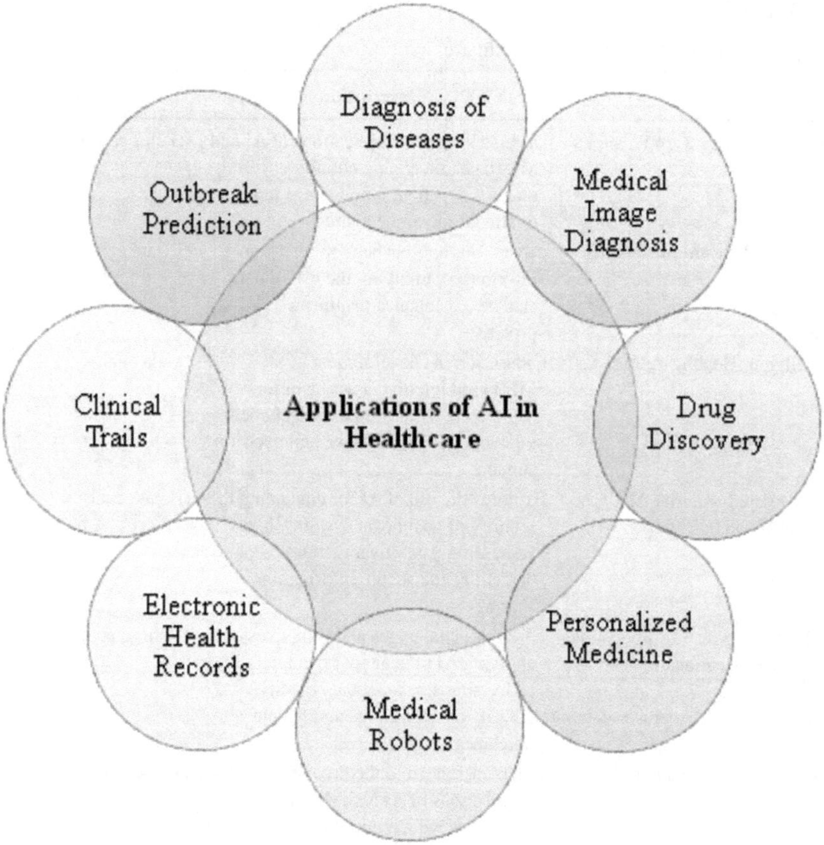

Diagnosis of Diseases
Medical Image Diagnosis
Drug Discovery
Personalized Medicine
Medical Robots
Electronic Health Records
Clinical Trails
Outbreak Prediction
Applications of AI in Healthcare

FIGURE 3.2 Applications of AI in healthcare.

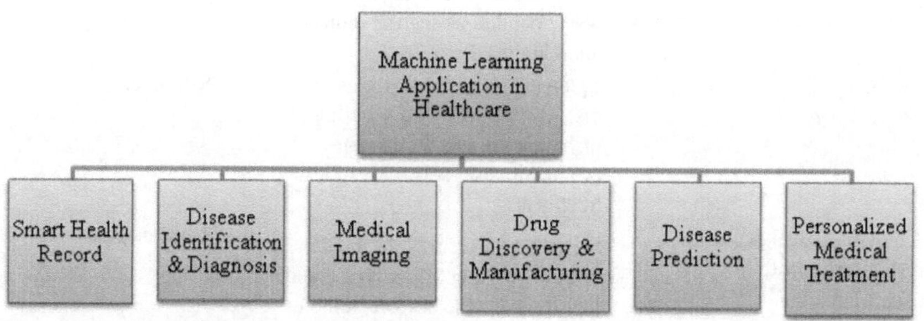

FIGURE 3.3 Applications of ML in healthcare.

a) **AI-Assisted Diagnostics and Decision Support**

Providing AI and ML-informed algorithms can prove extremely beneficial for the medical diagnostics (Toh and Brody, 2021). With the help of analyzing patient data, medical imaging, and also clinical records, these algorithms participate in the diagnostic procedures and treatment planning. Since AI can uncover new and never-before-used therapy routes, as well as predict patient's behavior, more accurate decisions are made.

b) **Drug Discovery and Development**

ML and AI allow for the sifting through of the massive databases that are in a constant search for potentially useable pharmacological agents. Such approaches can make the drug discovery a lot more efficient by predicting molecular interactions, assessing medication efficacy and also decreasing the number of potential test compounds (Tsoniotis, 2022). With the aid of AI, innovation in the pharmaceutical research is made faster by significantly reducing both the time and also costs associated with developing new drugs.

c) **Predictive Analytics for Public Health**

In the field of public health, predictive analytics based on ML and AI is used to predict the incidence of disease outbreaks and the development of relevant health trends. The analysis of data obtained from a wide variety of sources, including social media, environmental factors, and patient records, makes it possible for these technologies to make accurate predictions regarding potential health risks and to enable quick treatment of those risks (Ahmed and Ahmed, 2022). The utilization of such instruments is required for proactive management of public health.

d) **Telemedicine and Virtual Health Assistants**

With the help of telemedicine and virtual health aids, which are powered by AI, medical care is easier to access nowadays. Operation of AI-driven interfaces enables patients to get remote medical consultations, diagnoses, and also recommendations on the treatment (Kavitha et al., 2022). Such technologies encourage access to quality medical services by relieving most of the patients of the necessity of traveling long distances in order to reach healthcare facilities. It is particularly effective in poor and rural regions where the transportation may not be available.

3.3.1 Machine Learning Models for Healthcare in Smart Cities

Healthcare in smart cities is being revolutionized by ML algorithms. In order to decrease healthcare costs and process data more quickly, these models leverage a variety of computer paradigms. Table 3.3 gives the details about the computing paradigm studied so far.

a) **Cloud Computing for Healthcare Data Processing**

Cloud computing offers an infrastructure that is both adaptable and powerful, making it ideal for the management of large amounts of medical data. The use of ML algorithms for the analysis of medical data carried out on

TABLE 3.3
Comparison of Computing Paradigms

Computing Paradigm	Advantages	Use Case/Application	References
IoT-Based Smart Healthcare	Enhanced patient monitoring and personalized care	Remote health monitoring, disease prediction	(Hallur et al.)
Machine Learning in Healthcare Informatics	Data-driven insights, process optimization	Health records analysis, resource allocation	(Jiwani et al.)
Machine Learning-Based Healthcare Assistant	Decision support, patient interaction	Virtual medical assistants, symptom analysis	(Mala et al.)
AI-Assisted Security Analysis in Healthcare	Enhanced data security, fraud detection	Protected health information sharing	(Haque et al.)
AI Challenges in Smart Healthcare	Improved patient outcomes, predictive analytics	Personalized treatment, disease management	(Kumari et al.)
AI and ML in Healthcare	Advanced diagnostics, treatment optimization	Disease prediction, patient care	(Ahmed et al.)
AI for Brain Disorder Diagnosis	Accurate diagnosis, early intervention	Neurological disorder detection	(Mir et al.)
Machine Learning for Disease Assessment	Early detection, personalized medicine	Disease progression prediction	(Saha et al.)
Ubiquitous Healthcare Monitoring with ML	Real-time monitoring, preventive care	Remote patient monitoring, health analytics	(Motwani et al.)

cloud servers provides the door for quicker diagnosis and the formulation of treatment plans (Kumar et al., 2022). It is possible for healthcare organizations to improve their data-processing capabilities by making use of extensive computational resources that are available on demand.

b) **Fog Computing and Its Advantages in Latency-Sensitive Scenarios**

Fog computing moves computation closer to the data source, mitigating cloud computing's latency issues (Mir et al., 2022). For time-sensitive medical applications, fog computing's edge processing benefits guarantee lightning-fast responses. In the context of remote patient monitoring and emergency response systems, this is of paramount importance.

c) **Mist Computing and Its Proximity to Data Sources**

When using mist computing, data is processed even more locally than when using fog computing, which was already very local (Saha and Islam, 2023). As a result of the fact that data processing takes place directly on the devices themselves, fog computing offers both of these advantages. The use of mist computing has the potential to enhance real-time patient monitoring and diagnostics, which will result in a reduction in the amount of time needed to provide care.

d) **Incorporating Incremental/Federated Learning for Cost-Effective Solutions**

Federated learning models that integrate incremental gains are required for any healthcare solutions that are both affordable and protect the personal information of patients. In incremental learning, rather than enduring a full retraining session, model predictions are continuously improved by incorporating newly collected data (Motwani et al., 2022). Federation learning enables the training of models to take place across a large number of nodes without requiring the revelation of individual patient data.

3.3.2 Block Chain Integration for Secure Health Data Management

Healthcare data security and patient privacy are two areas where block chain technology is gaining traction. Block chain improves the security of medical records through providing an immutable and decentralized ledger, allowing for safe data sharing between authorized parties (John et al., 2023). When data privacy is a major concern, as it is in smart cities, this integration becomes even more useful.

a) **Explainable AI for Enhanced Healthcare Decision-Making**

   Explainable AI models are becoming vital in healthcare as they offer transparent insights into the decision-making process. In life-or-death medical situations, knowing how AI reached a result is crucial. Better patient outcomes can be achieved thanks to explainable AI, which allows healthcare workers to trust and evaluate AI-driven judgments.

b) **Human–AI Collaboration for Improved Diagnostics**

   When AI systems and medical experts work together, patient diagnoses improve. Large amounts of medical data can be processed by AI algorithms, with preliminary results being sent for evaluation and validation by medical personnel. Together, AI and human professionals may learn in a dynamic feedback loop, ensuring thorough diagnoses (Rassia, 2022).

c) **Ethics and Bias Mitigation in AI-Driven Healthcare**

   In AI-driven healthcare, it is crucial to examine ethical implications and eliminate bias. Unfair or discriminating AI results could be the result of using biased training data (Nelgadevi and Jacob, 2020). To guarantee that AI solutions improve universal healthcare access and treatment, strong mechanisms must be put in place to detect and eliminate biases.

d) **Network Paradigms for Healthcare Data**

   Optimizing healthcare data management and protecting personal health information in smart cities requires the incorporation of cutting-edge network paradigms.

3.4 Introduction to Software-Defined Networking (SDN)

When it comes to managing networks, software-defined networking (SDN) is a game-changer because it allows for centralized control and programmability of network infrastructure (Hussain et al., 2021a, 2021b). With SDN, managers can dynamically manage the network using software-defined controllers because the control plane is separated from the data plane (Banu, 2021; Hussain et al., 2022a, 2022b). SDN improves network adaptability, scalability, and agility, which is especially useful for smart city healthcare infrastructure.

a) **SDN's Role in Healthcare Applications and Network Awareness**

Healthcare applications in smart cities can greatly benefit from SDN. To adapt to changes in data traffic and application needs, the network can be reconfigured on the fly and in real time (Hussain et al., 2021b). Network awareness provided by SDN can direct vital medical data through optimized pathways in healthcare contexts where low latency and high dependability are required. The result is better quality of service for healthcare applications and more efficient data transmission.

b) **Ensuring Security and Privacy Using SDN and Block Chain Integration**

Privacy of the data and security is paramount in the healthcare industry. By merging block chain technologies with the SDN, more robust solutions can be obtained. Because of block chain's immutability and also decentralization, the data integrity is maintained from any tampering (Ciaburro, 2021). With SDN, the network administrators can regulate the users' access to and manipulation of data traffic as well as track network activities in real time (Hussain et al., 2024). The integration increases the security and also privacy compliance for the transmission and storage of healthcare data in smart cities.

c) **Ethical Considerations and Future Trends**

Further analysis is required due to increasing trends and ethical considerations about the usage of AI and ML in healthcare settings within smart cities.

d) **Ethical Challenges in Using AI and ML for Healthcare Decisions**

When AI and ML are being used in medical decision-making, ethical issues come up. First of all, in the creation of automated decision-making systems, primary attention should be aimed at the patient's health and safety (Kumari et al., 2022). Ethical issues require in-depth analyses of such complexities as algorithmic bias, the danger of erroneous diagnosing, and also the need for human intervention. To make sure that the AI-based conclusions are reasonable, ethical, and medical standards need to be taken into consideration.

e) **Transparency, Fairness, and Accountability in Healthcare AI**

Being open, equal, and responsible is essential to the success of AI-powered healthcare systems. AI healthcare models should allow both clinicians and patients to freely participate in the decision-making process. Being equitable ensures that AI-powered healthcare systems won't propagate discriminatory practices or preexisting biases (Tsoniotis, 2022). A mechanism for assigning blame must be in place when something goes wrong. By following these guidelines, ethical standards in AI-assisted healthcare are preserved.

3.5 Future Trends in AI-Powered Healthcare Technology

Trends in AI-enhanced healthcare in the future show great potential to revolutionize current medical procedures and improve health outcomes. Improved disease diagnosis through the use of cutting-edge diagnostic algorithms could pave the way for early intervention and individualized treatment strategies. Health risks and trends may be predicted by predictive analytics, allowing for preventative healthcare management.

Access to healthcare in rural areas may be enhanced via telemedicine and AI-powered remote monitoring (Subha, 2023). The potential for AI to transform treatment techniques lies in its ability to integrate with genomics and precision medicine. These tendencies point to the AI's ability to significantly alter smart city healthcare.

a) **Incorporating Responsible AI in Smart City Healthcare**

   Integrating AI safely into smart city healthcare systems calls for a holistic strategy. Regulatory organizations, healthcare providers, and AI researchers and developers should work together to create a set of morally sound rules and standards for AI in healthcare. If we want AI systems to be trustworthy, accurate, and compliant with ethical standards, we must constantly test and evaluate them. Integrating AI responsibly into smart city healthcare requires verifying that AI-driven decisions are in line with medical expertise and putting patient welfare first.

b) **Case Studies and Real-World Examples**

   Case studies from the real world, showcasing successful implementations and novel solutions, provide light on the practical impact of ML and AI in healthcare within smart cities.

c) **Real-World Cases Showcasing the Impact of ML and AI in Healthcare**

   The transformational power of ML and AI in healthcare is demonstrated by several real-world examples. There is evidence that AI-powered diagnostic systems may correctly detect diseases in medical imaging, paving the way for quicker and more precise diagnosis. Predicting when a patient in an intensive care unit would need medical attention has been made possible with the help of ML algorithms (Zamponi and Barbierato, 2022). AI-driven chatbots have enhanced patient engagement and provided personalized health advice. These examples show how ML and AI are being applied in a variety of ways to enhance health outcomes.

d) **Successful Implementations of SDN and Block Chain for Healthcare Data Security**

   The effective application of block chain technology and SDN for healthcare data security underscores the significance of these technologies in safeguarding patients' private medical records. SDN allows healthcare networks to be dynamically configured, enhancing security and network awareness (Hussain et al., 2022c). Block chain technology ensures data security and privacy and makes it feasible for healthcare professionals to securely and transparently share medical records. These technologies solve important security issues and increase the dependability of the healthcare infrastructure.

3.6 Case Study: Smart Healthcare City Implementation

This case study examines how a Smart Healthcare City was effectively implemented, demonstrating how the integration of ML, AI, SDN, and Block chain technology has revolutionized healthcare services, improved patient outcomes, and ensured data security.

Together, healthcare organizations, IT companies, and local governments developed Smart Healthcare City. The plan was to build a system that uses cutting-edge innovation to improve healthcare delivery, streamline operations, and put patients' needs first.

- **Healthcare Monitoring and Predictive Analysis**
  ML and AI algorithms were implemented to monitor residents' vitals in real time. Wearable technology and Internet of Things (IoT) sensors were used to collect data on health, everyday activities, and sleep habits (Mutlutürk, 2022). Using advanced analytics, patterns indicating health risks were found, enabling prompt treatment. For example, a resident's declining heart rate pattern notified medical personnel and prompted immediate treatment.
- **Personalized Treatment Plans**
  Electronic health information and treatment outcomes were analyzed by AI-powered systems, and individualized treatment plans were generated. Precision medicine was improved thanks to ML algorithms' predictions of how different treatments will affect individual patients. The recommendations given to doctors were backed up by data, allowing them to make better choices.
- **Secure and Interoperable Data Sharing**
  To build a reliable and adaptable network, SDN technology was used. Information collected from a wide variety of healthcare settings, such as hospitals, clinics, and wearable devices, was safely shared with qualified professionals in the healthcare industry. With SDN, sensitive data could be dynamically isolated, which reduces security threats.
- **Block Chain-Enabled Data Integrity**
  The integration of block chain helped guarantee the security and confidentiality of patient information. All patient information, medical history, and medicines were securely recorded in an unalterable ledger. By allowing patients to decide who might view their records, the healthcare system became more open and trustworthy.

The Smart Healthcare City initiative has a significant positive impact on patient outcomes as well as healthcare delivery. Readmissions to hospitals decreased by 15% as a result of prompt treatments made feasible by the use of AI-driven predictive analysis. Because their treatment plans were tailored to their unique medical histories, patients were generally happier (Mutlutürk, 2022).

The combination of SDN and block chain technology also increased data security and privacy. Unauthorized access attempts were decreased, and patients were aware of how their information would be handled. This resulted in a safer and more cooperative environment for data sharing that benefited the healthcare business.

The smart healthcare city project explores what is feasible in the healthcare industry by fusing block chain, SDN, AI, and ML. This case study can help your community modernize healthcare delivery through the use of cutting-edge IT.

The integration of ML and AI into healthcare systems within smart cities has resulted in a transformative change in patient outcomes, data management, and healthcare delivery. This chapter explores possible future methods for research, innovation, and collaboration; it also offers an overview of the key insights from previous sections and looks into the transformational effects of ML and AI on healthcare in smart cities.

We have covered a great deal in this chapter about medical AI and ML for future cities. We have examined how cutting-edge technologies are used by smart cities to enhance healthcare delivery, from early disease identification and customized treatment planning to remote patient monitoring and intelligent healthcare infrastructure management. Cloud, fog, and mist computing have shown promise in optimizing data processing for healthcare applications. SDN and block chain integration have resolved privacy and security concerns, protecting patient data.

AI and ML have completely changed healthcare in smart cities. Early disease identification, more focused treatment plans, and ongoing patient monitoring have all led to better patient outcomes and reduced healthcare costs. Large-scale medical data analysis has enhanced medical decision-making by giving healthcare professionals evidence-based understanding. The infrastructure of the smart city that has been put in place has also enhanced the general quality of treatment for patients.

It is imperative that comprehensive standards are implemented as quickly as possible to ensure the ethical and responsible use of AI in healthcare systems. Regulatory frameworks need to take data privacy, accountability, openness, and bias reduction into consideration. Governments, healthcare organizations, technology vendors, and researchers must work together to define norms that uphold patients' rights and promote AI innovation.

3.7 Conclusion and Future scope

In summary, this chapter has examined how ML and AI are incorporated into healthcare services in smart cities, offering insightful information about how these technologies can drastically change patient data management and healthcare delivery. When AI advances, there will be enough opportunity to enhance healthcare decision-making, patient engagement, and resource optimization. By adopting ethical AI practices, using teamwork, and encouraging a culture of continuous innovation, we may envision a future in which ML and AI transform healthcare within smart cities.

The long and winding road toward using ML and AI in medical care for smart cities is just getting started. Future work should focus further on developing AI-driven preventative interventions, streamlining the exchange of healthcare data across systems, and enhancing ML algorithms for more accurate disease forecasts. Clinicians, data scientists, ethicists, and legislators must work together to ensure that AI solutions are grounded in the needs of the real healthcare system.

REFERENCES

Ahmed, J. and Ahmed, M. "Machine learning and artificial intelligence in healthcare," *Empowering Artificial Intelligence Through Machine Learning*, pp. 43–56, 2022. doi:10.1201/9781003055129-3

Banu, A. "Artificial intelligence for sustainable health care advancements," *Artificial Intelligence, Machine Learning, and Data Science Technologies*, pp. 19–36, 2021. doi:10.1201/9781003153405-2

Chandra, S. and Mazumdar, S. "The implication of Artificial Intelligence and machine learning to incorporate intelligence in architecture of Smart Cities," *Emerging Technologies for Sustainable and Smart Energy*, pp. 157–184, 2022. doi:10.1201/b23013-9

Ciaburro, G. "Security Systems for smart cities based on acoustic sensors and Machine Learning Applications," *Studies in Computational Intelligence*, pp. 369–393, 2021. doi:10.1007/978-3-030-72065-0_20

Dhaya, R. and Kanthavel, R. "An analysis of machine learning for Smart Transportation System (STS)," *Explainable Artificial Intelligence for Smart Cities*, pp. 167–182, 2021. doi:10.1201/9781003172772-9

Hallur, S., Aithal, V., and Sangolli, V. "IOT based smart healthcare applications using artificial intelligence or machine learning algorithms," *Applications of Artificial Intelligence and Machine Learning in Healthcare*, 2022. doi:10.36647/aaimlh/2022.01.b1.ch005

Haque, N. I. and Rahman, M. A. "Artificial Intelligence-Assisted Security Analysis of Smart Healthcare Systems," *AI, Machine Learning and Deep Learning*, pp. 287–311, 2023. doi:10.1201/9781003187158-22

Hussain, M. W. Centralized traffic engineering. In *Towards Wireless Heterogeneity in 6G Networks*, pp. 180–193, (2024). CRC Press doi:10.1201/9781003369028

Hussain, M. W., and Roy, D.S. Enabling indirect link discovery between SDN switches. In *Proceedings of the International Conference on Computing and Communication Systems: I3CS 2020*, NEHU, Shillong, India(pp. 471–481), (2021a). Springer Singapore.

Hussain, M. W., Moulik, S., and Roy, D. S. A broadcast based link discovery scheme for minimizing messages in software defined networks. In *2021 IEEE Globecom Workshops (GC Wkshps)* (pp. 1–6), (2021b, December). IEEE, Madrid.

Hussain, M. W., and Roy, D. S. A counter-based profiling scheme for improving locality through data and reducer placement. In *Advances in Machine Learning for Big Data Analysis* (pp. 101–118), (2022a). Singapore: Springer Nature Singapore.

Hussain, M. W., and Roy, D.S. Intelligent node placement for improving traffic engineering in hybrid SDN. In *Advances in Communication, Devices and Networking: Proceedings of ICCDN 2020* (pp. 287–296), (2022b). Springer Singapore.

Hussain, M. W., Khan, M. S., Reddy, K. H. K., and Roy, D. S. "Extended indirect controller-legacy switch forwarding for link discovery in hybrid multi-controller SDN," *Computer Communications*, *189*, pp. 148–157, 2022c.

Hussain, M. W., and Roy, D. S. Performance optimization strategies for big data applications in distributed framework. In *Intelligent Technologies: Concepts, Applications, and Future Directions*, *2*, pp. 221–252, 2023. Singapore: Springer Nature Singapore.

Jiwani, N., Gupta, K., and Whig, P. "Machine learning approaches for analysis in Smart Healthcare Informatics," *Machine Learning and Artificial Intelligence in Healthcare Systems*, pp. 129–154, 2022. doi:10.1201/9781003265436-6

John, G. K., Sindhu, M. R., and Nambiar, T. N. P. "Renewable energy based hybrid power quality compensator based on Deep Learning Network for smart cities," *Artificial Intelligence and Machine Learning in Smart City Planning*, pp. 137–157, 2023. doi:10.1016/b978-0-323-99503-0.00017-x

Kavitha, M., Roobini, S., Prasanth, A., and Sujaritha, M. "Systematic view and impact of artificial intelligence in Smart Healthcare Systems, principles, challenges and applications," *Machine Learning and Artificial Intelligence in Healthcare Systems*, pp. 25–56, 2022. doi:10.1201/9781003265436-2

Kumar, K. P., Baskaran, P., and Thulasisingh, A. "Artificial Intelligence in healthcare analytics," *Applications of Artificial Intelligence and Machine Learning in Healthcare*, 2022. doi:10.36647/aaimlh/2022.01.b1.ch011

Kumari, R., Dubey, G., Dubey, N., and Pradhan, N., "Artificial Intelligence Challenges, principles, and applications in Smart Healthcare Systems," *Machine Learning and Artificial Intelligence in Healthcare Systems*, pp. 1–24, 2022. doi:10.1201/9781003265436-1

Mala, D. J. "Machine learning-based intelligent assistant for smart healthcare," *Machine Learning and Artificial Intelligence in Healthcare Systems*, pp. 265–286, 2022. doi:10.1201/9781003265436-12

Manjunath, T.D. and Bhowmik, B. "Quantum Machine Learning and recent advancements," *2023 International Conference on Artificial Intelligence and Smart Communication (AISC)*, 2023. (pp. 206–211). IEEE, Greater Noida, India, doi:10.1109/aisc56616.2023.10085586

Mir, W. A., Zamarrud, I., and Shaikh, T. A. "Smart approaches for diagnosis of brain disorders using artificial intelligence," *Machine Learning and Artificial Intelligence in Healthcare Systems*, pp. 155–172, 2022. doi:10.1201/9781003265436-7

Mohaghegh, S. D. "Artificial Intelligence and machine learning," *Smart Proxy Modeling*, pp. 1–6, 2022. doi:10.1201/9781003242581-1

Motwani, P. K., Shukla, P. K., and Pawar, M. "Ubiquitous and smart healthcare monitoring frameworks based on Machine Learning: A comprehensive review," *Artificial Intelligence in Medicine*, *134*, p. 102431, 2022. doi:10.1016/j.artmed.2022.102431

Mutlutürk, M. "Industry 4.0 for smart cities," *Artificial Intelligence Perspective for Smart Cities*, pp. 55–73, 2022. doi:10.1201/9781003230151-5.

Nelgadevi, M. and Jacob, G. "Air pollution-level estimation in smart cities using machine learning algorithms," *Proceedings of International Conference on Artificial Intelligence, Smart Grid and Smart City Applications*, pp. 343–352, 2020. doi:10.1007/978-3-030-24051-6_33

Padmavathi, K. "Machine learning and artificial intelligence techniques in Smart Health Care Systems," *Handbook of Green Engineering Technologies for Sustainable Smart Cities*, pp. 205–217, 2021. doi:10.1201/9781003093787-12

Pradhan, B., Hussain, M. W., Srivastava, G., Debbarma, M. K., Barik, R. K., and Lin, J. C. W. (2022). *A Neuro-Evolutionary Approach for Software Defined Wireless Network Traffic Classification*. IET Communications, London.

Procopiou, A. and Chen, T. M., "Explainable AI in machine/deep learning for intrusion detection in Intelligent Transportation Systems for smart cities," *Explainable Artificial Intelligence for Smart Cities*, pp. 297–321, 2021. doi:10.1201/9781003172772-17, CRC Press.

Rassia, S. T. "Unbuildable cities," *Springer Optimization and Its Applications*, pp. 41–49, 2022. doi:10.1007/978-3-030-84459-2_3

Reddy, K. H. K., Roy, D. S., Mishra, T. K., and Hussain, M. W. (Eds.). (2023). *Handbook of Research on Network-Enabled IoT Applications for Smart City Services*. IGI Global, USA.

Saha, S. and Islam, S. M. "Machine learning for disease assessment," *Artificial Intelligence for Disease Diagnosis and Prognosis in Smart Healthcare*, pp. 7–34, 2023. doi:10.1201/9781003251903-2

Saxena, A. and Chandra, S. "Correction to: Artificial Intelligence and machine learning in Healthcare," *Artificial Intelligence and Machine Learning in Healthcare*, 2021. doi:10.1007/978-981-16-0811-7_11

Sowmitha, R., Harshini, R. and Arjuna, S. "Artificial Intelligence in smart cities and Healthcare," *EAI Endorsed Transactions on Smart Cities*, *6*(3), 2022. doi:10.4108/eetsc.v6i3.2275

Sundaresan, S., Suresh Kumar, K., Nishanth, R., Harold Robinson, Y., and Jaya Kumar, A. "Artificial Intelligence and machine learning approaches for smart transportation in smart cities using Blockchain Architecture," *Blockchain for Smart Cities*, pp. 35–56, 2021. doi:10.1016/b978-0-12-824446-3.00009-0

Tejaswi, P. and Gnana Swathika, O. V. "Machine learning algorithms-based solar power forecasting in Smart Cities," *Artificial Intelligence and Machine Learning in Smart City Planning*, pp. 171–179, 2023. doi:10.1016/b978-0-323-99503-0.00001-6

Toh, C. and Brody, J. P. "Applications of machine learning in Healthcare," *Smart Manufacturing - When Artificial Intelligence Meets the Internet of Things*, 2021. doi:10.5772/intechopen.92297

Tsoniotis, N. "Smart cities as identities," *Springer Optimization and Its Applications*, pp. 51–62, 2022. doi:10.1007/978-3-030-84459-2_4

Yigitcanlar, T., and Cugurullo, F. "The sustainability of artificial intelligence: An urbanistic viewpoint from the lens of smart and sustainable cities," *Sustainability 12*(20), p. 8548, 2020.

Zamponi, M. E. and Barbierato, E. "The dual role of Artificial Intelligence in developing Smart Cities," *Smart Cities*, *5*(2), pp. 728–755, 2022. doi:10.3390/smartcities5020038

4

Comprehensive Survey of IoT, Machine Learning, and Reliability Engineering for Healthcare Applications

Suneel Kumar Rath and Madhusmita Sahu
C.V. Raman Global University, Bhubaneswar, Odisha, India

Shom Prasad Das
Birla Global University, Bhubaneswar, Odisha, India

4.1 Introduction

For identifying, preventing, and treating numerous diseases, healthcare systems have become increasingly reliant on software programs in recent years. There are a variety of medical services applications that are employed for computed tomography and nuclear medicine for treating and diagnosing disorders such as tumours, malignancies, heart ailments, and other anomalies within the human body. Because these are safety and critical systems, any failure or malfunction of equipment could cause a dangerous occurrence, resulting in increased disease or even death. Patients want hospitals to be extremely dependable and error-free. To be a highly dependable institution, all medical equipment, procedures, and processes must be of the highest quality. When equipment is tested as an independent subsystem as well as in conjunction with the hospital environment and other devices, it is critical to assure its reliability. As per IEEE software reliability is termed as, the capacity of a component or system to carry out its necessary roles under determined conditions over a predefined timeframe. In terms of software quality, dependability is critical. The capacity of a system to produce fault-free functioning is referred to as its reliability. It's a function of how many times a user of that software has encountered a problem. Because software is so complicated, metrics that can be utilized to estimate hardware reliability are unable to quantify software reliability. In an integrated context, traditional methods of reliability estimation, such as the mean time between failures, are ineffective. The reliability test focuses substantially more and more text-based because that particular system always needs to be tested in conjunction with multiple other different systems. Because the data is largely text, statistical analysis techniques can't be used right away. As a result, this method necessitates text analysis techniques including quantitative text analysis, facts,

DOI: 10.1201/9781032631738-4

relationships, and event extraction among others. A healthcare system is a set of processes, routes, and sub-processes, each of which ensures the conveyance of safe consideration administrations and stakeholder satisfaction. (1) The defect rate is a common way to express reliability. An opportunity for a malfunction in healthcare usually translates to a community of patients who are at risk of a medical error or an adverse event. (2) The most high-reliability company achieves a high level of dependability and safety despite operating in potentially dangerous circumstances. (3) For hardware and software medical equipment, reliability analysis methodologies are utilized. Over 30 years ago, reliability analysis of medical equipment and systems was recognized to be one of the most important aspects of reliability engineering in the healthcare system. For equipment estimation analysis, reliability engineering approaches are employed, which include fault-tolerant systems design, software reliability analysis, safety, availability, and study of medical equipment. The failure mode and effective analysis (FMEA) model is described. This is a strategy for assessing the relative impact of various failures that is methodical and proactive. A board's need to pursue the goal of zero preventable harm leads to modifications in leadership styles, greater transparency, and business investment plans. Over the last two decades, a lot of scholars have looked at the reliability expected of medical systems during the development and design stage, but there is less literature on the dependability identification and trend analysis of medical gadgets in hospitals. It's critical to guarantee the reliability of medical equipment when they're put to the test in the context of the hospital environment.

Medical care is one of the quickest enterprises to take on the Internet of Things (IoT) since coordinating IoT highlights into clinical gadgets further develops administration quality and viability, which is particularly significant for old patients with persistent circumstances and patients who require steady observation and management. Emergency notification systems and remote health monitoring are possible because of IoT devices. Heart rate monitors and blood pressure as well as more advanced monitoring systems for specific implants like electronic wristbands, pacemakers, and advanced hearing aids are examples of health monitoring devices. Machine learning (ML) is a field of artificial intelligence (AI) that uses statistical methods and data to emulate human learning behaviour (Hussain and Roy, 2023; Pradhan et al., 2022). The healthcare industry is one of the world's biggest and most active, relying heavily on manual regulation at all stages. The majority of clinical records relating to patient care are handwritten by specialists, with only a few reports generated by machines. This procedure increases the likelihood of misdiagnosis, putting a patient's life in jeopardy. The application of ML has been widely used in recent technology adoptions for automating manual activities. This chapter examines the utilization of ML techniques in medical systems automation. In general, reliability engineering has been employed in the field of healthcare informatics (Castro, 2009). For hardware and software medical equipment, reliability analysis methodologies are utilized. E.F. Taylor defined the investigation of clinical or medical instruments and devices as a primary item of reliability engineering in the medical services framework over 30 years ago. Methods for analyzing human reliability allow researchers to look into the likelihood of the risk factor for a final diagnosis and medical errors. However, in the healthcare system, these procedures are used and reviewed with caution. As a result, in particular healthcare system reliability analysis, the software and hardware have been primarily evaluated. In most works on healthcare or medical system reliability analysis, this type of particular tendency has been developed. For instance, in the paper by Taleb-Bendiab et al. (2006), several perspectives on software components' and different system hardware's safety and reliability are examined. Human blunders are viewed as a distinct issue in the healthcare system. In this field of research, human blunders in the medical or healthcare system are a separate feature (Cook and Woods, 2018). The first path is to assess the technological system's reliability (software and hardware mainly). Second, human reliability analysis methodologies are used to examine the probability of human errors. As a result, this healthcare system is made up of two non-intersecting pieces that do not form a whole. A framework for dependable patient monitoring in the context of a smart city has been established in the study by Nagarajan et al. (2021) using IoT. Their primary objective is to offer dependability based on federated learning, data security, privacy, and AI's social acceptability.

4.2 IoT Services and Applications for the Healthcare Sector

The implementation, development, publication, and deployment of numerous IoT services and healthcare applications are documented in Islam et al. (2015). This section includes a proposed request for IoT applications, a proposed idea for IoT in medical care organizations, and three applications that are described in another IoT outline (Fuqaha, et al., 2015): a nursing home patient monitoring system, a system for noticing and assistance with dietary issues, an indoor course structure for blind and ostensibly handicapped people, and a diabetes patient application.

4.2.1 Application Categories for IoT in Healthcare

Identification, tracking of items and people, autonomous data collecting, authentication of people, and sensing are all examples of IoT applications in healthcare. Movement following through stifle focuses, constant position following, similar to admittance to assigned regions, consistent stock area following, and materials/objects following are instances of following. Patient distinguishing proof to keep away from unfavourable episodes like some unacceptable medication, portion, timing, or therapy, electronic clinical record support in both in- and out-patient settings, and ID of children in clinics to try not to bungle are all examples of identification and authentication.

4.2.2 IoT-Powered Closed-Loop Medical Services

Patients are watched by IoT gadgets that send information to and get control from a telecheck administration centre, as detailed in Wears et al. (2006). The service centre is accessible to both healthcare and patient professionals (nurses and physicians at healthcare stations). The introduction of gathered information in the assistance centre allows for direct communication between patients and healthcare workers via mobile phones, like clinical treatment counsel to patients.

4.2.3 Monitoring System for Patients in Nursing Homes

The vital signs of patients are taken and relayed to several nursing stations. With that, patients have private rooms, and light and door sensors are used to track their activity levels and perhaps identify those who are depressed. A sensor is a linked microcontroller through USB that has been configured to a client for the application-level message queue telemetry transport (MQTT) convention (Cook et al., 1990), which depends on the transmission control protocol convention. Utilizing a wireless local area network, the MQTT client sends sensor information gathered to an MQTT merchant gadget. To get collected data of interest, MQTT servers associated with nursing stations buy into the MQTT agent. Specialists can remotely get to sensor information utilizing a portable broker of MQTT application that buys into information with the themes they're interested in.

4.2.4 Eating Disorders: Monitoring and Reduction Disorders

Patients with critical tremors or Parkinson's disease can use the app to eat without spilling their food. Hand movement instability detected by accelerometers is counteracted by a glove with little vibrating motors. To offer the desired functionality, the sensors of the accelerometer and vibrating motors must contact each other with the shortest possible latency. Subsequently, for an inconsequential direct relationship between vibrating motors and accelerometers without the cooperation of an MQTT dealer, the data distribution service convention, a merchant-less distribute buy-in convention for continuous M2 communications (Bogner et al., 1994), is the right arrangement. We should introduce an entryway to decipher DDS text into MQTT and distribute text sent utilizing Wi-Fi to an MQTT specialist gadget to consolidate this usefulness with the nursing objections.

4.2.5 Blind and Visually Impaired People's In-Car Navigation System

Users can get real-time location services (RTLSs) from a constellation of transceivers. A user-held device connects to RTLS local server and obtains a confirmation token to get to RTLS services using the multicast DNS (MDNS) protocol. Data distribution service is used by the RTLS nodes to exchange data packets in a timely fashion. The acquired data from the RTLS nodes can be relayed to the RTLS server, which can then estimate the user's current location. The nearby RTLS server can overlay the situation on an Internet-associated server's floor plan to give material route data to clients, permitting them to keep away from obstructions and other actual development requirements revealed by past framework clients.

4.2.6 Diabetes Patients' Insulin Dosage Administration

GoCap, an IoT gadget created by a firm, can help diabetic people. The GoCap is a trading cap for a prefilled insulin pen that monitors the different measures of insulin utilized every day and when it was given. The data is shipped off a telephone or an associated glucometer through Bluetooth. The goal is to give healthcare providers a continual stream of essential data in an easy-to-understand manner so that possible problems can be identified and addressed before they become so serious that patients need to be admitted to the hospital (Baum, 2013).

4.3 Analysis of the Healthcare Systems' Reliability

It is possible to identify two separate paths in healthcare system dependability analysis by reviewing prior work, as shown in Figure 4.1. Equipment assessment and doctor activity analysis are done using reliability engineering approaches. The fault-tolerant system design, analysis of software reliability, safety, availability, and medical instruments analysis are all part of the first portion of these methodologies. The human reliability analysis methods are used in the second half of the methods.

In the medical system, two tiers of reliability engineering (Rath et al., 2023a, 2023b) techniques will be applied (Figure 4.2). The first step is to conduct a system design reliability analysis:

(a) Resilient architecture of the system refers to fault-prevention strategies and procedures for the expounded item.
(b) Fault tolerance is an important feature for obtaining high dependability in many critical applications, and it can be accomplished by utilizing repetitive hardware or software.
(c) Unlike software, hardware is not subject to wear and tear and can be simply replicated. In addition, software systems are typically normally repaired during the testing system so their dependability works on over the reliability improve over time.
(d) Human dependability examination is a method for forestalling specialist mistakes or bumbles in the medical care framework.

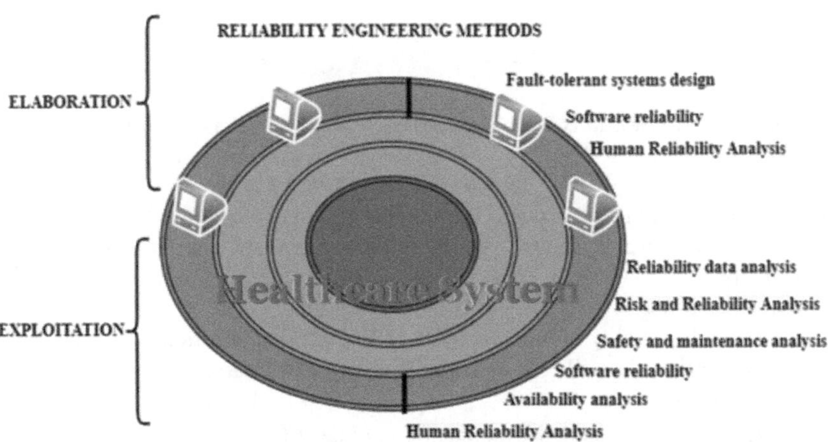

FIGURE 4.1 Design and implementation of the healthcare system using reliability engineering approaches.

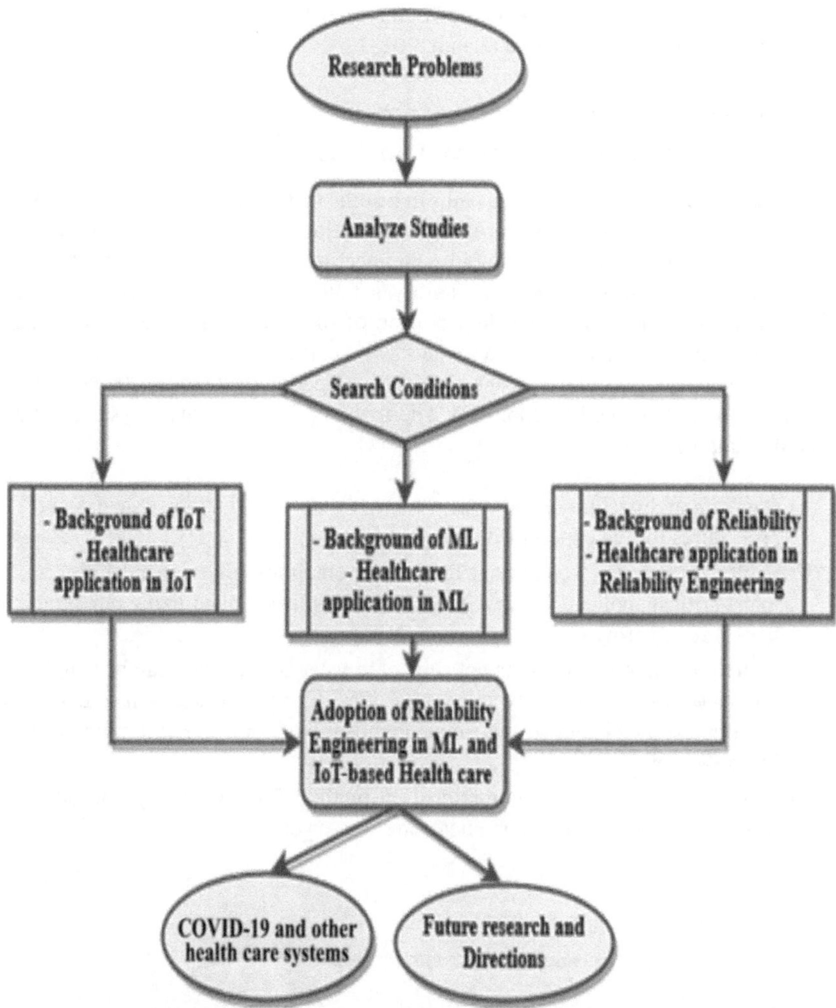

FIGURE 4.2 Approach to conduct a comprehensive study on healthcare applications of IoT, reliability engineering, and ML.

The use of the healthcare system is the second stage of exploitation. They're identical to the previous level's methods and algorithms, but they're for real-world object exploitation:

(a) Reliability quality information (Rat, et.al, 2021) examination is utilized for the control of new keeps and the consistency of information in electronic prosperity records.
(b) Risk and dependability examination is utilized to gauge the working of a medical services framework's hardware and gadgets.
(c) Safety and support examination of data assets is utilized for the control of gadgets and programming.

(d) Availability investigation is utilized to quantify the right capability of a medical services framework and a portion of its parts.
(e) Human reliability is used for the control of devices and software. Because dependability can be generally construed as a system's capacity to perform its intended function, it is a quantitative metric that is relevant in this context.

To get to the next level of the chances that the systems would operate sufficiently in tasks, extensive studies on reliability models and analytical techniques are conducted. The majority of computing system dependability models assume that the system can only be in two states. Many systems, especially those that are real-time, may contain more than two states in reality. If a few parts in an ongoing framework fall flat, the framework might in any case work, yet its presentation may suffer. Between flawless operating and fully failing systems, such a degradation condition exists. Many scholars have recently been concerned with the reliability of multi-state systems (MSS) to examine these sorts of systems (Zaitseva, 2003). Reliability engineering encompasses a wide range of methods.

Reliability block pictures, Markov model, Monte Carlo recreation, and fault tree examination are among the most extensively used methodologies. Many articles have looked at these strategies for various application problems. Some studies have evolved these fundamental methodologies and proposed novel solutions that integrate aspects of Reliability block pictures, the Markov model, Monte Carlo simulation, and fault tree analysis to exploit their benefits (Lisnianski & Levitin, 2003). Reliability engineering employs a variety of methodologies. A reliability engineering problem is an important analysis. The relative relevance of the many aspects and components that make up the system is a significant problem in reliability engineering. Indeed, determining which factors have the most impact on overall system performance allows for the identification of technological bottlenecks and the development of effective improvement of system strategies. In this case, the main important measurements are employed to assess the commitment of different components to framework execution (i.e., dependability, availability, and risk). The criticality of a specific aspect inside a system design is quantified using important measurements. They've been frequently utilized as tools for discovering system flaws and prioritizing operations aimed at improving reliability.

4.4 The Use of ML in Medicine

The healthcare industry generates a lot of heterogeneous information and data regularly, making traditional data analysis and processing problematic. Using ML and deep learning (DL) to help automate time-consuming operations and produce insights that are actionable. Furthermore, data sources such as medical information, environmental data, social media data, and genomes can be used to segment healthcare service information into various areas.

4.4.1 Health Information Technology (EHRs)

Medical clinics and other medical services suppliers utilize electronic health records (EHRs) to keep track of patients' medication histories and other details about their recovery. Manually extracting clinical characteristics from EHRs is a time-consuming operation, but ML-based solutions can help. Methods based on ML make it simple to retrieve the data needed to help with diagnosis. Various points of reference have been displayed to analyze diseases including lung infections, diabetes caused by COVID-19, and tumour cell progression using unorganized EHRs. EHRs' various unstructured records are mostly evaluated for the following two goals: predicting duration of stay and predicting death. In investigations, it has been discovered that when historical records are used to train, the prediction for the diagnosis process degrades. Stojanovic et al. (2016) reported a study in which they used advanced ML algorithms to predict significant healthcare quality metrics using EHRs. Diminished layered vector portrayals of patients' clinical systems and conditions are the focus of this research. Brisimi et al. (2018) created ML methods to estimate the likelihood of hospitalization because of the two most normal ongoing infections like coronary illness and diabetes. Expectations are completely based on patient clinical histories documented in EHRs. The number of digital information systems of medical data acquired in EHRs has skyrocketed in the preceding age. Shickel et al. (2017) reviewed existing research on the utilization of profound figuring out how clinical assignments utilize EHR data and found several flaws. Fuente et al. (2019) published a survey in which they used the Random Forest algorithm to study the behavioural patterns in patients' EHRs. Their research is primarily concerned with establishing a link between various diseases and the factors that influence them. When it comes to data-driven technologies for medical convenience, analytics is crucial. Harriman et al. (2019) provided a clear overview of how to use optimum DL techniques to manage and use data from EHRs. Data availability is increasing at an exponential rate, which may lower the requirement for data in ML algorithms. Performance, on the other hand, is sacrificed in exchange for computation time, which can be essential in medical crises.

4.4.2 Analysis of Medical Images Using ML

The application of ML algorithms to medical image investigation is well-established. These computational algorithms enable the effective extraction of critical data from picture tests generated by a variety of imaging modalities (like ultrasound imaging, computed tomography, magnetic resonance imaging, and positron emission tomography among others). Physicists can now modify existing AI calculations and examinations with new numerical thoughts thanks to recent breakthroughs in computing technology (Tsang, et al., 2020). The mechanically generated images allow for the detection of the underlying cause of illness as well as the localization of anomalies throughout the body. Important tasks in clinical picture analysis include segmentation, detection, reconstruction, localization (Lee et al., 2020), improvements, classification, and so on (Zebari et al., 2020). As a result, it's expected that a fully robotized keen framework for clinical picture examination will be able to deliver services including localization, segmentation, classification, and detection. Li et al. (2021) introduced a trial investigation using histopathological imaging to aid in the detection of lung cancer. The relevant features, support vector machine model, which they offered as the best classifier, had the highest accuracy, demonstrating the capability of assistant demonstrative models employing medical images. In a variety of ways, ML and AI have altered therapeutic methods. Rath et al. (2022a, 2022b) provide a comprehensive overview of how AI is changing the medical imaging landscape. Similarly, Umamaheswari and Geetha (2018) offer an approach for acute lymphoblastic leukaemia cell classification and segmentation. As a result, it is expected that a fully computerized canny framework for clinical picture investigation will be able to deliver utility including segmentation, detection, localization, and classification. Li et al. (2021) introduced an exploratory investigation based on histopathological imaging in computer-assisted lung cancer detection. The relief-support vector machine model, which they offered as the best classifier, accomplished the most elevated exactness, proving the potential of auxiliary indicative models employing medical images. Treatment processes have been modified by ML and AI in a variety of ways. Rath et al. (2022c) provide a comprehensive overview of how AI is transforming the medical picture landscape. Clinical pictures that have been examined are used to feed the system. Segmentation comes first for graphical analysis, followed by morphological administrators and Otsu's thresholding.

4.4.3 ML Applications in Healthcare

Later advancements and research in large-scale ML applications for medical services have cleared the way for more effective treatment options. Prognosis, diagnosis, and therapy are all three steps in the medication process. Expert clinicians and radiologists examine medical images during the diagnosis phase to determine potential hazards and treatments. Every day, a lot of medical information is gathered from a variety of little and enormous medical care offices, the data is scrutinized, and the results are documented in reports. Anyway, creating such reports necessitates competence, what's more, whenever taken care of by someone with less involvement with regions of emerging healthcare services, misdiagnosis or a critical synopsis may occur. Then again, generating text-type medical papers at organizational stages can be a time-consuming and exhausting effort for medical radiologists and experts, thus different researchers have used ML approaches to try to solve some specific challenges. A natural language processing approach was proposed by Zack et al. (2019) in response to a comment on radiology reports. Jing et al. (2017) revived a performing various tasks ML system for the programmed depiction and labelling of clinical radiological pictures in a similar project. Likewise, analysts and clinicians have discovered ways to combine approaches like recurrent neural networks, convolutional neural networks, and long short-term memory to make sense of robotized best-in-class engineering for prescient plan frameworks in localizing damaged body regions. Zhao et al. (2019) reported a study in which they built ML calculations for drug repositioning in the instances of melancholy and schizophrenia. Among the algorithms that have been tested, SVMs outperform others. A great many individuals have kicked the bucket because of the COVID-19 episode, which has caused a slew of issues. Since then, researchers and medical specialists have worked tirelessly to find new ways to save lives, with technology playing a significant role. Jamshidi et al. (2020) have compiled a list of several DL techniques for diagnosing and treating COVID-19 sufferers.

4.4.4 Machine Learning for Computer-Aided Detection (CAD)

ML has been generally utilized as a significant technique of the CAD conspire, i.e., computer-aided diagnosis/detection of injury competitors into specific classes of multidisciplinary innovation mixing components of AI/ML with pathology and radiology picture handling, with IBM's Watson serving as an excellent example. When time is of the essence, automatic medical image interpretation has proven to be quite useful in assisting radiologists and clinicians with clinical care. DL/ML procedures, for example, t-test, Fisher score discriminator, and chi-square test, as well as classic processes such as computer vision, predictive algorithms, and image processing methods, are all included in the workflow. Saygili (2021) used image processing and ML to investigate multiple categorization models for early PC helped conclusion and treatment of COVID-19. On a dataset of X-ray pictures, their proposed method had a remarkable accuracy of 99.02%. Similarly, Nagiub et al. (2018) used microscopic blood pictures to investigate the applicability of CNNs in computer-assisted leukaemia detection. The majority of the talk centres on human disease identification and apparent remedies employing the big name in technology, ML. He et al. (2018) have recommended a large investigation into hookworm invention in light of one of the most frequent infectious diseases that cause catastrophic outcomes in children, namely, hookworm. Their research includes an ML identification system for wireless capsule endoscopy (WCE) pictures that track hookworm-rounded examples and models at the same time.

4.4.5 Diagnosis and Prognosis of Disease

Early diagnosis and prediction of disease can save a person's life. Predictive ML approaches initiate finding and early visualization using medical data, reducing the time expected to follow-up on the infection for treatment. According to overviews, certain ML algorithms were successful in predicting cardiovascular risk utilizing clinical information (Yang et al., 2017), and research concluded that ML proficiency improved visualization and analysis consistency. The inherent use of ML-based approaches for cancer visualization and analysis, as well as the detection of other diseases such as dengue fever, virulent infections, heart issues, hepatitis, diabetes, malaria, and other diseases, has proven to be capable (Chaitra et al., 2020). Major depressive disorder (MDD) is a term that refers to a group of mood disorders that can be diagnosed by biological psychiatry. It has become increasingly popular among today's youth. Its diagnosis necessitates determining the underlying reason. Using heart rate variability serum proteome analysis data, Kim et al. (2017) investigated MDD and used ML to categorize peripheral biomarkers. Akbulut et al. (2018) published an orderly review that demonstrates how ML can help with a variety of cognitive diagnosis processes. Following this, Akbulut et al. (2018) suggested several ML approaches for observing and gauging fatal wellbeing status utilizing maternal clinical history. Over the years, ML has seen a lot of development. Clinical professionals' burden has been decreased due to the decision support offered by ML models. Karhade et al. (2018) used a Bayes Point algorithm to predict minimum 5-year survival in patients with spinopelvic chordoma diseases. Even though the ML algorithm was created expressly for this unusual pathology, its precision was not harmed. Abdar et al. (2019) presented ML approaches for coronary artery disease diagnosis. In particular COVID-19 patients, Burdick, et al. (2020) used ML to predict and diagnose respiratory decomposition. Hashem et al. (2020) made prescient models for the recognizable proof of constant liver problems, as well as hepatocellular carcinoma. An introduction and their exploration of the early discovery of Parkinson's illness (Magesh, et al., 2020), and demonstrative models for *E. coli* contamination, numerous sclerosis, and different sicknesses have likewise been laid out.

4.4.6 Data from Clinical Time Series and ML

A collection of statistical/numerical features tracked over time is called time-series data. Clinical time-series data is a collection of medical imaging observations that are collected regularly to trace the progress of key data points of interest. The application of medical time-series ML modelling includes health status prediction in intensive care units utilizing long-short term memory networks and convolutional neural networks (CNNs), death rate expectation of patients with traumatic brain injury, and appraisal of pulse, intracranial pressure, which is one of the main indications of cerebrovascular auto guideline in TBI patients. According to recent studies, combining data from time series using multivariate model preferences greatly improves the predictability of forecasting tasks such as prognosis, diagnosis, and suggestion. ML time-series models on glucose prediction were benchmarked by Xie and Wang (2020). For the modelling of a predictive system, Pezoulas et al. (2021) collected time-series data from microarrays expressing genes. The created model identifies possible Kawasaki disease biomarkers. To function well, every ML program requires a lot of information. Data administration, on the other hand, is regarded as a time-consuming but necessary task. Nancy et al. (2017) used a bio factual mining approach to efficiently classify and manage time-series information with unpredictable time spans utilizing a bio factual mining approach. Similarly, Froc et al. (2021) compiled a list of clinical qualities of urinary lot endometriosis because of a year of information from 232 patients.

4.4.7 Processing of Speech and Audio in Medicine

Concerned specialists in healthcare settings must prepare massive volumes of documentation, such as different reports like clinical, imaging, and discharge applications, which takes a long time and is physically demanding for professionals. (Wallace, 2018) noted how, given the existing heavy strain on specialists, documentation is an extra weight that consumes half of their time, lessening patient commitment time. Clinical discourse and sound handling moan help in this normal situation, which is burdening for clinicians and genuinely unattached for patients who need consideration. Its uses include interaction-free speech communication, transcript automation, clinical note synthesis, and correspondence in the event of a staff shortage, among others.

4.4.8 In Prognosis: ML

The process of predicting a disease's future outcome based on medical trials is referred to as prognosis. The procedure includes identifying potential dangers as well as determining disease pre-stages and survival chances. According to Collins and Yao (2018), multimodal patient data feeds ML models that help with prognosis. A recent study into the possible utilizations of ML in the medical anticipation process emphasizes the need for customized medicine, a still-developing subject. Strong validation procedures and the utilization of AI are expected to deliver the translational impact of customized medicine. For severe dengue prognosis, Davi et al. (2019) introduced an ML algorithm based on human genomic markers. Liu et al.'s (2019) ML models show that partial clinical scores and MRI data can predict brain illness prognosis.ML/DL techniques are also used to create a variety of other predictive systems. ML, on the other hand, can be used to choose characteristics in stroke prognosis. An exchange learning system for bladder disease guess was presented by Wang et al. (2020). Cai et al. (2020) looked into ML models for assessing and quantifying COVID-19 patient severity and prognosis. Finally, Zack et al. (2019) utilized AI strategies to foresee the guess of percutaneous coronary intervention, while He et al. checked out at intense renal injury forecast after heart demise and liver transplantation.

4.5 Security and Privacy

In the healthcare arena, IoT is used to provide tailored services, such as customized and speedy access to healthcare, which was previously unthinkable. Both technology and healthcare equipment collaborate in these applications to provide a wide range of services. Health-related IoT innovation is expected to represent around 40% of all IoT-related innovation by 2021, more than some other market areas, with a portion of the overall industry of USD 136.8 billion (Kaur, et al., 2020). Such advancements in this field are revolutionary, but they should be implemented with caution due to the issues that health-related data poses in terms of security, privacy, and sensitivity. Upstream transmission of corrupted information not only degrades the performance of the underlying data aggregation algorithm. It makes the fundamental organizations helpless against an assortment of including denial of service, security threats, eavesdropping, sinkhole Sybil, and sleep deprivation attacks. Because of the persistent development of the business and the rising number and intricacy of possible programming and equipment weaknesses, these dangers keep on being a test. Moreover, medical care information containing delicate and classified data, like individual data, family ancestry, electronic clinical records, and genomic information, should be kept hidden. Around 72% of noxious traffic was projected to be coordinated toward medical care information (Williams et al., 2016). It is subsequently basic to shield such data from programmers by carrying out protection and security arrangements, both truly and online. Low security, misconfigured gadgets, and organization settings are among the different issues that should be tended to. Besides, information from these many kinds of gadgets is normally heterogeneous and is habitually kept up with by outsiders, making information administration, security, and protection a troublesome cycle. Additionally, because of the asset requirements of IoT gadgets, traditional security arrangements are not a suitable other option. Planning lightweight and energy-productive information total methodologies that safeguard, yet additionally guarantee, the security, data's secrecy, and privacy is an intriguing subject to investigate further.

4.6 Research Methodology and Results

In this part, the methodology of a topical study of modern IoT-based models in healthcare domains based on reliability engineering, IoT, and ML is provided. This study provides a comprehensive overview of current research in machine learning (ML) and reliability engineering as they pertain to ensuring the reliability of IoT systems. It highlights the diverse methodologies used in reliability engineering, illustrated in

Figure 4.2. The discussion begins with an introduction to machine learning, reliability engineering (Rath et al., 2023), and IoT technologies. It then explores healthcare applications that leverage these advancements. Additionally, the study presents a case analysis of COVID-19, demonstrating the application of these technologies. Finally, it examines the convergence and adaptability of these technologies, addressing the associated challenges and proposed solutions.

4.7 Directions for Future Research

Various concerns connected to the privacy, security, and resilience of ML in the medical services environment are covered in this part, which requires active study attention.

4.7.1 The Edge of Machine Learning

As of late, there has been an exponential development in the use of ML in healthcare applications. Traditional approaches have been transformed by ML research, which has settled on the brilliant and energy-useful utilization of wearable gadgets, and other IoT sensors. There is a proceeding with popularity expected for upgraded ML models prepared on edge gadgets as savvy urban communities and movable clinical gadgets, for example, oxygen concentrators, convenient ventilators, and MRI machines, arise. This has some drawbacks, such as a shortage of accessible equipment and high computational handling abilities. The field of ML in edge devices is still in its infancy, and researchers must pay attention to it.

4.7.2 The Annotation of Datasets

The training and inference result of AI frameworks is heavily reliant on labelled datasets. This necessitates medical specialists and physiologists manually annotating medical information (such as clinical reports and photo signals), which consumes a significant amount of their time. The range of useful clinical information featured with exact names will evaluate the execution of ML or DL models (Rath et al., 2022d) and uncover blocks that could have slipped by everyone's notice already. As a result, manually classifying data is demanding, time-consuming, and energy-intensive. To inscribe this limitation, automatic approaches such as dynamic learning ought to be utilized and created.

4.7.3 ML and Distributed Data Management

Data is generated discretely in healthcare systems, i.e., information is handled from different offices inside an emergency clinic and afterward disseminated to different medical clinics all through the country. This puts a strain on data exchange and management, especially when utilizing ML models, for clinical analysis. Models for ML and DL are created with the assumption that all analytical data is freely accessible and centralized. These flaws in information interchange management require the attention of developers and researchers who can work together to address distributed data and ML administration.

4.7.4 ML That Is Both Fair and Responsible

In their analysis of the resilience and security of ML/DL approaches, Qayyum et al. (2020) concluded that the models' outputs are biased and unreliable. For life-basic applications in medical care frameworks, guaranteeing the precision and fairness of forecasts is crucial. Trading away these models' accuracy and accountability could lead to cynical outcomes and put patients' health in danger. Several instances with little data have an impact on the ML/DL models' ability to make accurate predictions. Taking into mind the meaning of fair judgment and interpretability, models can be tuned to be more resilient and avoid prior clinical record misjudgments. In this area, more research is needed to develop dynamic approaches for ensuring safety and reducing flaws.

4.7.5 Machine Learning with a Model-Centric Approach

The utilization of ML and AI in healthcare has both benefits and drawbacks. In clinical terms, failure to recognize Latif's flaws might be fatal. Typically, the advantages of these models convince one that information, once plentiful, can deal with speculation creation without the requirement for clinical expert approval and translation, bringing about inevitable issues. To stay away from these obstacles, it's basic to foster a consolidated information-driven technique that consolidates theory and model-based approaches to accomplish controlled accuracy in these explores. Further research is needed in areas such as producing technically exact, robust, secure, and responsible ML deliverables.

4.8 Conclusions

We have given a thorough outline of ML and reliability engineering analytics in the IoT healthcare domain in this chapter. To identify research gaps, we conducted a thorough review of the writing and picked the most important and current overviews. Also the application of IoT, ML, and reliability engineering in the larger context of developing smart cities and healthcare systems is explained in this chapter. Moreover, we've gathered total and state-of-the-art writing on ML-based reliability engineering analytics in IoT smart health. Their strengths and weaknesses were also discussed in detail. This gave peruses knowledge of the space and permitted them to start their examination by picking a subject from the pool of strategies advertised. Different exploration concerns and obstructions were talked about, and the specialists were urged to seek after them further. Besides, different issues that emerged because of the arising and cross-space models of IoT, like the Internet of Nano-Things and Web of Things, were entirely examined to understand a widespread IoT vision, a dream that effectively coordinates this innovation in practically all spaces and will ideally prosper our regular routines in the years to come.

REFERENCES

Abdar, M., Książek, W., Acharya, U. R., Tan, R. S., Makarenkov, V., & Pławiak, P. (2019). A new machine learning technique for an accurate diagnosis of coronary artery disease. *Computer Methods and Programs in Biomedicine*, *179*, 104992.

Abdelsalam, E. M. N., Hussain, K. F., Omar, N. M., & Ali, Q. T. (2018). Computer aided leukemia detection using microscopic blood image based machine learning "Convolutional neural network". *Clinical Lymphoma, Myeloma and Leukemia*, *18*, S297.

Akbulut, A., Ertugrul, E., & Topcu, V. (2018). Fetal health status prediction based on maternal clinical history using machine learning techniques. *Computer Methods and Programs in Biomedicine*, *163*, 87–100.

Al-Fuqaha, A., Guizani, M., Mohammadi, M., Aledhari, M., & Ayyash, M. (2015). Internet of things: A survey on enabling technologies, protocols, and applications. *IEEE Communications Surveys & Tutorials*, *17*(4), 2347–2376.v

Baum, S. (2013). A remote monitor embedded in insulin pen caps could help personalize diabetes treatment, https://medcitynews.com/2013/06/a-remote-monitor-embedded-in-insulin-pen-caps-could-help-personalize-diabetes-treatment/.

Brisimi, T. S., Xu, T., Wang, T., Dai, W., Adams, W. G., & Paschalidis, I. C. (2018). Predicting chronic disease hospitalizations from electronic health records: An interpretable classification approach. *Proceedings of the IEEE*, *106*(4), 690–707.

Burdick, H., Lam, C., Mataraso, S., Siefkas, A., Braden, G., Dellinger, R. P., … Das, R. (2020). Prediction of respiratory decompensation in Covid-19 patients using machine learning: The READY trial. *Computers in Biology and Medicine*, *124*, 103949.

Cai, W., Liu, T., Xue, X., Luo, G., Wang, X., Shen, Y., … Liang, T. (2020). CT quantification and machine-learning models for assessment of disease severity and prognosis of COVID-19 patients. *Academic Radiology*, *27*(12), 1665–1678.

Castro, D. (2009, October). Meeting national and international goals for improving health care: The role of information technology in medical research. In *2009 Atlanta Conference on Science and Innovation Policy* (pp. 1–9). IEEE.

Chaitra, N., Vijaya, P. A., & Deshpande, G. (2020). Diagnostic prediction of autism spectrum disorder using complex network measures in a machine learning framework. *Biomedical Signal Processing and Control*, *62*, 102099.

Collins, A., Yao, Y. (2018). Machine Learning Approaches: Data Integration for Disease Prediction and Prognosis. In: Yao, Y. (eds) *Applied Computational Genomics. Translational Bioinformatics*, vol *13*. Springer, Singapore. https://doi.org/10.1007/978-981-13-1071-3_10.

Cook, R. I., & Woods, D. D. (2018). Operating at the sharp end: the complexity of human error. In *Human error in medicine* (pp. 255–310). CRC Press.

Davi, C., Pastor, A., Oliveira, T., de Lima Neto, F. B., Braga-Neto, U., Bigham, A. W., … Acioli-Santos, B. (2019). Severe dengue prognosis using human genome data and machine learning. *IEEE Transactions on Biomedical Engineering*, *66*(10), 2861–2868.

De la Fuente, C., Urrutia, A., & Chavez, E. (2019). Using the random forest algorithm for searching behavior patterns in electronic health records. *IEEE Latin America Transactions*, *17*(05), 875–881.

Froc, E., Dubernard, G., Bendifallah, S., Hermouet, E., Rubod-Dit-Guillet, C., Canis, M., … Philip, C. A. (2021). Clinical characteristics of urinary tract endometriosis: A one-year national series of 232 patients from 31 endometriosis expert centers (by the FRIENDS group). *European Journal of Obstetrics & Gynecology and Reproductive Biology*, *264*, 155–161.

Harerimana, G., Kim, J. W., Yoo, H., & Jang, B. (2019). Deep learning for electronic health records analytics. *IEEE Access*, *7*, 101245–101259.

Hashem, S., ElHefnawi, M., Habashy, S., El-Adawy, M., Esmat, G., Elakel, W., … Shousha, H. I. (2020). Machine learning prediction models for diagnosing hepatocellular carcinoma with HCV-related chronic liver disease. *Computer Methods and Programs in Biomedicine, 196*, 105551.

He, J. Y., Wu, X., Jiang, Y. G., Peng, Q., & Jain, R. (2018). Hookworm detection in wireless capsule endoscopy images with deep learning. *IEEE Transactions on Image Processing, 27*(5), 2379–2392.

Hussain, M. W., & Roy, D. S. (2023). Performance optimization strategies for big data applications in distributed framework. In *Intelligent Technologies: Concepts, Applications, and Future Directions*, Volume *2* (pp. 221–252). Singapore: Springer Nature Singapore.

Islam, S. R., Kwak, D., Kabir, M. H., Hossain, M., & Kwak, K. S. (2015). The internet of things for health care: A comprehensive survey. *IEEE Access, 3*, 678–708.

Jamshidi, M., Lalbakhsh, A., Talla, J., Peroutka, Z., Hadjilooei, F., Lalbakhsh, P., … Mohyuddin, W. (2020). Artificial intelligence and COVID-19: Deep learning approaches for diagnosis and treatment. *IEEE Access, 8*, 109581–109595.

Jing, B., Xie, P., & Xing, E. (2017). On the automatic generation of medical imaging reports. *arXiv preprint arXiv: 1711.08195.*

Karhade, A. V., Thio, Q., Ogink, P., Kim, J., Lozano-Calderon, S., Raskin, K., & Schwab, J. H. (2018). Development of machine learning algorithms for prediction of 5-year spinal chordoma survival. *World neurosurgery, 119*, e842–e847.

Kaur, H., Atif, M., & Chauhan, R. (2020). An internet of healthcare things (IoHT)-based healthcare monitoring system. In *Advances in Intelligent Computing and Communication: Proceedings of ICAC 2019* (pp. 475–482). Springer Singapore.

Kim, E. Y., Lee, M. Y., Kim, S. H., Ha, K., Kim, K. P., & Ahn, Y. M. (2017). Diagnosis of major depressive disorder by combining multimodal information from heart rate dynamics and serum proteomics using machine-learning algorithm. *Progress in Neuro-Psychopharmacology and Biological Psychiatry, 76*, 65–71.

Lee, S., Wei, S., White, V., Bain, P. A., Baker, C., & Li, J. (2020). Classification of opioid usage through semi-supervised learning for total joint replacement patients. *IEEE Journal of Biomedical and Health Informatics, 25*(1), 189–200.

Li, M., Ma, X., Chen, C., Yuan, Y., Zhang, S., Yan, Z., … Ma, M. (2021). Research on the auxiliary classification and diagnosis of lung cancer subtypes based on histopathological images. *IEEE Access, 9*, 53687–53707.

Lisnianski, A., & Levitin, G. (2003). *Multi-state System Reliability: Assessment, Optimization and Applications*. World scientific.

Liu, M., Zhang, J., Lian, C., & Shen, D. (2019). Weakly supervised deep learning for brain disease prognosis using MRI and incomplete clinical scores. *IEEE transactions on cybernetics, 50*(7), 3381–3392.

Magesh, P. R., Myloth, R. D., & Tom, R. J. (2020). An explainable machine learning model for early detection of Parkinson's disease using LIME on DaTSCAN imagery. *Computers in Biology and Medicine, 126*, 104041.

Nagarajan, S. M., Deverajan, G. G., Chatterjee, P., Alnumay, W., & Ghosh, U. (2021). Effective task scheduling algorithm with deep learning for Internet of Health Things (IoHT) in sustainable smart cities. *Sustainable Cities and Society, 71*, 102945.

Nancy, J. Y., Khanna, N. H., & Kannan, A. (2017). A bio-statistical mining approach for classifying multivariate clinical time series data observed at irregular intervals. *Expert Systems with Applications, 78*, 283–300.

Pezoulas, V. C., Papaloukas, C., Veyssiere, M., Goules, A., Tzioufas, A. G., Soumelis, V., & Fotiadis, D. I. (2021). A computational workflow for the detection of candidate diagnostic biomarkers of Kawasaki disease using time-series gene expression data. *Computational and Structural Biotechnology Journal, 19*, 3058–3068.

Pradhan, B., Hussain, M. W., Srivastava, G., Debbarma, M. K., Barik, R. K., & Lin, J. C. W. (2022). A neuro-evolutionary approach for software defined wireless network traffic classification. *IET Communications*.

Qayyum, A., Qadir, J., Bilal, M., & Al-Fuqaha, A. (2020). Secure and robust machine learning for healthcare: A survey. *IEEE Reviews in Biomedical Engineering, 14*, 156–180.

Rath, S. K., Sahu, M., Das, S. P., Bisoy, S. K., & Sain, M. (2022a). A comparative analysis of SVM and ELM classification on software reliability prediction model. *Electronics, 11*(17), 2707.

Rath, S. K., Sahu, M., Das, S. P., & Mohapatra, S. K. (2022b, March). Hybrid Software Reliability Prediction Model Using Feature Selection and Support Vector Classifier. In *2022 International Conference on Emerging Smart Computing and Informatics (ESCI)* (pp. 1–4). IEEE.

Rath, S. K., Sahu, M., Das, S. P., & Pradhan, J. (2022c, February). An Improved Software Reliability Prediction Model by Using Feature Selection and Extreme Learning Machine. In *International Conference on Metaheuristics in Software Engineering and its Application* (pp. 43–55). Cham: Springer International Publishing.

Rath, S. K., Sahu, M., Das, S. P., & Pradhan, J. (2022d, February). Survey on Machine Learning Techniques for Software Reliability Accuracy Prediction. In *International Conference on Metaheuristics in Software Engineering and its Application* (pp. 43–55). Cham: Springer International Publishing.

Rath, S. K., Sahu, M. K., & Das, S. P. (2023a). IoT and Machine Learning Applications for Industrial Reliability Frameworks. In *Handbook of Research on Intelligent Decision Support System for IoT-Enabling Technologies: Opportunities, Challenges and Applications*, ISBN: 979-8-89113-249-8, https://doi.org/10.52305/QUGV2734 (pp. 73–94). Nova science publishers.

Rath, S. K., Sahu, M. K., & Das, S. P. (2023b). Applications of machine learning in industrial reliability model. In *Handbook of Research on Applications of AI, Digital Twin, and Internet of Things for Sustainable Development* (pp. 30–46). IGI Global.

Reddy, K. H. K., Roy, D. S., Mishra, T. K., & Hussain, M. W. (Eds.). (2023). *Handbook of Research on Network-Enabled IoT Applications for Smart City Services*. IGI Global.

Saygılı, A. (2021). A new approach for computer-aided detection of coronavirus (COVID-19) from CT and X-ray images using machine learning methods. *Applied Soft Computing, 105*, 107323.

Stojanovic, J., Gligorijevic, D., Radosavljevic, V., Djuric, N., Grbovic, M., & Obradovic, Z. (2016). Modeling healthcare quality via compact representations of electronic health records. *IEEE/ACM Transactions on Computational Biology and Bioinformatics, 14*(3), 545–554.

Taleb-Bendiab, A., England, D., Randles, M., Miseldine, P., & Murphy, K. (2006). A principled approach to the design of healthcare systems: Autonomy vs. governance. *Reliability Engineering & System Safety, 91*(12), 1576–1585.

Taylor, E. F. (1972, January). The reliability engineer in the health care system. In *Proc IEEE the 18th Annual Reliability & Maintainability Symposium* (pp. 245–248).

Tsang, G., Zhou, S. M., & Xie, X. (2020). Modeling large sparse data for feature selection: hospital admission predictions of the dementia patients using primary care electronic health records. *IEEE Journal of Translational Engineering in Health and Medicine, 9*, 1–13.

Umamaheswari, D. S. G. D., & Geetha, S. (2018, June). Segmentation and classification of acute lymphoblastic leukemia cells tooled with digital image processing and ML techniques. In *2018 Second International Conference on Intelligent Computing and Control Systems (ICICCS)* (pp. 1336–1341). IEEE.

Wallace, D. S. (2018). The role of speech recognition in clinical documentation. *Nuance Commun.*

Wang, G., Zhang, G., Choi, K. S., Lam, K. M., & Lu, J. (2020). Output based transfer learning with least squares support vector machine and its application in bladder cancer prognosis. *Neurocomputing*, *387*, 279–292.

Xie, J., & Wang, Q. (2020). Benchmarking machine learning algorithms on blood glucose prediction for type I diabetes in comparison with classical time-series models. *IEEE Transactions on Biomedical Engineering*, *67*(11), 3101–3124.

Yang, S., Wei, R., Guo, J., & Xu, L. (2017). Semantic inference on clinical documents: Combining machine learning algorithms with an inference engine for effective clinical diagnosis and treatment. *IEEE Access*, *5*, 3529–3546.

Zack, C. J., Senecal, C., Kinar, Y., Metzger, Y., Bar-Sinai, Y., Widmer, R. J., … Gulati, R. (2019). Leveraging machine learning techniques to forecast patient prognosis after percutaneous coronary intervention. *Cardiovascular Interventions*, *12*(14), 1304–1311.

Zaitseva, E. (2003). Dynamic reliability indices for multi-state system. *Journal of Dynamical Systems and Geometric Theories*, *1*(2), 213–222.

Zebari, D. A., Zeebaree, D. Q., Abdulazeez, A. M., Haron, H., & Hamed, H. N. A. (2020). Improved threshold based and trainable fully automated segmentation for breast cancer boundary and pectoral muscle in mammogram images. *IEEE Access*, *8*, 203097–203116.

Zech, J., Pain, M., Titano, J., Badgeley, M., Schefflein, J., Su, A., … Oermann, E. K. (2018). Natural language–based machine learning models for the annotation of clinical radiology reports. *Radiology*, *287*(2), 570–580.

Zhao, K., & So, H. C. (2018). Drug repositioning for schizophrenia and depression/anxiety disorders: a machine learning approach leveraging expression data. *IEEE Journal of Biomedical and Health Informatics*, *23*(3), 1304–1315.

5

Artificial Intelligence–based Solutions for Optimized Data Routing through Multi-Hop Healthcare Sensor Networks

Kuldeep Singh
Guru Nanak Dev University, Amritsar, India

Jyoteesh Malhotra
National Institute of Technology, Delhi, India

Bhanu Priya
Lovely Professional University, Phagwara, India

Abhishek Sharma
National Institute of Technology, Hamirpur, India

Manjit Singh and Butta Singh
Guru Nanak Dev University Regional Centre, Jalandhar, India

5.1 Introduction

During the contemporary age, the Internet of Things (IoT)-enabled mechanisms have started revolutionizing the healthcare field to resolve numerous health-related troubles using cloud and fog computing services. These technologies are assuring methods for uninterrupted and real-time monitoring of the health of patients via wearable IoT devices (Yuehong et al., 2016; Reddy et al., 2023). Generally, these IoT devices could sense various types of physiological signals, involving EEG, ECG, pulse, blood pressure, temperature, motion or position, etc. All these sensing devices form a wireless body area network (WBAN) (Negra et al., 2016; Su et al., 2013), which acts as an appropriate key for making a robust and scalable IoT network of a healthcare system. In WBAN, the patients wear different sensing devices, which are wirelessly connected to a wearable coordinator node (CN). The role of the CN is to relay sensed signals to the access point or edge devices. An example of a WBAN consisting of a patient wearing a variety of sensing devices and a CN is shown in Figure 5.1. Usually, these WBAN CNs of multiple patients form a wireless sensor network (WSN).

DOI: 10.1201/9781032631738-5

Depending upon the application scenario of a single patient staying at home, office, or moving outside, a source CN may communicate directly to the cloud through the internet, which could be termed single-hop communication. In other scenarios, e.g., hospital environment, a source CN could not be able to communicate directly via internet because of hardware limitations, poor coverage, or bandwidth limitations due to simultaneous transmission by multiple users (Su et al., 2013; Sobral et al., 2019). Therefore, these nodes could route data through a routing path of multiple CN nodes in a sensor network, which could be termed multi-hop communication. The process of determining a suitable routing path to transfer sensed data is accomplished by a routing protocol (Sobral et al., 2019). It confirms secure, reliable, and error-free transmission of sensed signals from sensing devices to edge devices or access points so that these signals can reach cloud servers properly for providing real-time healthcare solutions (Sobral et al., 2019).

For real-time IoT-healthcare applications in case of multiple users, the healthcare WSN comprises WBANs of multiple patients having their individual coordinating nodes. These large-scale networks are extremely complex in nature. These wireless sensor networks (abbreviated as WSNs) are generally deployed within the wireless environment, which encounters dynamic changes, unreliability, and asymmetry issues (Al-Anbagi et al., 2014; Di Marco et al., 2016). The sensor or coordinating nodes in these networks could be constrained by various factors such as dynamically changing communication environment, limited battery power, limited memory, limited bandwidth for data communication, and limited computing capability (Chelloug, 2015; Marietta & Chandra Mohan, 2020). Another significant problem is the network sensor nodes' dense connectivity, which arises from the reduced sensing range compared to the radio range and their dense distribution (Airehrour et al., 2016). The final and foremost problem is the asymmetrical and inconsistent wireless connections between the sensor nodes, which lowers the sensor network's overall performance (Di Marco et al., 2016; Rani et al., 2015). All of these problems make it difficult to implement energy-aware and quality-of-service (QoS) aware routing in healthcare WSNs, resulting in the need for algorithms that are naturally scalable, compatible, energy-effective, and secure (Di Marco et al., 2016; Al-Fuqaha et al., 2015).

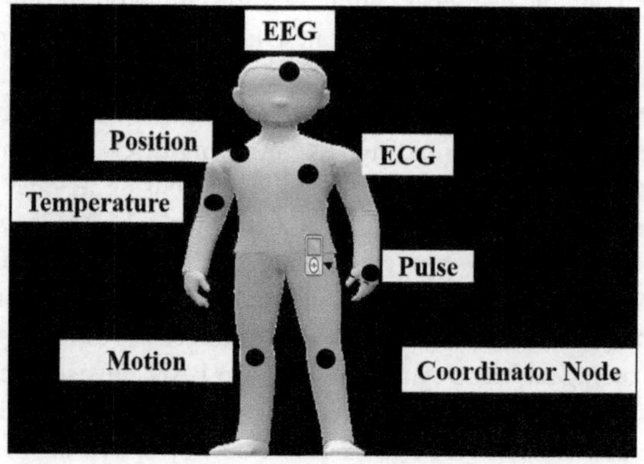

FIGURE 5.1 General architecture of a WBAN: a patient wearing body sensors.

Nowadays, the reinforcement learning (RL) approach (Yau et al., 2015; Liang et al., 2008; Al-Rawi et al., 2015) has earned huge consideration for solutions to several issues in WSNs to improve their overall network performance. Usually, the RL-based Q-learning algorithms are used to perform efficient routing by considering the link cost estimation of wireless links. Additionally, these estimates are based on physical and MAC (medium access control) layer metrics, including the strength of received signals at a given node based on received signal strength indicator (RSSI), rate of lost or failed packets, residual energy of nodes, the total time for each packet to move to the destination node, etc. (Di Marco et al., 2016). The present study also presents two routing algorithms based on RL for energy-effective and QoS-sensitive routing in WSNs using wireless link cost estimation strategies in smart healthcare scenarios in the context of smart cities. These algorithms include the fuzzy real-time search (Fuzzy RTS) algorithm and the fuzzy adaptive tree (Fuzzy AT) algorithm. Both of these algorithms make use of some of the physical and MAC layer parameters of sensor nodes, which include RSSI, remaining energy of each node, packet loss rate, and total time for packets in their reception at the destination node, for estimation of cost of a wireless connection between two given sensor nodes in WSN.

The major contributions presented in this chapter are enumerated as follows:

- This work presents the architecture of single-hop and multi-hop healthcare IoT networks and also discusses the need for optimized routing in multi-hop IoT sensor network scenarios for their implementation in smart cities.
- This work gives a comprehensive literature review of existing routing techniques for energy-effective and real-time routing in different kinds of WSNs.
- The usage of traditional RL-based routing strategies is also elaborated in this chapter.
- This work presents fuzzy logic-based energy-efficient routing algorithms, which are based on RL's Q-learning strategy. These algorithms include Fuzzy RTS and Fuzzy AT approaches.
- The appropriateness of these algorithms has been analyzed through simulation results, so that these algorithms may ensure QoS-aware and energy-effective routing in different IoT sensor networks of smart healthcare systems.
- The other existing fuzzy logic-based optimized routing algorithms are also discussed in detail in this chapter.

This chapter is systematized into different sections. Section 5.1 delivers a general overview of WBANs, healthcare IoT networks, and various constraints in data routing in these data-driven networks. The architectures of healthcare IoT systems are discussed in Section 5.2, which include single-hop and multi-hop healthcare networks. Section 5.3 provides information about routing in multi-hop healthcare networks. The existing routing solutions are comprehensively discussed in Section 5.4. In addition, Section 5.5 gives a brief overview of traditional routing algorithms based on RL for multi-hop healthcare systems. Similarly, fuzzy link cost estimation-based routing algorithms, i.e., Fuzzy RTS and Fuzzy AT are discussed in Section 1.6. The performance comparison of the given fuzzy logic-based algorithms has been exhibited in Section 1.7. Conclusively, Section 1.8 presents the deduction about major findings and the future possibilities of the research work presented in this chapter.

5.2 Architectures of Healthcare IoT Systems

As mentioned earlier, WBANs are one of the most appropriate technologies for the construction of scalable, and robust IoT-enabled healthcare systems (refer Figure 5.1) (Negra et al., 2016). These WBANs are used for real-time monitoring of a patient's body to detect any significant change in his/her sensed physiological signals. These signals may include EEG signals for neurological and mental disorders, ECG signals for cardiac diseases, glucose levels for diabetes, blood pressure, pulse rate, temperature, body position and motion, etc. (Islam et al., 2015). These are gathered by a variety of wearable sensing devices that can be worn over clothing, on patient's body directly as well as underneath his/her skin (Su et al., 2013). All of these signals are collected by the CN, which further transfers them to the cloud through the internet. Based on a patient's medical background, these healthcare systems analyze these signals for detecting the occurrence of various mental or physical disorders and send alert messages and health statistics reports to the families of the patients as well as the doctors. In this way, these healthcare systems may help in the detection and prediction of various disorders occurring in a patient. Depending on different application scenarios and types of routing of sensed data, these healthcare systems can be categorized into two classes, namely, single-hop systems and multi-hop systems.

5.2.1 Single-Hop Healthcare System

The single-hop healthcare system is based on single-hop communication for direct delivery of detected data of the patients to the final destination node of given network. The general architecture of a single-hop system is shown in Figure 5.2. This type of system could be applicable for a single patient residing at home or office, or during travelling. In this system, each WBAN CN for a patient has direct access to the internet. It transmits its collected biological signals from wearable body sensors to nearby fog/edge devices through Zigbee, Bluetooth, or Wi-Fi technologies. These edge devices may include smartphones, smart routers or access points, laptops or personal computers, etc. These devices transfer received signals to the cloud through the internet using an IoT gateway. Depending on the computational capabilities of the edge devices, the sensed signals may be locally processed on them, and the analyzed outputs along with processed signals could be sent to the cloud to store them. On the other hand, these signals could also be examined on cloud servers. This system conveys about detected states of the disease or disorder under-diagnosis to the respective patients, caregivers or family of the patients, and clinicians or doctors in nearby hospitals or ambulance services in case of emergency.

5.2.2 Multi-Hop Healthcare System

In certain application scenarios, e.g., hospital scenario, there may exist a large group of patients seeking access to the internet for transfer of data to the cloud or local server of the hospital. However, due to the hardware limitations of the CNs and other supporting network devices, it may be difficult to provide direct internet access to each patient individually (Sobral et al., 2019). Therefore, multi-hop healthcare system or framework comes into play to deal with such situations. Figure 5.3 shows the overview of a multi-hop healthcare system consisting of various groups of patients. In this system, the sensed body signals of a source patient (S) are forwarded to the access point (AP) through a routing path of intermediate CNs of other WBANs using Zigbee technology, which is a low-power and high-transmission range communication

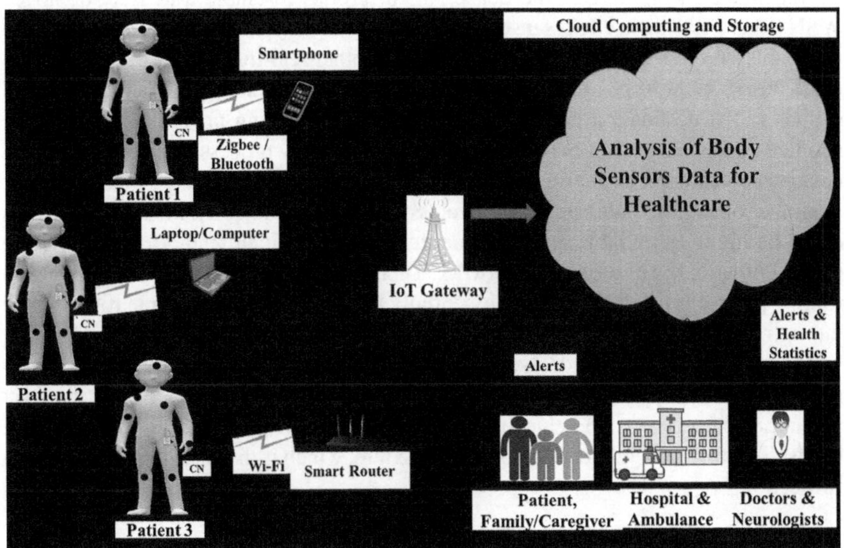

FIGURE 5.2 The overview of single-hop healthcare system.

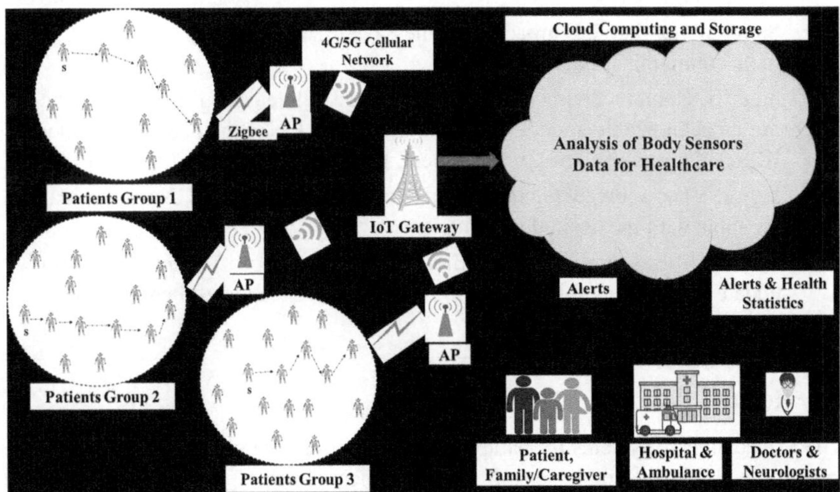

FIGURE 5.3 An illustration of multi-hop healthcare system.

technology (Chen et al., 2011). Furthermore, the received signals at AP are transferred to either the cloud through the internet or the local server of the hospital, where they are processed and analyzed. The analysis results and alerts are communicated to the respective users as mentioned in Section 5. 2.1.

5.3 Routing in Multi-Hop Healthcare System

As illustrated in Figure 5.3, the dense patient groups resemble a densely deployed WSN. These healthcare IoT sensor networks are usually set in highly dynamic and unreliable wireless environments of hospitals or other real-time scenarios (Al-Anbagi et al., 2014). In this type of environment, if a source node S intends to transfer detected signals to the destination node AP, then a multi-hop routing procedure needs to be adopted to achieve greater network coverage. The routing process transfers the sensed data packets through a routing path consisting of several other nodes. There may exist a number of routing paths made of wireless links among adjacent nodes. These links could be highly unreliable and asymmetric in nature, which leads to degrading the general functioning of the sensor network. Therefore, energy-effective and QoS-aware routing protocols or algorithms are essentially needed to select a suitable routing path through evaluation of link cost of wireless links. By avoiding congestion, using the least amount of energy, and delaying packet delivery as little as possible, a proper routing path makes it possible to transport data packets to the target node with the least amount of packet loss. To achieve successful delivery of packets, a routing protocol needs to perform a neighbour discovery procedure, which is discussed in the following subsection.

5.3.1 The Process of Neighbour Discovery

- Step I: One CN of a WBAN makes a routing table to store the information of neighbouring CNs.
- Step II: After that, CN broadcasts a message to search nearby neighbour CNs in its communication range.
- Step III: Upon receiving a broadcast message, all neighbouring nodes transmit an acknowledgement message to the source CN, which consists of their ID, residual energy level of the battery, location, RSSI, packet loss rate, etc.
- Step IV: The source CN makes entries of the neighbouring CNs in the routing table with the desired information.
- Step V: After a predetermined time period, Steps II to IV are repeated to update the routing table, so that the sensed signals can be routed efficiently.

5.4 Related Work

The IoT healthcare systems for patients suffering from different diseases or disorders are equipped with wearable sensor devices, which can transfer sensed data to edge devices. The sensed data received at these fog layer devices could be processed locally or transferred to cloud servers for further processing. For a single-user application, there exists a direct link between wearable sensor devices and sink node or access point through which data is to be transferred. But the problem arises in the case of multi-user applications, where data could be transferred to the access point through techniques routing based on multiple hops. In multiuser applications, WBANs of individual users make WSNs. These networks are generally deployed in unreliable, dynamically fluctuating and irregular wireless environments. Due to these issues, the effective routing of sensed data in these types of WSNs becomes a difficult task. Consequently, there is a strong necessity for a competent routing algorithm which could resolve these constraints in the given network and improve their inclusive performance with reference to energy effectiveness and quality of service (QoS).

The research community has presented a variety of algorithms, which are used for multipath or multi-hop routing in healthcare WSNs (Chan et al., 2020). In this concern, to ensure optimized routing in healthcare systems, Cicioğlu and Calhan et al. (2019) presented a software-defined network (SDN)-based WBAN energy-aware routing method. This approach used the concept of HUB or CNs for communication among various WBANs and access points. It decided on an optimized routing path by considering the node battery level and signal-to-noise ratio of neighbouring nodes. This SDN-based architecture illustrated superior performance for energy-aware routing in terms of energy consumption, throughput, delay, etc. In addition, Su et al. (2013) proposed a mobility-aided energy balance routing protocol for IoT healthcare applications. This routing protocol considered the energy and movement information of neighbouring CNs for initiating routing procedure to select the most appropriate neighbour for forwarding sensed biomedical data. Similarly, Sarwesh et al. (2017) also suggested an energy-effective network design for IoT healthcare networks. This architecture employed a routing protocol based on the monitored energy of neighbouring nodes to select a suitable path in WSN for forwarding data.

In the same concern, Chen and Weng (2012) described a minimum transmission power consumption routing (MTPCR) protocol to ensure energy-efficient routing. It utilized the information from neighbouring nodes to analyze power consumption. The link maintenance procedure was adopted to ensure the sustainability of link bandwidth. The activation of this procedure was decided with the help of node density. The implementation results of this protocol revealed its effectiveness with lower power consumption and good bandwidth as compared to ad-hoc on-demand distance vector (AODV), dynamic source routing (DSR), and other similar procedures. Similarly, Shokouhifar and Jalali (2015) described application-specific low-power routing (ASLPR) protocol for improving the lifetime of the network and lessening its energy consumption. Simulated annealing and genetic algorithm techniques were used in this protocol for the optimization of control parameters. This protocol showed better performance than that of the conventional low energy adaptive clustering hierarchy (LEACH) protocol.

Furthermore, Mohanty and Kabat (2016) presented an energy-effective consistent multipath transmission protocol to route data in healthcare WSNs. This approach adjusted the transmission rate at each middle node by considering the probability of congestion. It also used the concept of partitioned buffering at each node, hop-by-hop recovery of packet loss, and the response of delivered packets to ensure its reliability. In the same concern, Elappila et al. (2018) recommended a survival path routing protocol for healthcare networks with heavy traffic of simultaneous transmission of data from multiple sensor nodes. This protocol considered three different factors for the selection of subsequent nodes in the routing path, including signal-to-interference-and-noise ratio (SINR), survivability factor of the routing path from a subsequent node to the final node, along with congestion level at the subsequent node to be selected. It disclosed optimum performance for throughput, delay, packet delivery ratio, and remaining energy for healthcare IoT networks. Additionally, Nayyar and Singh (2020) presented an energy-competent routing procedure driven by ant colony optimization (ACO) for dynamically changing WSN environments. This protocol performed neighbour discovery procedure using link knowledge, the transmission of packets using exponentially weighted moving average technique and acknowledgement of delivered packets. It provided better performance for end-to-end delivery of data packets than that of basic ACO, DSR, and other traditional routing algorithms.

In this process of a comprehensive review of existing techniques for routing optimization in multi-hop healthcare networks, few recently published approaches have also been taken into consideration. In this regard, Javid and Mirzaei (2021) presented a multi-objective generic algorithm-based reliable routing procedure for secure data delivery in healthcare networks. This approach provided an enhanced network lifetime, delivery rate, and a minimum delay in data routing. Similarly, Chanak and Banerjee (2020) discussed a priority-based routing approach to ensure congestion-free routing in IoT-enabled WSNs for different healthcare applications. Moreover, Masood et al. (2023) raised the issue of privacy preservation in WSNs and discussed the idea of energy-efficient multipath routing approach for healthcare data. This approach provided results with higher throughput, less end-to-end delay, optimally lower energy depletion, and high packet delivery rate. A similar multipath routing approach in WBANs was also provided by Akbar et al. (2022), which ensured energy-efficient and reliable routing through the division of a network into different clusters. This approach also considered optimal packet routing with maximum throughput, an increased packet delivery rate, low value of end-to-end delay and minimum energy requirements.

To explore the usage of fuzzy logic for routing optimization in healthcare IoT networks, Hosseinzadeh et al. (2023) provided a fuzzy logic-based secure hierarchical routing approach, which made use of a firefly algorithm to confirm energy-efficient multilevel routing in healthcare IoT networks. This approach achieved better network longevity, packet delivery rate, and energy values than contemporary energy-efficient multi-level secure routing and enhanced balanced energy-efficient network-integrated super heterogeneous routing protocols. Another fuzzy logic-based approach by Shahbaz et al. (2021) presented the use of a firefly algorithm with fuzzy logic to ensure multipath routing in WSNs, which surpasses other current routing techniques for energy depletion, end-to-end delay, network lifetime, and packet loss rate. Similarly, Nasri et al. (2021) provided a fuzzy logic-based cross-layer routing protocol for energy-competent routing in wireless IoT networks. This method offered several advantages for data routing in cloud environments during pandemic times, such as COVID-19, which include better throughput, less energy depletion, less end-to-end delay, and better network lifetime than that of traditional LEACH-based protocols. A similar fuzzy logic-based approach presented by Geethalakshmi et al. (2023) made use of fuzzy-induced north-west corner technique to obtain an optimized routing path in wearable biomedical sensor networks, which offered minimum transportation cost and high node lifetime. Apart from this, Thangaramya et al. (2019) and Akbari and Tabatabaei (2020) also offered fuzzy logic-based optimized solutions for energy-competent routing in different types of WSNs.

The thorough study of literature related to various routing algorithms reveals that optimized routing is a crucial process for ensuring real-time and effective delivery of biomedical signals in data-driven healthcare IoT systems. A simple routing algorithm may require only one or two network parameters to select an optimum routing path. However, energy-effective routing in multi-hop data-driven healthcare IoT sensor networks depends on multiple parameters, which may include RSSI, drop rate of packets, total time packets take to move to the intended end node, and the energy level at each sensor node. To decide about optimized routing by considering multiple factors, fuzzy logic-based decision-making is an effective choice (Al-Kiyumi et al., 2018).

Therefore, the present work proposes two routing algorithms to realize QoS-aware and energy-effective routing in IoT sensor networks of healthcare systems, which uses link cost estimation driven by fuzzy logic. These algorithms are the modified versions of conventional routing algorithms based on RL, namely real-time search (Zhang & Fromherz, 2004) and adaptive tree (Zhang & Huang, 2006a), which are discussed in detail in the following section.

5.5 Traditional Routing Algorithms Based on Reinforcement Learning for Multi-Hop Healthcare System

During contemporary times, the RL approach (Liang et al., 2008; Al-Rawi et al., 2015), a well-known method of artificial intelligence (AI), has been taken into consideration for ensuring optimized routing in WSNs (Hosseinzadeh et al., 2023) (Hussain et al., 2023). The majority of these RL algorithms make use of unsupervised, online learning concepts like Q-learning. When interacting with other agents in WSNs, an agent tries to learn about the operational environment (Kiani et al., 2015). A sensor node learns as part of an award process in order to select the optimum course of action. With expertise in WSNs, it optimizes its long-term benefits in this manner (Kumar & Krishna, 2018). A well-known RL technique for WSN routing issues is the Q-learning algorithm (Kosunalp et al., 2016). On the basis of different actions performed for a certain condition of the node and surroundings, a sensor node in a sensor network uses Q-learning to update the rewards it has received on a regular basis. Real-time search and adaptive tree algorithms are two of the well-known Q-learning-based algorithms that may be very helpful in routing optimization of healthcare sensor networks. Both of these algorithms are briefly debated in the subsequent subsections.

5.5.1 Real-Time Search Routing Algorithm

In a WSN, the real-time search-based adaptive routing method developed by Zhang and Fromherz (2004) determines the routes by determining each network node's next-best hop (Zungeru et al., 2012). This intelligent routing technique assumes that it is simple to describe the cost function for respective routing nodes if the routing criteria for a message, such as its destination and QoS requirements, are known. Here, a cost function is characterized by the Q value, which indicates the lowest cost essential for going from the current network node to the target node (Zhang & Fromherz, 2004).

The preliminary Q value for a specific node in a distributed WSN is unknown. Depending on the sort of communication that will be transmitted from source to destination, its value is assessed. A node also maintains the NQ values, commonly known as the Q values of its nearby nodes. These NQ values are originally approximated based on the neighbouring nodes' attribute values, and they are updated as soon as neighbours send packets (Zhang & Fromherz, 2004). As shown in Figure 5.4, three steps make up RL-based search adaptive routing strategy: initialization, forwarding, and confirmation. Learning through reinforcement occurs in three levels. The current Q value of a node in relation to the destination node is reported for each packet that is transmitted from that node. Every node in the network begins a learning process upon the arrival of every packet, and the node's Q value is changed in accordance with equation 5.1 (Zhang & Fromherz, 2004). For learning rate α, $0 < \alpha \leq 1$; local cost function $o_m > 0$ and n neighbours of a given node, its updated Q-value can be obtained by the following equation 5.1.

$$Q_m = (1-\alpha)Q_m + \alpha\left(o_m + \min NQ_m(n)\right) \quad (5.1)$$

Afterward, the second step of the forwarding stage in the given routing strategy comes into action. This is the main improvement step, which selects the closest node to which a packet should be sent based on its current estimated value. The node with the current packet transmits it to the nearby node that provides the best NQ value for the present node in this sort of search-based routing method. All co-neighbouring nodes, involving the chosen receipt node, observe the packet when it is transmitted and utilize the Q value that was sent along with it.

Finally, immediate packet confirmation is utilized during the confirmation step. The consequent NQ value is reorganized to the greatest cost amid the neighbouring nodes, guaranteeing that node v should not be chosen in the succeeding time, if a packet sent from sent node v is not obtained by the next superlative neighbouring node or target point for a predetermined time period due to a failed node or fallacious and uneven wireless connection. For uneven, fluctuating, and unstable wireless networks, this idea is essential. Via the link cost function C, the NQ value is renewed through subsequent equation (5.2).

$$NQ(v) = \max NQ(n) + C \quad (5.2)$$

where $C = e^{\frac{l_u}{r_u}}$

In this case, r_u is the total quantity of packets obtained from node u, while l_u is the quantity of packets that vanished to node u (Zhang & Fromherz, 2004).

5.5.2 Adaptive Tree Routing Algorithm

Zhang and Huang (2006a, 2006b) introduced an adaptive tree-based routing system that is also based on RL techniques. Instead of dealing with node failure or base station mobility, this tree-based approach can keep the top connection to the base station within a certain sensor network. This algorithm is crucial for accomplishing load balancing as well as for reducing and managing network congestion. Regardless of the search-based routing approach used, the sink node must be known at the initialization step of the adaptive tree-based routing protocol. Similar to real-time search algorithm, three phases make up the adaptive routing technique employed in this algorithm, namely, initialization, forwarding, and confirmation (refer to Figure 5.4). Q-learning occurs at all three stages using equation (5.1).

During the startup phase, a starting spanning tree established at the sink node is generated. A reference to the parent node, which is the nearby node with the lowest NQ value, is included in all nodes save the sink node. During the forwarding step, the parent node receives the packets that have been received. Depending on the lowest NQ value of the nearby nodes, the parent of the present node may vary. The sink node which transmits with a Q value equal to zero (0) for every packet it receives will also only relay each detected data packet once. When implicit packet confirmation is utilized when a packet is not obtained within a predetermined amount of time, the intended receiving node's NQ value is updated. To ensure that this node won't be chosen again, the matching NQ value for the receiving node is changed to the highest value among its neighbours (Zhang & Huang, 2006b). Equation (5.2) is used to update the NQ value for receiving node v with the link cost function C (refer to equation (5.3)).

Search-based and adaptive tree-based routing techniques have a major drawback in that their cost function is solely dependent on the quantity of packets that are received and lost at the intended node. However, other physical layer parameters, namely, RSSI, remaining energy, and/or packet receiving time at the destination node should also be taken into consideration for obtaining the cost of wireless link among the nodes to ensure energy efficient and QoS conscious routing in healthcare IoT sensor networks.

Keeping in mind the above-mentioned issues in traditionally recognized RL-based algorithms, i.e., real-time search and adaptive tree, this chapter discusses the use of fuzzy logic-based approaches proposed by Singh and Malhotra (2018, 2019). These approaches provide modifications in the traditional real-time search and adaptive tree algorithms and present new algorithms based on fuzzy logic and RL, namely, Fuzzy RTS routing algorithm (Singh & Malhotra, 2019) and Fuzzy AT routing algorithm (Singh & Malhotra, 2018). These algorithms were proposed to ensure energy-effective and QoS-sensitive routing in healthcare WSNs and are discussed thoroughly in the following section.

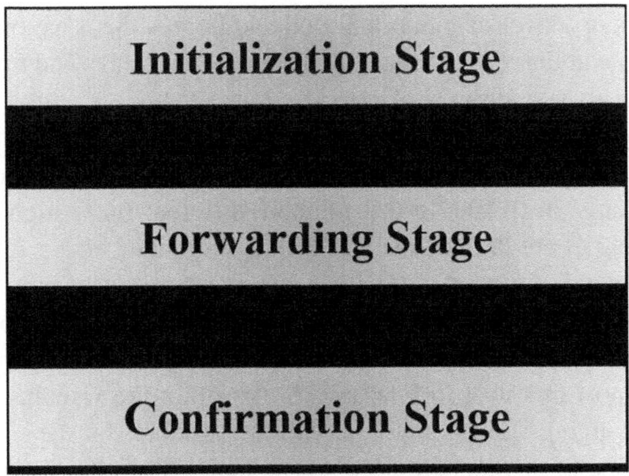

FIGURE 5.4 Different stages in RL-based adaptive routing strategies.

5.6 Fuzzy Logic and Reinforcement Learning–Based Routing Algorithms for Healthcare Sensor Networks

This section discusses the basic concepts of the development of RL-driven Fuzzy RTS and Fuzzy AT algorithms to achieve optimized routing in healthcare IoT networks. These networks will be the basic building blocks of IoT healthcare frameworks for remote healthcare and patient monitoring services in different real-time scenarios such as hospitals. Both of these algorithms are briefly illustrated in the following subsections.

5.6.1 Fuzzy Real-Time Search Algorithm

In fuzzy real-time search algorithm (also known as Fuzzy RTS) (Singh & Malhotra, 2019), the RL-based real-time search policy is combined with fuzzy link cost estimates for energy-effective and QoS-sensitive routing in WSNs, which is a vital component of IoT. This technique is essentially a more innovative version of the conventional real-time search-based adaptive routing algorithm introduced by Zhang and Fromherz (2004). This algorithm is based on the selection of a fuzzy logic-based link cost estimator to deal with faulty and irregular wireless connections between sensor nodes and to enhance network performance.

In order to estimate the Q value of a specific sensor node and the NQ values of neighbouring nodes, this method also employs a similar learning process, where RL takes place throughout the initialization, forwarding, and confirmation stages. In this algorithm, the link cost function C mentioned in equation (5.2) of real-time search algorithm has been substituted with the term LC_{fuzzy}, which is fuzzy logic-based link cost estimation.

$$NQ(v) = \max NQ(n) + LC_{fuzzy} \tag{5.3}$$

This fuzzy link cost was found from fuzzy link cost estimator, which makes use of residual energy of the current source node, packet loss rate and RSSI input parameters. These three parameters play a significant role in effective routing in WSNs because the remaining energy level of individual node addresses the issue of load balancing, the packet loss rate at unreliable links guarantees fewer delays and reliable communication, and RSSI gives assurance of error-free packet delivery through routes with a lower probability of link failure. These parameters are fed to the Mamdani-type fuzzy inference system, where fuzzy IF–THEN regulations are developed to provide fuzzy link cost in the range of 0–100. In this method, different fuzzy input parameters and fuzzy link cost output are defined using the Gaussian membership function with specific ranges. A general outline of fuzzy logic-based estimation of link cost is illustrated in Figure 5.5. Out of the four fuzzy input variables shown in this figure, the first three variables are employed in Fuzzy RTS algorithm. The fuzzy input and output variables for the estimation of link cost in Fuzzy RTS algorithm are visualized in Figure 5.6. Additionally, this figure shows ranges of various variables on the *x*-axis of provided plots and the degree of membership (DoM) oscillating from 0 to 1 on the *y*-axis.

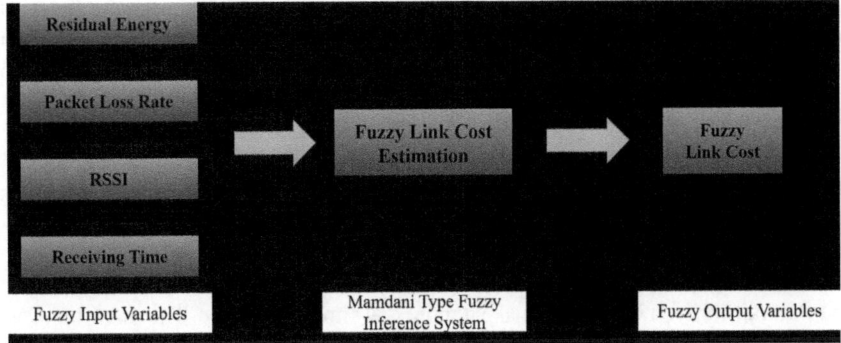

FIGURE 5.5 Fuzzy logic-based link cost estimation for RL-based enhanced routing in WSNs.

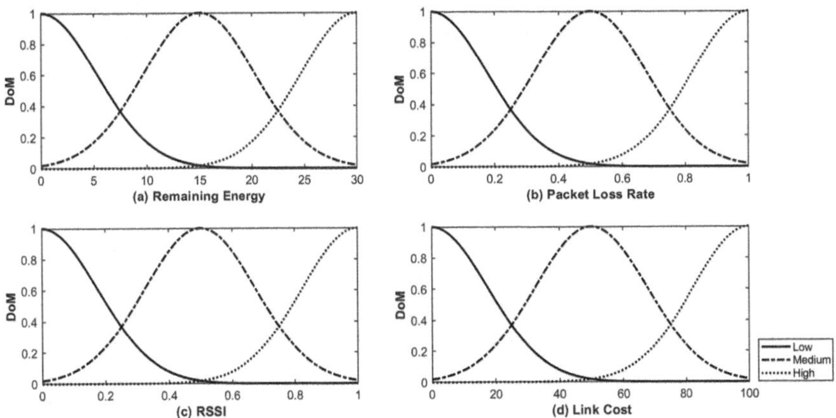

FIGURE 5.6 (a)–(c) Fuzzy input variables and (d) fuzzy output variable for link cost estimation in Fuzzy RTS algorithm.

5.6.2 Fuzzy Adaptive Tree Algorithm

For energy-effective and QoS-conscious routing in IoT networks of multi-hop healthcare systems, Fuzzy AT algorithm combines RL-based adaptive tree routing strategy and fuzzy logic-based estimation of link cost. This approach is basically an improved version of the adaptive tree routing procedure presented by Zhang and Huang (2006a, 2006b). Similar to Fuzzy RTS algorithm, the use of fuzzy logic-driven link cost estimator in Fuzzy AT algorithm is the key feature, which assists in dealing with the unstable and asymmetric character of wireless communications between sensor nodes and for increasing network performance.

Just like Fuzzy RTS algorithm, this method also makes use of Q-learning approach of RL in different stages, namely, initialization, forwarding, and confirmation. In this algorithm, the fuzzy link cost function (LC_{Fuzzy}) is calculated using physical layer factors, including remaining energy, packet loss rate, RSSI, and complete time spent in reception of packets at the end node, termed receiving time. An overview of link cost estimation using fuzzy logic-based method is demonstrated in Figure 5.5. This idea of fuzzy link cost improves network performance by providing an optimum routing path for the error-free transmission of data packets across an unstable and dynamic wireless medium.

In dense and heterogeneous WSNs, a Mamdani-type fuzzy inference system with triangular-type membership functions for input as well as output fuzzy variables is considered to estimate the superiority of inconsistent and uneven wireless communications amid sensor nodes. This technique considers total packet receiving time at the sink node in addition to remaining energy, packet loss rate, and RSSI to diminish packet transmission delays and make it more real-time compatible. The fuzzy link cost estimator receives these input attributes and outputs the link cost as an output attribute based on fuzzy IF–THEN logic. This link cost assessment ensures that the node being chosen for routing in sensor networks is suitable. Figure 5.7 displays the fuzzy input and output variables for the Fuzzy AT algorithm's connection cost estimation. Additionally, this figure shows ranges of various variables on the x-axis of given plots and their corresponding DoM extending from 0 to 1 on the y-axis.

5.7 Results and Discussion

This section gives the performances of Fuzzy RTS and Fuzzy AT algorithms, which are compared and analyzed to obtain optimal routing solutions for reliable and error-free routing in healthcare sensor networks. The performance analysis of these algorithms was done using MATLAB-based routing modelling application simulation environment (RMASE) framework (Zhang & Huang 2006a), which was realized in the probabilistic wireless network simulator (Prowler) (Simon, 2003).

During the implementation of these RL-based algorithms by Singh and Malhotra (2018, 2019), normal radio model and Rayleigh fading model were selected in prowler for Fuzzy RTS and Fuzzy AT, respectively. In order to create a densely populated

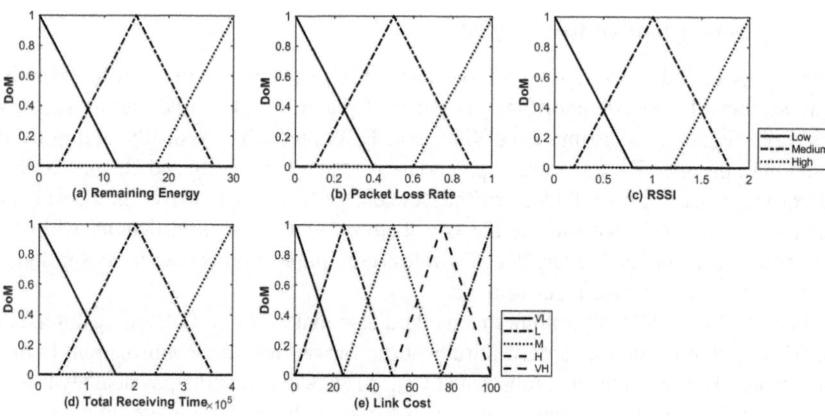

FIGURE 5.7 (a)–(d) Fuzzy input variables and (e) fuzzy output variable for link cost estimation in Fuzzy AT algorithm.

network architecture, 100 sensor nodes were sited in an area of 100 square meters. Source nodes were seen as dynamic nodes in a dynamic environment, whereas destination nodes were regarded as mobile nodes. The static centres were assumed to be the centres of the source and destination nodes with a node radius of 1 meter. In order to effectively validate the network's energy depletion, node battery life, and energy efficacy for the specified routing algorithms, every sensor node's starting energy was kept high, which was taken as 30 joules in this work. The packet transmission rate with a value of 1 packet per second with each packet having 960 bits was opted in this work to reduce network complexity and to appropriately achieve simulation results. The time reserved for the simulation of the algorithms in the given network was considered as 100 s.

To appraise the functioning of given routing algorithms in dense, asymmetric, and erratic WSNs, authors have chosen the following performance metrics, which are proposed by Singh and Malhotra (2018, 2019) for the Fuzzy RTS and Fuzzy AT algorithms.

- Throughput (p/s): It determines the quantity of packets which are obtained at the terminus node per second. The unit of measurement is packets per second (p/s).
- Latency (ms): In WSNs, latency is defined as the end-to-end delay that happens through the communication of a packet of sensed data from the initial to the destination or sink node. It is measured in milliseconds (ms).
- Energy consumption (J): It provides a measurement of the overall energy used by various nodes along the routing way amid the source and the destination nodes in the wireless network throughout the course of the implementation. This term is measured in joules (J).
- Energy efficiency (kb/J): The ratio of the net quantity of packets supplied at the ultimate terminus node to the net energy spent by a specific sensor node inside the sensor network is known as energy efficiency. This term is measured in kbits/Joules (kb/J).

While making the comparative analysis of Fuzzy RTS and AT algorithms, their performances in terms of mean values of specified performance measures have been illustrated in Table 5.1. Moreover, Figure 5.8 illustrates the assessment of the functioning of Fuzzy RTS and Fuzzy AT algorithms with respect to throughput, latency, energy consumption, and energy efficiency. Figure 5.8(a) shows the higher value of throughput for Fuzzy RTS as compared to that of Fuzzy AT. As given in Table 5.1, the average value of throughput in case of Fuzzy RTS is 1.8 p/s. This value can be equivalented to

TABLE 5.1

Average Values of Throughput, Latency, Energy Consumption, and Energy Efficiency for Fuzzy RTS and Fuzzy AT Algorithms

Fuzzy RL Algorithms	Throughput (p/s)	Latency (ms)	Energy Consumption (J)	Energy Efficiency (kb/J)
Fuzzy RTS	1.8025	283.2	14.0793	1.5345
Fuzzy AT	1.2917	122.7	8.3236	1.8451

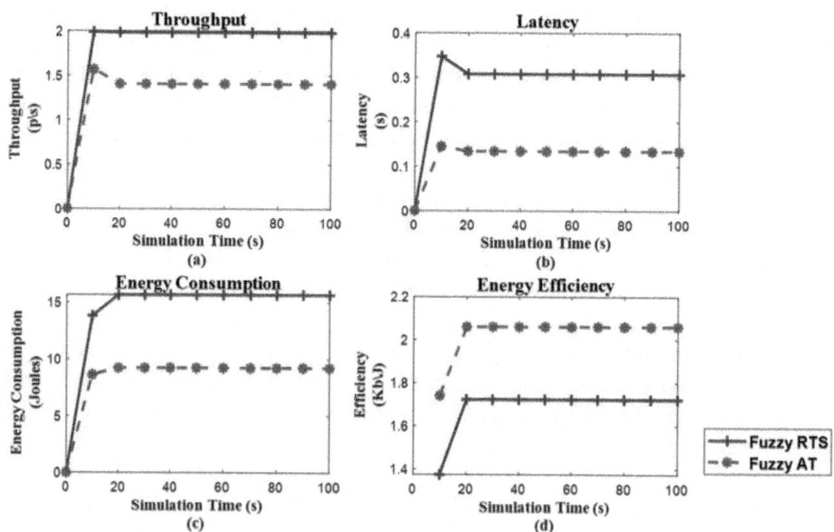

FIGURE 5.8 Performance comparison of Fuzzy RTS and Fuzzy AT in terms of (a) throughput, (b) latency, (c) energy consumption, and (d) energy efficiency.

approximately 1728 bits/s (1 packet = 960 bits). On the other hand, Fuzzy AT provides an average throughput of *1.3 p/s*, which is equivalent to *1248 bits/s* approximately.

The latency values of both algorithms are compared in Figure 5.8(b). As per this figure, Fuzzy AT offers very little latency for transmission of sensed data packets than that of Fuzzy RTS algorithm. As per Table 5.1, the average values of latency for Fuzzy AT and Fuzzy RTS are 122.7 and 283.2 ms, respectively. As shown in Figures 5.8(c) and (d), efficiency, Fuzzy AT again shows enhanced performance with respect to energy depletion and energy efficiency than that of Fuzzy RTS. It is visible from Table 5.1 that the energy consumption and energy efficiency values for Fuzzy AT are 8.3236 J and 1.8451 kb/J, respectively. Conversely, these values for Fuzzy RTS algorithm are 14.0793 J and 1.5345 kb/J, respectively.

Thus, it is evident from this discussion that Fuzzy RTS algorithm performs better in terms of higher value of throughput only, which is approximately 1.4 times higher than that of Fuzzy AT. On the other hand, Fuzzy AT algorithm performs better for routing optimization in multi-hop healthcare WSNs in terms of a lesser value of latency, lesser value of energy consumption, higher value of energy efficiency, and an optimum value of throughput in order to confirm free of errors delivery of packets of detected data to the final sink node.

Furthermore, the given Fuzzy AT and Fuzzy RTS techniques are also compared with other recent fuzzy logic-based routing methods in Table 5.2. This table gives the overview of different fuzzy logic-based routing algorithms, fuzzy input variables, the associated routing technologies and the results of given algorithms for energy consumption, energy efficiency, end-to-end delay, packet delivery rate, etc. As per this table, the given Fuzzy RTS (Singh & Malhotra, 2019) and Fuzzy AT (Singh & Malhotra, 2018) algorithms made use of Q-learning-based RL strategies, which were optimized using fuzzy logic-based link cost estimation for energy-effective routing.

TABLE 5.2

Comparative Study of Different Fuzzy Logic-Based Approaches for Optimized Routing in IoT Wireless Sensor Networks

References	Algorithm Name	Fuzzy Input Variables	Supporting Techniques	Results
Singh & Malhotra (2018)	Fuzzy adaptive tree	Residual energy, packet loss rate, RSSI, packet receiving time	Reinforcement learning (Q-learning)	Energy consumption = 8.3236 J Energy efficiency = 1.8451 Kb/J Latency = 122.7 ms
Thangaramya et al. (2019)	Energy-aware cluster and neuro-fuzzy based routing algorithm	Cluster current energy, distance between cluster and sink, distance between node and cluster, cluster degree	Convolutional neural networks	Energy consumption = 0.15 J (after 1600 rounds)
Singh & Malhotra (2019)	Fuzzy real-time search	Residual energy, packet loss rate, RSSI	Reinforcement learning (Q-learning)	Energy consumption = 14.0793 J Energy efficiency = 1.5345 Kb/J Latency = 283.2 ms
Akbari & Tabatabaei (2020)	Fuzzy logic and reinforcement learning-based reliable routing method	Distance to sink node, available bandwidth, battery level energy	Reinforcement learning	Medium access delay= > 0.002 s End-to-end delay = < 0.025 s Energy consumption = 0.00020 J
Nasri et al. (2021)	Fuzzy-based routing protocol (FRP-LEACH)	Residual energy, cluster energy, distance of node and cluster node	LEACH	Energy consumption= 200 J, End-to-end delay= 106 ms
Shahbaz et al. (2021)	Multipath routing through the firefly algorithm and fuzzy logic	Residual energy, distance from cluster nodes to base station, traffic in cluster node	Firefly algorithm	Energy consumption= >400 J, End-to-end delay = 8 ms (approx.) Network lifetime = 700 s
Hosseinzadeh et al. (2023)	Fuzzy logic-based secure hierarchical routing scheme using the firefly algorithm (FSRF)	Direct trust: packet delivery ratio, packet transfer frequency, packet reception frequency, and the consumed energy ratio Indirect trust of recommended nodes	Firefly algorithm	Energy consumption = < 80J, Packet delivered = 10 p Packet delivery rate= 0.98 (approx.)

Similarly, the routing approach proposed by Akbari and Tabatabaei (2020), also made use of RL for energy-effective routing having a least end-to-end delay of less than 0.025 s only. On the other hand, hierarchical and multipath routing algorithms suggested by Shahbaz et al. (2021) and Hosseinzadeh et al. (2023) discussed the usage of the firefly algorithm for optimized routing in WSNs.

In the same concern, the routing approach provided by Nasri et al. (2021) discussed the usage of fuzzy logic for optimization of LEACH routing protocol, which offered end-to-end delay of 106 ms only. In addition, Thangaramya et al. (2019) presented a neuro-fuzzy routing approach which made use of fuzzy logic in combination with convolutional neural networks for energy-competent routing requirements in IoT networks.

The simulation analysis of the given Fuzzy RTS and Fuzzy AT algorithms and detailed discussion of other fuzzy logic-based routing approaches clearly reveal that the use of fuzzy logic-based techniques is crucial for IoT healthcare sensor networks to provide energy-effective routing. These types of approaches are useful in ensuring secure and error-free delivery of healthcare data in multi-hop routing scenarios.

5.8 Conclusion

The present work discusses two routing algorithms, namely, Fuzzy RTS and Fuzzy AT routing algorithms to ensure optimized routing in dynamically fluctuating and erratic sensor networks with multi-hop healthcare systems. These algorithms make use of fuzzy logic-based link cost estimation among sensor nodes, which was attained from numerous parameters, namely, remaining energy, rate of dropped packets, RSSI, and receiving time of packets at the final end node of the IoT network. The performance of these algorithms has been assessed and evaluated on the basis of various performance measures. The simulation outcomes disclose that Fuzzy AT appears to be a better choice for routing optimization in healthcare WSNs due to its effective performance in terms of minimum latency of 122.7 ms, minimum energy consumption of 8.32 J, maximum energy efficiency of 1.85 Kb/J, and an optimum throughput of 1.3 p/s (approximately equal to 1248 bits/s). Thus, for dynamically fluctuating, irregular, and erratic WSN environments, the Fuzzy AT algorithm appears a suitable RL-based routing algorithm for delivering energy-effective, error-free, consistent, and QoS-sensitive routing. Apart from this, this chapter also presents other existing fuzzy logic-based solutions, which could be used for real-time and energy-competent routing in multi-hop WSNs. These solutions also offer a key solution for optimized routing in IoT-enabled and AI-based data-driven smart healthcare systems in the context of smart city scenarios.

Although fuzzy logic-based techniques offer several benefits for routing optimization in unstable and dynamic WSN environments, their efficacy may be limited by a limited number of fuzzy IF–THEN rules. These rules depend on a small number of fuzzy input variables, and more variables can result in the creation of more complex rules. Due to the possibility of redundant or incorrect wireless links being recommended in the routing paths, this complexity could lead to the inconsistent delivery of data packets. In order to provide more dependable and realistic routing paths for safe and error-free data routing, machine learning algorithms must be integrated. This is because of the reason that machine learning algorithms can adjust to a range of real-time routing conditions based on previously gathered data.

REFERENCES

Airehrour, D., Gutierrez, J., & Ray, S. K. (2016). Secure routing for internet of things: A survey. *Journal of Network and Computer Applications*, *66*, 198–213.

Akbar, S., Mehdi, M. M., Jamal, M. H., Raza, I., Hussain, S. A., Breñosa, J., … Ashraf, I. (2022, November). Multipath routing in wireless body area sensor network for healthcare monitoring. In *Healthcare* (Vol. *10*, No. 11, p. 2297). MDPI.

Akbari, Y., & Tabatabaei, S. (2020). A new method to find a high reliable route in IoT by using reinforcement learning and fuzzy logic. *Wireless Personal Communications*, *112*(2), 967–983.

Al-Anbagi, I., Erol-Kantarci, M., & Mouftah, H. T. (2014). A survey on cross-layer quality-of-service approaches in WSNs for delay and reliability-aware applications. *IEEE Communications Surveys & Tutorials*, *18*(1), 525–552.

Al-Fuqaha, A., Guizani, M., Mohammadi, M., Aledhari, M., & Ayyash, M. (2015). Internet of things: A survey on enabling technologies, protocols, and applications. *IEEE communications surveys & tutorials*, *17*(4), 2347–2376.

Al-Kiyumi, R. M., Foh, C. H., Vural, S., Chatzimisios, P., & Tafazolli, R. (2018). Fuzzy logic-based routing algorithm for lifetime enhancement in heterogeneous wireless sensor networks. *IEEE Transactions on Green Communications and Networking*, *2*(2), 517–532.

Al-Rawi, H. A., Ng, M. A., & Yau, K. L. A. (2015). Application of reinforcement learning to routing in distributed wireless networks: a review. *Artificial Intelligence Review*, *43*, 381–416.

Chan, L., Gomez Chavez, K., Rudolph, H., & Hourani, A. (2020). Hierarchical routing protocols for wireless sensor network: A compressive survey. *Wireless Networks*, *26*, 3291–3314.

Chanak, P., & Banerjee, I. (2020). Congestion free routing mechanism for IoT-enabled wireless sensor networks for smart healthcare applications. *IEEE Transactions on Consumer Electronics*, *66*(3), 223–232.

Chelloug, S. A. (2015). Energy-efficient content-based routing in internet of things. *Journal of Computer and Communications*, *3*(12), 9.

Chen, C. W., & Weng, C. C. (2012). A power efficiency routing and maintenance protocol in wireless multi-hop networks. *Journal of Systems and Software*, *85*(1), 62–76.

Chen, M., Gonzalez, S., Vasilakos, A., Cao, H., & Leung, V. C. (2011). Body area networks: A survey. *Mobile networks and applications*, *16*, 171–193.

Cicioğlu, M., & Çalhan, A. (2019). SDN-based wireless body area network routing algorithm for healthcare architecture. *Etri Journal*, *41*(4), 452–464.

Di Marco, P., Athanasiou, G., Mekikis, P. V., & Fischione, C. (2016). MAC-aware routing metrics for the internet of things. *Computer Communications*, *74*, 77–86.

Elappila, M., Chinara, S., & Parhi, D. R. (2018). Survivable path routing in WSN for IoT applications. *Pervasive and Mobile Computing*, *43*, 49–63.

Geethalakshmi, M., Venkatesh, J., Mageswari, R. U., Mahalakshmi, A., Anand, J., & Partheepan, R. (2023, January). Fuzzy based route optimization in wearable bio-medical wireless sensor network. In *AIP Conference Proceedings* (Vol. *2523*, No. 1). AIP Publishing.

Hosseinzadeh, M., Yoo, J., Ali, S., Lansky, J., Mildeova, S., Yousefpoor, M. S., … Tightiz, L. (2023). A fuzzy logic-based secure hierarchical routing scheme using firefly algorithm in Internet of Things for healthcare. *Scientific Reports*, *13*(1), 11058.

Hussain, M. W., & Roy, D. S. (2023). Performance Optimization Strategies for Big Data Applications in Distributed Framework. In *Intelligent Technologies: Concepts,*

Applications, and Future Directions, Volume 2 (pp. 221–252). Singapore: Springer Nature Singapore.

Islam, S. R., Kwak, D., Kabir, M. H., Hossain, M., & Kwak, K. S. (2015). The internet of things for health care: a comprehensive survey. *IEEE Access*, *3*, 678–708.

Javid, S., & Mirzaei, A. (2021). Presenting a reliable routing approach in iot healthcare using the multiobjective-based multiagent approach. *Wireless Communications and Mobile Computing*, *2021*, 1–20.

Kiani, F., Amiri, E., Zamani, M., Khodadadi, T., & Abdul Manaf, A. (2015). Efficient intelligent energy routing protocol in wireless sensor networks. *International Journal of Distributed Sensor Networks*, *11*(3), 618072.

Kosunalp, S., Chu, Y., Mitchell, P. D., Grace, D., & Clarke, T. (2016). Use of Q-learning approaches for practical medium access control in wireless sensor networks. *Engineering Applications of Artificial Intelligence*, *55*, 146–154.

Kumar, T. P., & Krishna, P. V. (2018). Power modelling of sensors for IoT using reinforcement learning. *International Journal of Advanced Intelligence Paradigms*, *10*(1–2), 3–22.

Liang, X., Balasingham, I., & Byun, S. S. (2008, October). A reinforcement learning based routing protocol with QoS support for biomedical sensor networks. In *2008 First International Symposium on Applied Sciences on Biomedical and Communication Technologies* (pp. 1–5). IEEE, Aalborg, Denmark.

Marietta, J., & Chandra Mohan, B. (2020). A review on routing in internet of things. *Wireless Personal Communications*, *111*, 209–233.

Masood, J. A. I. S., Jeyaselvi, M., Senthamarai, N., Koteswari, S., Sathya, M., & Chakravarthy, N. K. (2023). Privacy preservation in wireless sensor network using energy efficient multipath routing for healthcare data. *Measurement: Sensors*, *29*, 100867.

Mohanty, P., & Kabat, M. R. (2016). Energy efficient reliable multi-path data transmission in WSN for healthcare application. *International journal of wireless Information Networks*, *23*(2), 162–172.

Nasri, M., Helali, A., & Maaref, H. (2021). Energy-efficient fuzzy logic-based cross-layer hierarchical routing protocol for wireless Internet-of-Things sensor networks. *International Journal of Communication Systems*, *34*(9), e4808.

Nayyar, A., & Singh, R. (2020). IEEMARP-a novel energy efficient multipath routing protocol based on ant Colony optimization (ACO) for dynamic sensor networks. *Multimedia Tools and Applications*, *79*, 35221–35252.

Negra, R., Jemili, I., & Belghith, A. (2016). Wireless body area networks: Applications and technologies. *Procedia Computer Science*, *83*, 1274–1281.

Rani, S., Talwar, R., Malhotra, J., Ahmed, S. H., Sarkar, M., & Song, H. (2015). A novel scheme for an energy efficient Internet of Things based on wireless sensor networks. *Sensors*, *15*(11), 28603–28626.

Reddy, K. H. K., Roy, D. S., Mishra, T. K., & Hussain, M. W. (Eds.). (2023). *Handbook of Research on Network-Enabled IoT Applications for Smart City Services*. IGI Global.

Sarwesh, P., Shet, N. S. V., & Chandrasekaran, K. (2017). Energy efficient network design for IoT healthcare applications. *Internet of Things and Big Data Technologies for Next Generation Healthcare*, *23*, 35–61.

Shahbaz, A. N., Barati, H., & Barati, A. (2021). Multipath routing through the firefly algorithm and fuzzy logic in wireless sensor networks. *Peer-to-Peer Networking and Applications*, *14*(2), 541–558.

Shokouhifar, M., & Jalali, A. (2015). A new evolutionary based application specific routing protocol for clustered wireless sensor networks. *AEU-International Journal of Electronics and Communications*, *69*(1), 432–441.

Simon, G. (2003). Prowler: Probabilistic Wireless Network Simulator. Retrieved February 3, 2023, from http://www.isis.vanderbilt.edu/projects/nest/prowler/

Singh, K., & Malhotra, J. (2018). Fuzzy link cost estimation based adaptive tree algorithm for routing optimization in wireless sensor networks using reinforcement learning. *International Journal of Sensors Wireless Communications and Control*, *8*(3), 151–164.

Singh, K., & Malhotra, J. (2019). Reinforcement learning-based real time search algorithm for routing optimisation in wireless sensor networks using fuzzy link cost estimation. *International Journal of Communication Networks and Distributed Systems*, *22*(4), 363–384.

Sobral, J. V., Rodrigues, J. J., Rabêlo, R. A., Saleem, K., & Furtado, V. (2019). LOADng-IoT: An enhanced routing protocol for internet of things applications over low power networks. *Sensors*, *19*(1), 150.

Su, H., Wang, Z., & An, S. (2013). MAEB: Routing protocol for iot healthcare. *Advances in Internet of Things*, *3 (2)*, 8–15.

Thangaramya, K., Kulothungan, K., Logambigai, R., Selvi, M., Ganapathy, S., & Kannan, A. (2019). Energy aware cluster and neuro-fuzzy based routing algorithm for wireless sensor networks in IoT. *Computer Networks*, *151*, 211–223.

Yau, K. L. A., Goh, H. G., Chieng, D., & Kwong, K. H. (2015). Application of reinforcement learning to wireless sensor networks: models and algorithms. *Computing*, *97*, 1045–1075.

Yuehong, Y. I. N., Zeng, Y., Chen, X., & Fan, Y. (2016). The internet of things in healthcare: An overview. *Journal of Industrial Information Integration*, *1*, 3–13.

Zhang, Y., & Fromherz, M. (2004, July). Search-based adaptive routing strategies for sensor networks. In *AAAI04 workshop on Sensor Networks*. San Jose, California.

Zhang, Y., & Huang, Q. (2006a). A Learning-based Adaptive Routing Tree for Wireless Sensor Networks. *Journal of Communications*, *1*(2), 12–21.

Zhang, Y., & Huang, Q. (2006b, January). Adaptive tree: a learning-based meta-routing strategy for sensor networks. In *3rd IEEE Consumer Communications and Networking Conference*, Las Vegas, NV, USA (pp. 122–126).

Zhang, Y., Simon, G., & Balogh, G. (2006, May). High-level sensor network simulations for routing performance evaluations. In *Third International Conference on Networked Sensing Systems (INSS06)*, Rosemont, Illinois.

Zungeru, A. M., Ang, L. M., & Seng, K. P. (2012). Classical and swarm intelligence based routing protocols for wireless sensor networks: A survey and comparison. *Journal of Network and Computer Applications*, *35*(5), 1508–1536.

6

AIoMT: An AI-Based Network Selection Framework for Next-Generation-Enabled IoMT Network in Smart City

Bhanu Priya
Lovely Professional University, Phagwara, India

Jyoteesh Malhotra
National Institute of Technology, Delhi, India

Kuldeep Singh
Guru Nanak Dev University, Amritsar, India

Aadi Koshal
Amador Valley High School, Pleasanton, California, USA

6.1 Introduction

Internet of Medical Things (IoMT) has emerged as a viable and efficient solution in the COVID-19 pandemic which improves the efficiency and productivity of the healthcare system in Smart City by optimizing clinical workflows and information flows (Reddy et al., 2023). Due to the pandemic, it is anticipated that the worldwide telemedicine market will expand by 19.3% per year rather than the 15% annually that was initially anticipated for this time frame (Ugalmugale & Swain, 2020). This unstoppable rise in the IoMT industry is an indication of the expansion of diverse e-health scenarios and wide-ranging applications with stringent Quality of Service (QoS) requirements, which has placed an unprecedented strain on wireless networks. For instance, data-intensive applications require a large bandwidth to improve user experience whereas delay-sensitive applications demand a highly dependable network with low latency to allow accurate operations (Cisotto, Casarin, & Tomasin, 2020a) as elucidated in Figure 6.1. As a result, it is not possible to synchronize all characteristic smart healthcare applications to strictly rely on a single Radio access technology (RAT).

In this context, 5G heterogeneous networks (HetNets) have surfaced as a promising solution that maintains service through symbiotically integrating multiple radio access technologies. In addition, 5G HetNet offers multifaceted advantages such as 24x7 services, effective resource management, and improved scalability. In such a complex and dynamic environment, however, an ideal relationship that increases robustness against deviations to the users' advantage is essential (Hussain, 2024). Numerous RAT

DOI: 10.1201/9781032631738-6

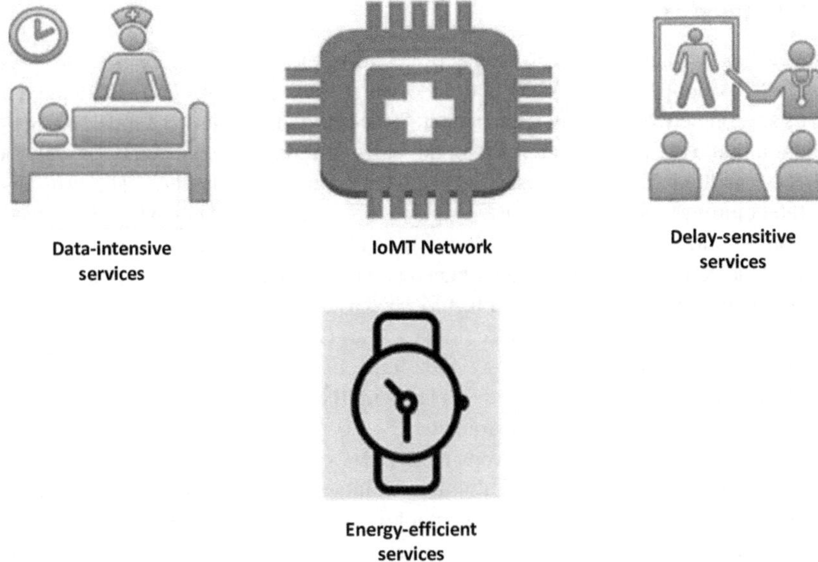

FIGURE 6.1 Next-generation IoMT services in Smart City.

selection procedures, including game theoretic approaches, optimization models, and multi-attribute decision-making (MADM), have been contributed to the current literature. Still, these methods suffer from drawbacks. Within this paradigm, a double deep reinforcement learning (DDRL)-based RAT selection framework has been developed, with the following contributions:

1. A layered software-defined wireless networking (SDWN)-based RAT selection framework has been proposed for the characteristic smart healthcare services namely data-intensive, delay-sensitive, and energy-efficient services in Smart City.
2. A DDRL-based approach has been employed to converge to the best RAT selection policy as per the niche requirements of considered healthcare services in Smart City.
3. Numerous simulations have been run in order to verify the proposed solution's performance and efficacy.

This Chapter is organized as follows. The recent literature regarding RAT selection methods is described in Section 6.2. The proposed system model is elaborated in Section 6.3 for a better comprehension of the proposed solution. The mathematical strategy for the specified problem's fine-grained association policy is described in more detail in Section 6.4. Section 1.5 elaborates on the result validating the proposed solution. Lastly, a succinct conclusion of the Chapter is presented.

6.2 Related Work

The current literature has a wide range of network selection strategies that have been put forth. Among them, MADM is the most preferred RAT selection technique that takes several network factors into account. Desogus et al. developed a traffic-oriented solution that associates with a RAT on the basis of reputation computed through the MADM method considering user feedback and network parameters. The proposed method employs utility function to compute a score related to the RAT under consideration for each type of service. Monteiro et al. (2019) presented a context-aware network selection solution for heterogeneous wireless networks. The proposal delineates a method based on contextual factors such as user and network preferences aiming to improve overall performance. Yadav et al. (2018) presented a MADM-based network selection method for biovital data transmission with a reduced frequency of handovers. Nevertheless, these methods fail with the increase in the network of interdependencies and the number of parameters.

Game theory, as showcased in Arabi et al. (2019), serves as a solution to the above-described challenge. This proposal aims to guarantee stable association among Internet of Things (IoT) devices and RATs in a complex and composite 5G network. In relation to this, preference functions that validate energy efficiency while respecting the RATs capacity and connectivity costs have been defined for both IoT devices and RATs. The concept of evolutionary game theory leveraged by Ma et al. (2020) guarantees an appropriate RAT selection that ensures load balancing. In correspondence to the same, a utility function that considers network parameters and network capacity is employed. Furthermore, Alizadeh & Vu (2019) employed an early acceptance algorithm to facilitate balanced RAT selection in 5G HetNets. However, the stability and adaptability of the game theoretic approaches are lacking in relation to the case.

Artificial intelligence (AI)-based algorithms serve as a promising RAT selection solution in a highly radical environment based on experience samples. Li & Wang (2022) developed a probabilistic optimization model for RAT association in healthcare IoT systems, improving data transmission efficiency. Through the integration of various network parameters and probabilities, the proposed solution dynamically associates with the most suitable RAT, considering critical healthcare data while ensuring reliability and security. Khan et al. (2022) implemented swarm-based optimization techniques for medical IoT networks, to ensure data transmission efficiency within healthcare systems. The proposal employed a swarm intelligence algorithm for optimizing connectivity in the medical IoT landscape. Patel et al. (2022) investigate the application of graph algorithms to optimize network selection in healthcare facilities. By leveraging graph-based methodologies, the study aims to enhance connectivity and data transmission efficiency within healthcare networks, potentially revolutionizing connectivity decisions in healthcare settings. Yang et al. (2023) introduced an adaptive network selection approach employing Q-learning specifically tailored for ambulatory healthcare. By leveraging Q-learning, it aims to dynamically optimize network choices, potentially enhancing connectivity and data transmission efficiency in mobile healthcare environments, promising improved patient care and data accessibility (Hussain and Roy, 2023; Pradhan et al., 2022). Sandoval et al. (2019) present a RAT selection framework based on a reinforcement learning model for smart city. According to the generated alerts, authors developed a well-defined reward function that takes into account the IoT and RAT preferences to optimize throughput while lowering energy consumption and connectivity costs.

Realizing the drawbacks of the present literature as mentioned in Table 6.1, this Chapter presents an intelligent framework based on the diversity of DDRL to converge to best RAT selection policy efficiently and quickly.

TABLE 6.1

Study of Existing Literature in Terms of Key Features and Drawbacks

References	Technique/Approach	Key Features	Drawbacks
Desogus et al. (2019)	Utility function	Utilizes network reputation calculated via multi-criteria approach considering service-specific utility functions	Limited to strict traffic requirements, potential complexity in computation
Monteiro et al. (2019)	Context-aware network selection (CANS)	Considers user preferences, cost, local network and terminal capabilities, displacement speed, device state	Complexity due to multiple characteristic parameters, potential challenges in defining utility functions
Yadav et al. (2018)	MADM-based network selection	Enables seamless biovital data transmission, minimal handovers	Issues with network interdependencies, lack of agreement on evaluation criteria
Arabi et al. (2019)	Game theory	Aims for stable association between IoT devices and RATs, defining preference functions for efficiency	Complexity in ensuring stable association, defining preference functions may be challenging
Ma et al. (2020)	Evolutionary game theory	Focuses on load balancing in 5G heterogeneous network using utility function	Challenges in achieving stable load balancing, potential complexity in utility function design
Alizadeh & Vu (2019)	Matching game theory	Establishes balanced association in 5G HetNets using early acceptance, improving speed and energy efficiency	Stability and adaptability concerns, potential limitations in extensive scalability
Li & Wang (2022)	Bayesian optimization	Efficient network resource allocation, probabilistic modeling	Complexity in handling high-dimensional spaces
Khan et al. (2022)	Swarm intelligence algorithms	Improved network efficiency, self-organization	Sensitivity to parameter settings and initial conditions

(Continued)

TABLE 6.1 (Continued)

References	Technique/Approach	Key Features	Drawbacks
Patel et al. (2022)	Graph-based approaches	Enhanced network scalability, adaptive routing	Scalability with increasing network complexity
Yang et al. (2023)	Q-learning	Improved network performance, adaptive learning	Exploration–exploitation trade-off, convergence issues
Sandoval et al. (2019)	AI-based algorithms	Reinforcement learning for RAT selection in smart cities, optimizing throughput, energy consumption, and costs	Incompatible in handling large state space

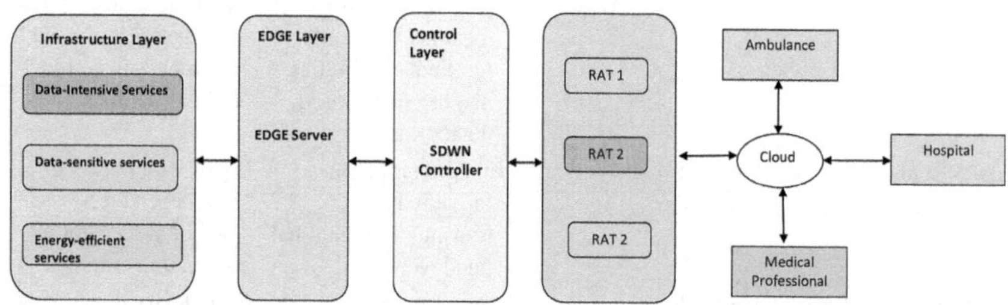

FIGURE 6.2 AIoMT: intelligent RAT selection framework for IoMT services in Smart City.

6.3 AI Framework Design

The system model for the suggested RAT selection solution has been described in this section for better understanding. The multi-objective issue has been developed with the goal of improving system performance while connecting users to the best RAT. The system under study takes into account an IoMT network comprising data-intensive, delay-sensitive, and energy-efficient service requests. The system model has two main functional entities, namely, infrastructure layer and SDWN layer as depicted in Figure 6.2. The infrastructure layer comprises distinct radio access technologies, namely, 5G, LTE, and LoRa. The presence of multiple RATs ensures efficient QoS provisioning in the considered scenario. The service request along with the network parameters measurements, dynamically sensed through IEEE 802.21 are delineated to the SDWN layer periodically for efficient RAT selection. The control layer encapsulates the SDWN controller which renders the best connection to k service requests associated with the considered IoMT network.

6.4 Mathematical Analysis

On the basis of network measurement status received from the infrastructure layer, the SDWN controller associates the service request to the appropriate RAT and the same can be defined with the help of integer linear optimization theory as:

$$z(k,j) = \begin{cases} 1, \text{if service request } k \text{ is associated to } RAT_j \\ 0, \text{otherwise} \end{cases} \tag{6.1}$$

where $z(k, j)$ depicts the binary indicator that indicates 1 if the service request k associates to RAT_j and 0 otherwise. Each RAT_j possesses the offered data rate B_j, delay D_j, PLR P_j and energy consumption EC_j. Similarly, each service request has been characterized with minimum data rate demand $B_{k,j}$, maximum tolerable delay $D_{k,j}$, PLR $P_{k,j}$, and energy consumption $EC_{k,j}$, respectively.

The AP selection problem β has been formulated as:

$$\beta : \max \text{UF} * y(k,j) \quad k \in \text{service request}, j \in \text{AP} \tag{6.2}$$

subject to:

$$b_{k,j} * y(k,j) \leqslant B_j \tag{6.3}$$

$$d_{k,j} * y(k,j) \geqslant D_j \tag{6.4}$$

$$P_{k,j} * y(k,j) \geqslant P_j \tag{6.5}$$

$$EC_{k,j} * y(k,j) \geqslant E_j \tag{6.6}$$

$$y(i,j) \leqslant 1 \tag{6.7}$$

The optimization problem delineated in equation (6.2) is formulated to maximize the total utility of the system. The constraints defined in equation (6.3) ensure that the data rate offered by the AP must be greater than the minimum data rate demand of client. While equations (6.4)–(6.6) guarantees that the delay, PLR, and energy consumption offered by the radio access point should not exceed the maximum threshold value. The constraint highlighted in equation (6.7) assigns single RAT to the requested service at a given time. The gain that the system receives by associating a client (i) with an appropriate AP (j) is measured by the q-score, i.e., utility function u(i, j) (Priya, 2015; Priya & Malhotra, 2021).

The definition of the same has been delineated as:

$$UF = w_B * U_B + w_D * U_D + w_{PLR} * U_{PLR} + w_{EC} * U_{EC} \tag{6.8}$$

$$U_B = \ln\left(B_j / b_{k,j}\right) \tag{6.9}$$

$$U_D = \ln\left(d_{k,j} / D_j\right) \tag{6.10}$$

$$U_{PLR} = \ln(g_{k,j} / G_j \tag{6.11}$$

$$U_{EC} = \ln\left(EC_{k,j} / EC_j\right) \tag{6.12}$$

Since the environment is radical and complex, the defined problem is modeled as a Markov decision process (MDP) M = (S, A, R, γ). In relation to this, the SDWN controller acts upon the state and returns a reward (R) in response to action (A). The definition of the same has been presented as:

1. **State space**: The SDWN controller has been modelled as a DDRL agent that accepts the service request as well as the network parameters as the state space.

$$S = \{k, B_j, D_j, PLR_j, EC_j\} \tag{6.13}$$

2. **Action space**: It accounts for the list of all RATs present in the considered IoMT network.

$$A = \{5G, LTE, LoRa\} \tag{6.14}$$

3. **Reward**: The reward to the DDRL agent, i.e., SDWN controller is defined as follows:

$$R = UF \tag{6.15}$$

Based on these definitions, the SDWN controller accepts the service request and network measurements as state. Accordingly, it selects the best RAT as an action and expects a reward in return for it.

6.5 Results and Discussion

To validate the effectiveness of the proposed method, numerous thorough simulations have been run. Primarily, the simulation environment has been presented, and then the weight computation with respect to the service has been presented. Afterward, the proposed scheme's convergence performance and a comparison with the other current schemes, including the DQN-based scheme (Sandoval et al., 2019; Priya & Malhotra, 2021; Van Hasselt et al., 2016), greedy (Sandoval et al., 2019), and random schemes (Priya & Malhotra, 2021) have been discussed.

6.5.1 Simulation Environment

The simulation scenario takes into account a multi-RAT network considering data-intensive, delay-sensitive, and energy-efficient service request as well as 5G, LTE, and LoRa radio access points. A discrete model has been used to characterize and analyze the network dynamics, including data rate, delay, and energy consumption to certain levels in order to simulate the aforementioned multi-RAT environment. The combined data rate-delay-PLR-energy consumption state must have a network parameter's minimum and maximum level, defined as one of all feasible combinations with an equal probability as mentioned in Table 6.2. Finally, the deep learning toolbox in MATLAB has been used to simulate the DDRL model (Van Hasselt et al., 2016). Table 6.3 lists the DDRL agent hyperparameters in brief.

TABLE 6.2

Simulation Setup Parameters

Parameters	Chosen Values
Considered RATs	[5G, LTE, LoRa]
Data rate	[100–900 Mbps],[75–300 Mbps], [0.3–50 Kbps]
Delay	[1–4 ms], [10–15 ms],[1.6–10s]
PLR	[1–10 per 10^6, 10–15 per 10^6, 10–40 per 10^6]
Energy consumption	[2.15 W, 0.370 W, 0.210 W]
Services	[Data-intensive, delay-sensitive, energy-efficient]

TABLE 6.3

List of DDRL Agent's Hyperparameters

Hyperparameters	Considered Values
Mini-batch size	32
Exploration rate (initial)	0.1
Exploration rate (final)	1.0
Discount factor	0.90
Learning rate	0.01
Double learning	On
Control policy	Epsilon-greedy policy
Optimization strategy	Adam

6.5.2 Service Preferences

To improve QoS in the network, the services in the smart health network must meet the stringent QoS requirements. Within this paradigm, the AHP approach has been utilized in this section to compute the preference weight for each considered parameter:

1. **Data-intensive services**: This class of service includes intra-procedural visualization, VR therapy, VR-goggled train surgeons, medical training, and physical therapy (Cisotto, Casarin, & Tomasin, 2020). Therefore, this class of service has rigorous criteria for high throughput and low latency as depicted in Figure 6.3(a).
2. **Delay-sensitive services**: Robotic surgery, brain –computer interaction, video consultation, wireless robotic care constitute the delay-sensitive services (Chkirbene et al., 2021). Within this paradigm, the most stringent requirements for this service class are low latency and high reliability as shown in Figure 6.3(b).
3. **Energy-efficient services**: Twin body area network and connected wearables are examples of energy-efficient services that must adhere to strict energy consumption guidelines (Wang et al., 2019). In Figure 6.3(c), the weights for the same are specified.

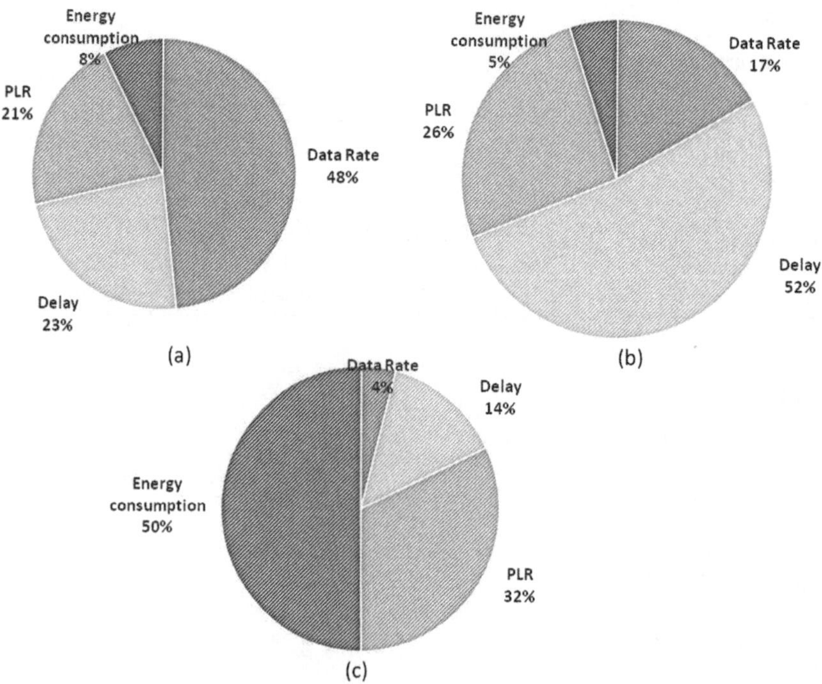

FIGURE 6.3 Service-specific weight measurement for (a) data-intensive, (b) delay-sensitive, and (c) energy-efficient services.

6.5.3 Performance Analysis

According to the reward variation in Figure 6.4, the starting exploration rate is set to 1 for the first 35 episodes in order to obtain a rough estimation of the policy picking random actions. The exploration rate is then reduced to be equal to 0.1 for each episode in order to quickly obtain optimal policy. The model is trained to recognize patterns of dependency between states and actions across the varied episodes, leading to higher rewards. The choice of suboptimal actions at each iteration with the probability of 0.01 ($\alpha = 0.90$) causes fluctuations that are still visible even after the curve has levelled off.

The incorporation of the DDRL allows a reduction in the overestimation error through the implementation of argmax operation leading to faster convergence of the proposed solution as elucidated in Figure 6.5. On the contrary, DQN-based scheme suffers from a catastrophic interference phenomenon that affects the stability resulting in slower convergence. The above-stated inferences can be verified from Figure 6.6, which underlines the efficiency of the proposed scheme as compared to DQN-based schemes, greedy, and random schemes by 7.65%, 25%, and 116.37%, respectively. The proposed DDQN-based approach facilitates higher reward as it sweeps the provided space to maximize reward values in lesser episodes. On the other hand, over-optimistic estimation in DQN-based scheme reduces the learning quality. Additionally, the oblivious RAT selection in the random scheme and the intemperate behaviour towards action value estimates in the greedy scheme, both contribute to their respective underperformance.

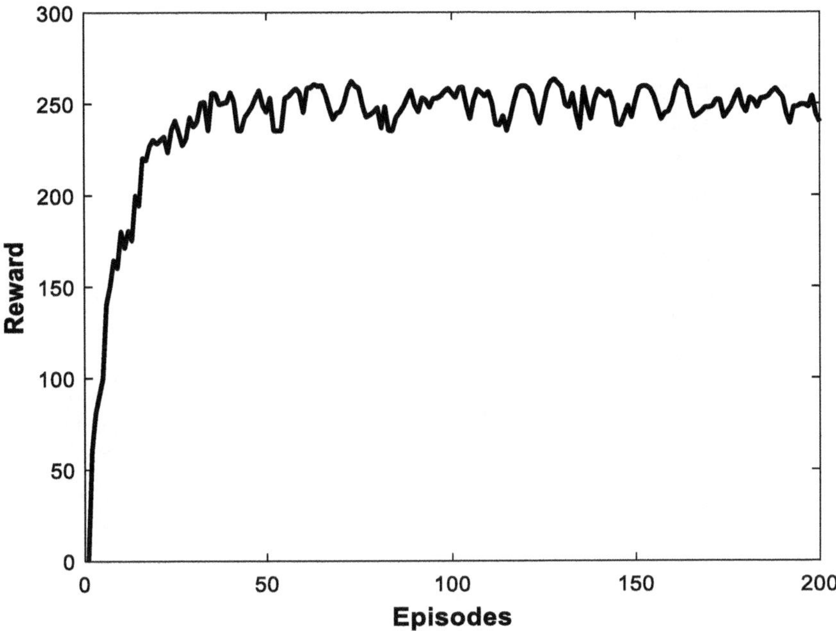

FIGURE 6.4 Reward vs. episodes trend in case of proposed solution.

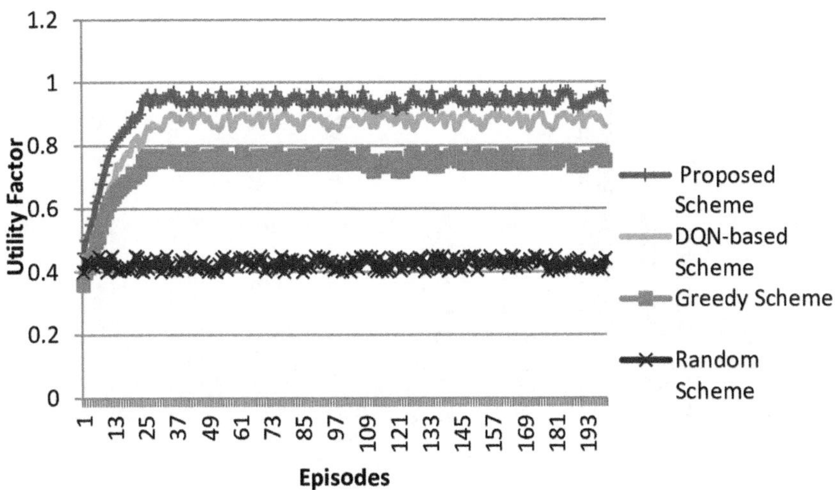

FIGURE 6.5 Convergence statistics of considered schemes.

It can be articulated from Figure 6.7 that 5G-NR has been the most preferred RAT for initial episodes. Subsequently, the RAT selection varies for each service between ten and thirty episodes because the proposed solution adheres to the exploitation policy for action selection that results in substantial rewards. After 30 episodes, the RAT selection for considered IoMT services finally stabilizes.

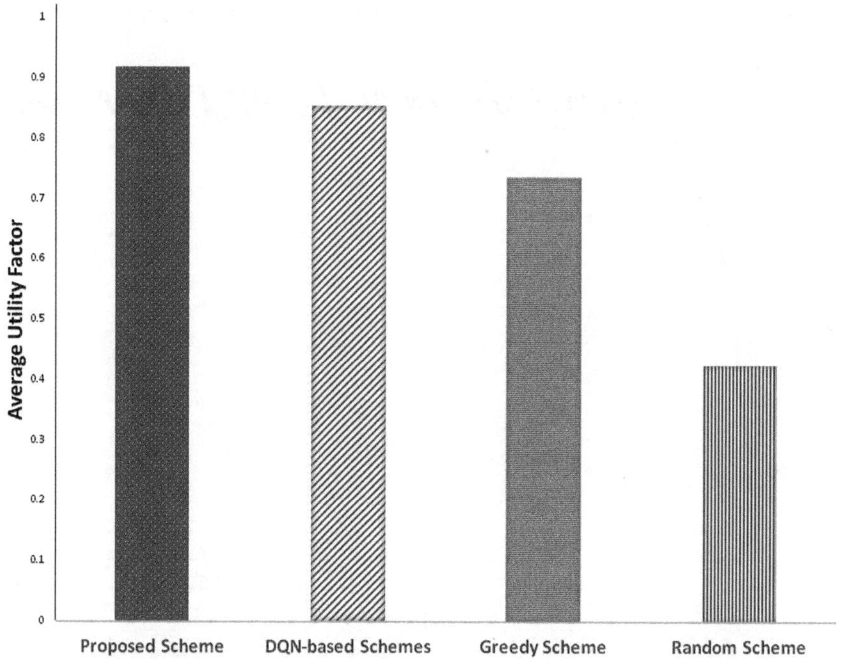

FIGURE 6.6 Comparison between considered schemes based on average utility factor.

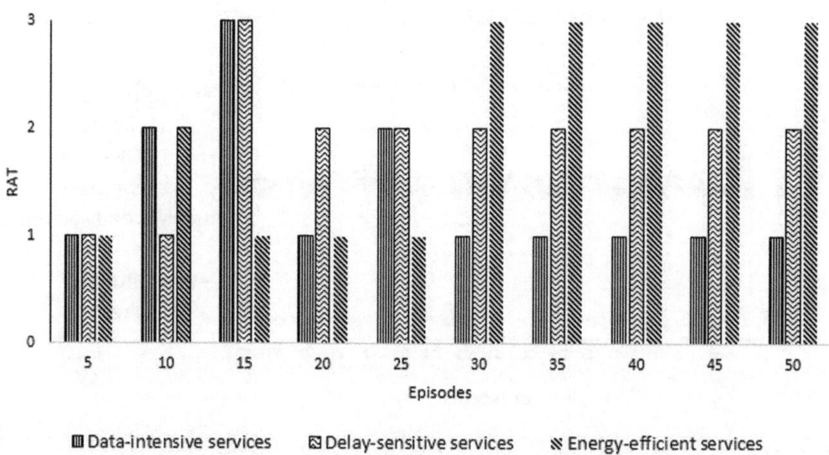

FIGURE 6.7 Trends in RAT selection attained prior to and following convergence.

6.6 Summary

The IoMT in Smart City has experienced substantial growth, which has brought to light the necessity for an efficient communication solution to enable smart healthcare services with stringent QoS requirements. Next-generation HetNets have emerged as a potential panacea to meet these needs since they support agility and adaptability in Smart City. Nevertheless, substantial QoS level maintenance in the smart healthcare is vital. As a solution, an AI-based RAT selection framework has been developed to select the best RAT in radical IoMT network reinforcing smart healthcare in Smart City. The AHP approach has been used to compute service preference weights in order to incorporate heterogeneity. The proposed technique converges to the best RAT association policy in fewer episodes, according to the analytical results proven by thorough simulations. Based on the findings of this study, it has been discovered that the proposed scheme has outperformed DRL, greedy, and random schemes by 7.65%, 25%, and 116.37% accordingly in terms of utility function modeled as q factor.

REFERENCES

Alizadeh, A., & Vu, M. (2019). Early acceptance matching game for user association in 5G cellular HetNets. In *Proceedings of IEEE Global Communications Conference (GLOBECOM)* (pp. 1–6). Waikoloa.

Arabi, S., Hammouti, H. E., Sabir, E., Elbiaze, H., & Sadik, M. (2019). RAT association for autonomic IoT systems. *IEEE Network, 33*(6), 1–8.

Chkirbene, Z. et al., (2021). "Deep reinforcement learning for network selection over heterogeneous health systems," *IEEE Transaction. Network Science Engineering, 9*(1), 258–270.

Cisotto, G., Casarin, E., & Tomasin, S. (2020). Requirements and enablers of advanced healthcare services over future cellular systems. *IEEE Communications Magazine, 58*(3), 76–81. https://doi.org/10.1109/MCOM.001.1900349

Desogus, C., Anedda, M., Murroni, M., & Muntean, G. M. (2019). A traffic type-based differentiated reputation algorithm for radio resource allocation during multi-service content delivery in 5G heterogeneous scenarios. *IEEE Access, 7*, 27720–27735.

Hussain, M. W. (2024). Centralized traffic engineering. In *Towards Wireless Heterogeneity in 6G Networks* (pp. 180–193). CRC Press https://doi.org/10.1201/9781003369028

Hussain, M. W., & Roy, D. S. (2023). Performance optimization strategies for big data applications in distributed framework. In *Intelligent Technologies: Concepts, Applications, and Future Directions*, Volume 2 (pp. 221–252). Singapore: Springer Nature Singapore.

Khan, S., et al. (2022). Swarm-based Optimization for Network Selection in Medical IoT. In *Proceedings of the International Conference on Healthcare Technologies* (pp. 45–56). Singapore: Springer Nature Singapore.

Li, Y., & Wang, Q. (2022). Probabilistic Optimization for Network Selection in Healthcare IoT Systems. *IEEE Transactions on Biomedical Engineering, 69*(3), 210–224.

Ma, M., et al. (2020). Heterogeneous network selection algorithm for novel 5G services based on evolutionary game. *IET Communications, 14*(2), 320–330. https://doi.org/10.1049/iet-com.2018.6290

Monteiro, A., Souto, E., Pazzi, R., & Nogueira, M. (2019). Context-aware network selection in heterogeneous wireless networks. *Computer Communications, 135*, 1–15. https://doi.org/10.1016/j.comcom.2018.11.006

Patel, A., et al. (2022). Optimizing Network Selection in Healthcare Facilities using Graph Algorithms. *Journal of Medical Networking*, *28*(2), 123–136.

Pradhan, B., Hussain, M. W., Srivastava, G., Debbarma, M. K., Barik, R. K., & Lin, J. C. W. (2022). *A Neuro-Evolutionary Approach for Software Defined Wireless Network Traffic Classification.* IET Communications. London.

Priya, B. (2015). Performance Analysis of SACOCDMA-FSO System Using MD Codes. *International Journal of Hybrid Information Technology*, *8*(5), 187–194.

Priya, B., & Malhotra, J. (2021). QAAs: QoS provisioned artificial intelligence framework for AP selection in next-generation wireless networks. *Telecommunication Systems, 76*, 233–249. https://doi.org/10.1007/s11235-020-00710-9

Reddy, K. H. K., Roy, D. S., Mishra, T. K., & Hussain, M. W. (2023). *Handbook of Research on Network-Enabled IoT Applications for Smart City Services*. USA, IGI Global.

Sandoval, R. M., et al. (2019). A reinforcement learning-based framework for the exploitation of multiple RATs in the IoT. *IEEE Access*, *7*, 123341–123354. https://doi.org/10.1109/ACCESS.2019.2938084

Ugalmugale, S., & Swain, R. (2020). Telemedicine market size by service (Tele-consulting, Tele-monitoring, Tele-education/training), by type (Telehospital, Telehome), by specialty (Cardiology, Gynecology, Neurology, Orthopedics, Dermatology, Mental Health), by delivery mode (Web/Mobile Telephonic, Visualized, Call Centers), Industry Analysis Report, Regional Outlook, Growth Potential, Price Trends, Competitive Market Share & Forecast, 2020–2026. *Global Market Insights*. Retrieved from https://www.gminsights.com/industry-analysis/telemedicine-market

Van Hasselt, H., Guez, A., & Silver, D. (2016). Deep reinforcement learning with double q-learning. In *Proceedings of the AAAI Conference on Artificial Intelligence* (Vol. *30*, No. 1). Arizona, USA.

Wang, X., et al. (2019). Intelligent user-centric network selection: A model-driven reinforcement learning framework. *IEEE Access*, *7*, 21645–21661.

Yadav, P., Agrawal, R., & Kashish, K. (2018). Heterogeneous network access for seamless data transmission in remote healthcare. *International Journal of Grid Distribution Computing*, *11*(8), 69–86.

Yang, H., et al. (2023). Adaptive Network Selection for Ambulatory Healthcare using Q-learning. In *Proceedings of the Conference on Healthcare Networking* (pp. 140–155).

7

Concurrent Clustering with Outlier Removal in Healthcare

M. Blessa Binolin Pepsi, V. Aishwharya, A. Shahina Fathima, and K. Vijaya Subasri
Mepco Schlenk Engineering College, Sivakasi, India

7.1 Introduction

In the context of smart cities and healthcare applications, clustering is usually done by identifying the common characteristics between the data points (Reddy et al., 2023). High intra-class similarity and low inter-class similarity are typical characteristics of an effective clustering strategy. The value of clustering (Xu and Wunch, 2005; Ma Hong et al., 2010) is mainly based on the similarity measure and discovering the hidden similar patterns. The distance metric (Ting et al., 2008) is an important term that describes identifying patterns in the provided data points. Many clustering methods are available, including distributed clustering, hierarchical clustering, density-based clustering, K-means clustering, centroid-based clustering, and K-means clustering. Many forms of clustering analysis, including binary, nominal, ordinal, interval-scaled variables, and ratio data, are performed for various data types. The three different distance measures used for numeric value calculation in the Manhattan Distance, Minkowski Distance, and Euclidean Distance are the three grouping techniques. This work partitioning clustering is the method employed for clustering in this instance. The term partitioning clustering means constructing various patterns and evaluating them by following some criteria. For example, we have used the K-means clustering technique (Masna Wati et al., 2022) for cluster analysis for different data points. Z-score is calculated by finding the mean and standardization of the sample. Clustering is usually the unsupervised learning technique where the class target for the data points is usually not available and the data points are not classified (Hussain and Roy, 2023). The class labels of each customer are known in classification and therefore it is mentioned as supervised learning. In clustering, we need to discover the data point groupings. The similarities between the data points and the dissimilarity between them are assessed often using distance measures or according to the value of the attribute describing the objects. Numerous fields, including biology, business, security, and most forms of online search, rely heavily on clustering. The real-life applications

DOI: 10.1201/9781032631738-7

based on clustering techniques are image processing, image recognition, and so on. A cluster label should be given to each point. In other words, the clustering method does not involve any anomalous data points. Unfortunately, especially in the case of the unsuspended task, this is not always the case. The performance of clustering is invariably hampered by potential anomalies or outliers. For instance, a few outliers can quickly ruin the K-means-derived cluster structure and produce strange Gaussian mixture model distributions. Some robust clustering (Yi et al., 2012; Elhamifar and Vidal, 2013) techniques have been presented to retrieve clean data when dealing with outliers or noisy data. The purpose of learning is to build a robust distance function that can fend off outliers, and the L1 norm is employed to reduce the negative impact of outliers on measures. We have implemented the COR technique in heart disease data set with regard to healthcare applications.

7.2 Related Work

We have considered the fields of robust clustering, consensus clustering, and outlier identification in this section and have highlighted the differences between our work and the current work.

7.2.1 Robust Clustering

A strong clustering technique can lessen the impact of outliers (Yi et al., 2012; Elhamifar and Vidal, 2013) approach is proposed. From the distance function aspect, to learn a robust metric, we use metric learning to draw similarities amidst two spots by including the outliers in the description; L1ethos plans the outliers for cluster examination as a scarce control. According to the element examination, the outlier has given certain weights through the cluster analysis process; low-rank representation takes the clean part as data and outliers.

From the design model fusion point of view, group clustering associates diverse partitions into an agreement one to deliver a powerful result. Even though such a robust cluster analysis approach decreases the drawback of outliers on the cluster framework, they fizzle to absolutely identify and discard outlier spots for clustering. Alternatively, every element is inclined with a cluster group.

7.2.2 Consensus Clustering

Consensus clustering (Liu et al., 2017; Lourenco et al., 2013) takes input as a set of fundamental divisions and combines one as output, as the partition of data-ensemble clustering (Ghosh and Strehl, 2003; Wu et al., 2017) is a combination problem. Many clustering techniques have been introduced in the past years; it has resulted in two groupings using many kinds of fundamental division inputs. An analysis of a category's basic partition into a co-association matrix counts the recurrent occurrence of two instances of the same class. In this manner, the graph partition problem is formed from a consensus clustering analysis.

7.2.3 Outlier Detection

Data points that are significantly different from the current data points are typically used to identify outliers. Without external supervision, some criteria are there to seek the deviation of the outlier candidates differing from the normal or available data points in the cluster. Numerous algorithms have been projected on the basis of different hypotheses, whose task is to allot an outlier score for every available cluster data point. It usually returns the results of top k-candidates as outliers. There are various methods that represent the outlier candidates such as the local outlier factor (LOF) (Breunig et al., 2000) based on distance, outlier factor based on local distance (LODF) (Hutter et al., 2009), or connectivity-based outlier factor (COF) (Woo et al., 2017), angle-based outlier factor (ABOD), outlier based on frequent pattern that is called to be frequent pattern-based Fp outlier, and outlier detection based on Bi-sampling that is Bi-sampling-based outlier detection (BSOD). The other detection techniques for outliers are ensemble-based iForest, the PCA oversampling based on eigenvectors, and NMF text outlier clustering. Deep learning methods are also available for detecting the outliers in the cluster. They include single class SVM and, also they include generative adversarial network-based method which produces the result as effective recognition of outliers which uses the transformation which is non-linear and is learned for projecting the hidden space from the original data. However, uncertain data points in the cluster are not appropriate for this approach, it is only suitable and it is usually used to train the model for clear data points for the prediction of new data to check and analyze whether the data points are highly dissimilar which is considered as outliers which are dissimilar from the hitch we are addressing here. In this work, we are analyzing cluster technique and detection of the outliers which partition the entire data sets into various clusters by grouping every data point, many clusters are created, but only one outlier set is generated. However, some pioneering works provide and show a new direction for cluster joining and for detecting the data points which are highly dissimilar to the available or existing data points that are considered to be outliers. None of the algorithms are amenable to the practical implementation of the sets of data with a lot of rows and columns, but they clearly explain by means of hypothetical interests. Additionally K-means has a spherical make-up supposition and the space limit of the original feature's ability to analyze difficult data. In this study, we use holoentropy-based partitioning to convert the original feature space into a binary space (Guha et al., 1999; Wu and Wang, 2013) and thereby achieving the simultaneous cluster analysis and finding the points that are highly dissimilar from the available or existing data points which is considered to be an outlier.

Holoentropy: Holoentropy is the term that usually describes the establishment of a relationship between each individual data point and the cluster. It is the term used for partitioning the original space into a binary space. It is typically based on outlier detection metrics and information theory. It usually handles the data that are categorical and it takes the entropy and the entire correlation for detecting the data points that are highly dissimilar to the existing data points that are essentially outliers within the data set.

7.3 Objective Function

Here, COR's objective function is presented, which has two inputs: the outliers (o) and the number of clusters (K). A small number of outliers can threaten the cluster structure, and these outliers want to be recognized by the cluster boundary. It resembles a chicken-and-egg scenario since cluster analysis and detection of outliers are interdependent. Consensus clustering (Lourenco, et al., 2013; Fred and Jain, 2005) is used to reduce the negative impacts of outliers and avoid issues in joint clustering and outlier identification. In order to convert the element from the original feature range into division range, it fuses many fundamental divisions made from the data for a robust fusion. These motivate us to generate a lot of fundamental partitions. This technique is comparable to how consensus clustering generates fundamental partitions.

Let X represent the feature data matrix with n by d rows. Think about using a label vector to represent the class of K object subsets that make up the partition of X into K exact clusters $\pi = \left(L_{\Pi}\left(x_1\right) \; \cdots L_{\pi}\left(x_n\right)\right)$, $1 \leq 1 \leq n$, where L is the constant $1 \leq 1 \leq n$, $L_{\pi}\left(x_l\right)$ maps to a K label in the set of 1, 2, ..., K. Some basic partitioning techniques, like K-means clustering, can use various cluster numbers to get r basic partitions $\Pi = \left\{\pi_i\right\}$, $1 \leq i \leq r$. Let K_i stand for cluster number and $R = \sum_{i=1}^{\Upsilon} K_i$. Following that, a binary matrix $B = \left\{b_l\right\}$, $1 \leq 1 \leq n$ able to be produced. We determine the dissimilarity by first normalizing the squared Euclidean distance. The suspicious spots are also readily discernible, and each set of data in the divider space has its own cluster structure. Even if these basic partitions were made with the faulty K-means clustering and are adversely affected by outliers, the data in the divider space have a significantly right cluster structure and are valuable for outlier detection. It is crucial to emphasize that the most basic partitions can be created without the use of a particular algorithm. K-means is advised to create results for the sake of simplicity and effectiveness.

This attempted to reduce the data set's holoentropy by eliminating any outliers. Here, we'll take into account the cluster organization of the entire data collection, therefore, reducing each cluster's holoentropy makes more sense. As a result, only the clusters – and not the entire data set – become compact when the outliers are eliminated. We therefore provide the objective function for COR as follows, based on each cluster's holoentropy:

$$\min_{\pi} \sum_{k} k = \mathrm{p_k HL}\left(\mathrm{C_k}\right) \tag{7.1}$$

where HL (.) is the holoentropy and the cluster measure with k clusters included is π.

7.3.1 Cluster Analysis

Cluster analysis usually takes place by partitioning all data points into subsets. Each subset consists of data points that are considered to be a cluster which has more similarity between them within the alike cluster and more dissimilarity between the other data points located in other clusters. The group of clusters resulting from cluster analysis is commonly known as clustering (Xu and Wunch, 2005; Ma Hong et al., 2010).

At the same time, the cluster generated as a result of one clustering technique may not be the same as the cluster generated as a result of other clustering techniques. The partitioning between data points is performed using algorithms, not by humans. Clustering can also be called automatic classification as its quality is to build and preserve a low inter-cluster relationship while maintaining a strong intra-cluster relationship additionally, here the groupings can be found automatically. The term data segmentation is also used here as the data points are segmented into various clusters. The outlier detection is done by finding and analyzing the cluster. In classification, the supervised learning algorithm is used as it has class labels for all the data points. There are different methods to analyze clusters. Some of them are partitioning methods, in this method, we usually find clusters that are mutually exclusive and of spherical shape. It is also based on distance. To represent cluster centre, it may use mean or medoid. This partitioning method has mostly given effective results for small-to-medium-sized data sets. The other method commonly used is a hierarchical method in which clustering is performed as a hierarchical decomposition. The negative aspect of the hierarchical method is that it cannot deal with erroneous merges or splits and it can take in other practices like micro-clustering or "linkages" object is considered. The other most commonly used method is density-based methods, through which arbitrarily shaped clusters can be found. The separation of low-density regions is done through clustering the dense regions of objects in space. The term cluster density is nothing but each data point available in the A cluster needs to have the fewest possible data points in its "neighbourhood". In this method, it may filter the data points that are highly dissimilar and are considered to be an outlier. The other method which is used is known as a grid-based method which uses a data structure which is considered to be a multi-resolution data structure. Because most approaches rely on, it requires relatively little time or quick processing. The grid-based technique accounts for grid size rather than just the number of data objects.

7.3.2 K-Means Clustering

The K-means cluster technique is frequently used to analyze data points by calculating the distance between each data point and the centroid after selecting a random data point to serve as the cluster's centroid. Partitioning the objects into non-empty sets K is one of the four crucial procedures that must be done. Calculate the cluster centroid and use it as the current position's starting point. Just place each data point in the cluster that has the closest seed point, then repeat step 2 until the values of the data points that fit into the cluster remain unchanged. The centroid is nothing more than the cluster's centre point, which is also its mean. Consider the data collection D, which contains N Euclidean objects, because the few data points have the potential to alter the mean value from which the centroid can be derived in subsequent repetitions. Since centroids need to be more effective, the above-mentioned challenge with the assignment of starting data points must be solved in order to boost the K-means' scalability. In order to increase the K-mean clustering algorithm's effectiveness for vast numbers of data points. The other option is to employ a technique called filtering, which often makes use of a geographic hierarchical data index to reduce costs when computing data point means. Investigating the concept of micro-clustering is another crucial strategy. Micro-clustering simply refers to the organization of close things.

7.4 Proposed System

System design's job is to provide hardware and software components what a large system need. After the system requirements study is finished, the design activity begins. Systems design is the process of defining the components, including architecture with modules, components, their interfaces, and data, depending on the desires that have been proposed. Explaining the plan of action is what the proposed system entails and how you intend to carry out this. Figure 7.1 briefly states the steps involved in the proposed system.

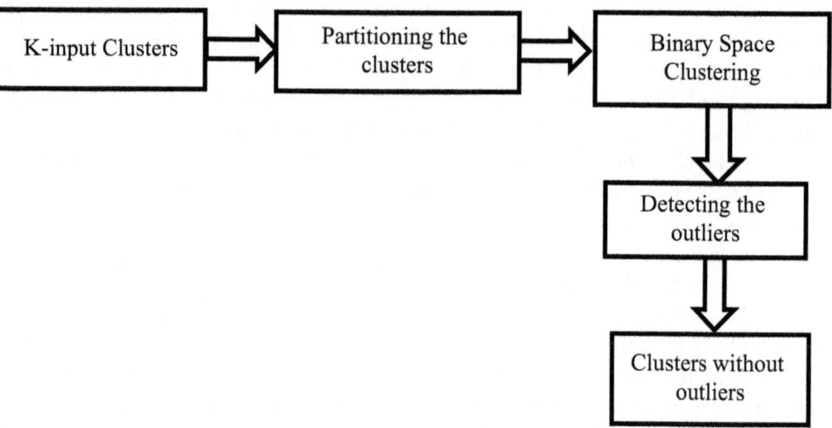

FIGURE 7.1 Architecture flow of the proposed work.

ALGORITHM 1. Outlier Removal Using Clustering Algorithm

Data matrix X is the input;
K is the number of clusters.
O: Outliers
r: number of fundamental partitions

Expected K clusters C1, CK, and the outlier set O are the output.

1. 1: Make the basic partitions of r from X;
2. Create B and B', the binary matrices;
3. K centroids are loaded from [B B'];
4. Redo
5. In steps 4 and 5, calculate the distance between each point in [B B'] and its closest centroid, then redo.
6. Mark the o spots that are the furthest apart as possible outliers;
7. Position the remaining n–o points on the centroids that are closest to them.
8. Adjust the centroids until the goal value remains constant by applying the arithmetic mean.

In terms of temporal complexity and convergence, we examine Algorithm 1's property. Create r fundamental division in line 1, which are typically concluded by K-means clustering (Fahim et al., 2006; Huang, 1998) with various cluster numbers. It takes O (rtKnd) to complete this step, where K and t_0 are the average cluster and replication counts, respectively. The conventional K-means algorithm, in lines 5–8, has a time complexity of O (tKnR) and has a dimension of R=, *i*=1-*γ*-, *k-i*, which is the binary matrices B and B's dimension. The fact that only R components in [B B'] are non-zero must be emphasized. We find the o points with the largest distances (*n*), as opposed to sorting the n points such that line 6 can be completed using O.

That parallel computation is used to construct r basic partitions, greatly reducing the execution time. Moreover, as compared to the total number of point's n, the values of t_0, t, r, and R are quite tiny. Because of this, our algorithm's time complexity is nearly linear in relation to the number of points, which makes scaling up for large-scale data clustering with outliers simple. The following theorem further guarantees that Algorithm 1 will eventually reach a local optimum.

Theorem 1:

If the binary matrix B has no inliers and K-means is applied to it, we have

$$\max\sum_{k=1}^{K} p_k \sum_{i=1}^{r}\sum_{j=1}^{K_I} p_{k,ij} \log p_{k,ij} \leftrightarrow \min\sum_{k=1}^{K}\sum_{b_l \in C_k} f\left(b_l, m_k\right) \tag{7.2}$$

the kth centroid, and m_k as well as the distance function.

$$f\left(b_l, m_k\right) = \sum_{i=1}^{r}\sum_{j=1}^{Ki} D_{kl}\left(b_{k,ij} \parallel m_{k,ij}\right) \tag{7.3}$$

Here, the KL divergence is denoted by *Dkl* (.||.).

Proof. The Bregman divergence indicates that we have DKL (s||t) = H(t)–H(s) + $\left(s-t\right)^T$ ∇H(t),
where t and s are two vectors of comparable sizes. Next, we start on the right side.

$$\begin{aligned}\sum_{k=1}^{K}\sum_{b_l \in c_k} f\left(b_{l,mk}\right) &= \sum_{k=1}^{K}\sum_{b_l \in c_k}\sum_{i=1}^{r}\sum_{j=1}^{K_i}\left(H\left(m_{k,ij}\right) - H\left(b_{l,ij}\right) + \left(b_{l,ij} - m_{k,ij}\right)^T \nabla H\left(m_{k,ij}\right)\right) \\ &= \sum_{k=1}^{K}\left|C_k\right| \sum_{i=1}^{r}\sum_{j=1}^{K_i} H\left(m_{k,ij}\right) - \sum_{k=1}^{K}\sum_{b_l \in C_k}\sum_{i=1}^{r}\sum_{j=1}^{K_i} H\left(b_{l,ij}\right)\end{aligned} \tag{7.4}$$

Due to $\sum_{b_l \in C_K}\left(b_{l,ij} - m_{k,ij}\right) = 0$, the above-mentioned equation is valid, and the second portion is distinct by the binary matrix B, with Lemma 1 clearly visible.

Remark 1.

The K-means on the binary matrix B have an equivalent connection, as demonstrated by Theorem 1. By doing this, part of this challenging problem can be successfully solved with the simple K-means clustering method by utilizing KL-divergence on each dimension.

$$b_l' = \left(b_{l,1}',\ldots,b_{l,i}',\ ,\ldots,\ b_{l,r}',\right),\ \text{with}$$

$$b_{l,i}' = \left(b_{l,i1}',\ldots,b_{l,ij}',\ldots,b_{l,iKi}'\right),\ \text{and}$$

$$b_{l,ij}' = \{\begin{matrix} 0, if\ L_{\pi_i}\left(x_l\right) = j, \\ 1, \quad \text{otherwise} \end{matrix}$$

It is also derivable from B'. When contrasted to B, B' can be thought of as the binary matrix B flipped. Actually, the 1-of-Ki and (Ki-1)-of-Ki coding of the original data are represented by B and B', respectively. We can define m' k based on B, and then we obtain $m_{k,ij}' = 1\text{-}\ m_{k,ij} = 1 - p_{k,ij}$. By applying the following theorem, using the binary matrices B and B' as our foundation, we transform the problem into a unified K-means system.

Theorem 2:

If K-means is applied to the binary matrix [B B'] with n-o inliers, we obtain,

$$\min_{\Pi} \sum_{k=1}^{k} p_k HL\left(C_k\right) \Leftrightarrow \min \sum_{k=1}^{k} \sum_{b_l \in c_k} \left(f\left(b_l, m_k\right) + \ f\left(\tilde{b}_l, \tilde{m}_l \right) \right) \tag{7.5}$$

Remark 2.

To model 1 $p_{k,ij}$, the problem can be fully expressed by introducing the binary matrix B', which is a turnover of B, and applying K-means clustering on the linked binary matrix [B B'] in Theorem 2. The benefits stem not only from the well-organized mathematical formulation of the issue but also from the successful use of K-means, which is suitable for massive data clustering with outlier termination.

We then analyze the properties of Algorithm 1 in terms of convergence and time complexity. R basic divisions are first created in line 1, after which they are typically clustered using K-means with different cluster numbers. This phase takes O (rt'Knd) to finish, where t_0 and K are the cluster and ordinary repetition numbers, respectively.

Theorem 3

The local optimum of Algorithm 1 is reached, due to K-means' excellent convergence, hence the proof is valid.

7.5 Discussion

In this section, cluster analysis and outlier detection methods are compared with the classical methods.

Cluster analysis comparison: The goal of a classic cluster analysis method is to divide a set of data points from the data set into disjoint groups of different sets, meaning that each data point in the cluster should have a strong association with every other set of data points. Typically, the data set assigns a hard label or a soft label to each data point. Despite the fact that robust clustering (Yi et al., 2012; Elhamifar and Vidal, 2013) is proposed to reduce the outlier data points impact, these methods cannot explicitly identify outliers such that each data point including similar data points and dissimilar data points must be included in the clustering process. The problem we analyze here is that the data points that are highly similar are known as inliers and are taken into account for the clustering process and therefore the separation of outliers occurs. It assigns the label only for the outliers not for inliers and therefore the data points without labels are mentioned as outliers. This is an example of non-exhaustive clustering, where some data points may belong to many groups simultaneously.

Comparison with outlier removal: Comparison combined with outlier detection is a popular subject of research, and significant attempts have been made to make it flourish in many ways. Only some carry out cluster analysis and outlier detection at the same time. When we take a pairwise distance matrix as input, Lagrangian relaxation (LP) (Pang et al., 2014) devises the problem similarly to K-means but uses integer programming. In addition to having a very sophisticated algorithm, LP finds it difficult to set this limit in real-world situations, which causes LP to return impractical answers because of this, we have neglected to report LP's performance in the experimental portion. To the best of our knowledge, the first data is clustered while also removing outliers from the partition space. Our COR algorithm illustrates the close relationship between the fields of outlier identification and cluster evaluation by beginning with the goal function with regard to outliers identification and solving it using a clustering tool.

7.5.1 Experimental Results

Data sets: Numerous data sets from various fields are used in order to completely test our COR technique. They include gene expression data, high-dimensional text data, high-dimensional image data, and multivariate data. These data sets can be accessed at UCI. Here, the smallest class is treated as an anomaly. In the original data sets, the three smallest classes are recognized as the outliers for *E. coli*.

7.5.1.1 Description of Data Set

1) **KDD CUP**: The International Knowledge Discovery and Data Mining Tools Competition was launched in tandem with KDD-99, the Fifth International Conference on Knowledge Discovery and Data Mining, and was based on the data gathering process. The competition's objective was to create a prediction model or network intrusion detector that could differentiate between "good" connections, which were regular, and "bad" connections, which were intrusions or attacks. This database contains a standard set of auditable

data with several examples of simulated breaches in a military network environment. There are 43 columns and 2,56,036 rows in it.

2) **Shuttle**: There are 14,500 test data sets and 43,500 training data sets in the shuttle data set. It has nine different qualities. Validation set: the cases in the original data set were arranged chronologically, and this chronological arrangement may possibly be significant for categorization. This wasn't considered important for Stat Log's objectives; thus, a piece of the original data set was deleted for validation and the instances' order was randomly generated.
3) **Glass**: There are 214 instances, and there are 10 qualities. Nothing is lacking from the available attributes.
4) **Heart disease data set**: This 1988 data set consists of four databases: Hungary, Switzerland, Cleveland, and Long Beach V. It contains 76 properties, including the one that was predicted; however, only 14 of them are listed in the published research, and none of them describe using all of them.

The patient's cardiac health is mentioned in the "target" field. Zero denotes no disease, whereas one denotes one. There are 18,494 columns in it.

7.5.1.2 Competitive Techniques

K-means and K-means are used for comparisons. For our COR technique, K-means is used to generate 100 fundamental divisions with cluster sizes ranging from 2 to 2K. The distance function for the outliers and partition is then coupled with K-means. K and o, which stand for the actual numbers of clusters and outliers, respectively, are used to make fair comparisons.

Supplied to COR and K-means. The outlier set is the cluster set produced by the K-means algorithm that has the fewest items; the cluster number for K-means is equal to the actual number plus one. We use a number of approaches, such as LOF (Elhamifar and Vidal, 2013) COF, LODF, FABOD (Pagh and Pham, 2012), iForest (Ting et al., 2008), OPCA (Wang et al., 2013), and TONMF (Woo et al., 2017), for comparisons, to identify outliers. The following are the settings for the above outlier detection parameters: In COF, LODF, LOF, and FABOD, the neighbour number is 50; in iForest, the subsampling The forgetting number is 50, while the size and tree numbers are 200 and 100.is set for the rank and two additional factors to 0.1 in OPCA and 10, 10, and 0.1 in TONMF. Every code is put into practice by using Python. After 20 iterations of the algorithms, the average value and standard deviation are obtained back.

7.5.1.3 Measures for Validation

Despite being an unsupervised task, clustering (Xu and Wunch, 2005; Ma Hong et al., 2010) with outlier removal (Kroger et al., 2010; Li et al., 2015) allows us to assess performance using label information by applying the ground truth. Four metrics are applied to the combined outlier identification and clustering in order to evaluate the efficacy of cluster validity and outlier detection. The outlier set is considered to be a distinct cluster in the ground truth.

Normalized Mutual Information (NMI) and Normalized Rand Index (Rn) (Chen et al., 2009), which originate from information theory and statistics, respectively, are two frequently used external assessments for cluster validity.

Following a normalizing process to create the range [0, 1], Rn counts the co-occurrence pairs that are accessible in the same class with a normalization. NMI then computes the mutual information between the resulting partition and the ground truth.

$$\mathrm{NMI} = \frac{\sum_{i,j} n_{i,j} \log \frac{n \cdot n_{ij}}{n_{i+} \cdot n_{+j}}}{\sqrt{\left(\sum_{i} n_i + \log \frac{n_{i+}}{n}\right)\left(\sum_{j} n_j + \log \frac{n_{+j}}{n}\right)}} \tag{7.6}$$

In binary classification, the F-measure and the Jaccard index are frequently utilized. Here, the two classes are outliers and inliers, it is used to gauge the effectiveness of outlier detection.

$$\mathrm{Jaccard} = \frac{\left|o \cap o^*\right|}{\left|o \cup o^*\right|} \tag{7.7}$$

$$\text{F- measure} = 2^* \frac{(\text{precision.recall})}{(\text{precision} + \text{recall})} \tag{7.8}$$

To evaluate overall effectiveness among all the employed data sets, we offer the following score.

$$\mathrm{Score}(A_i) = \sum_{j} \frac{P(A_i, D_j)}{\max_i P(A_i, D_j)} \tag{7.9}$$

7.5.2 Algorithmic Performance

Here, we contrast the effectiveness of COR with that of K-means and outlier detection methods. In relation to Figures 7.2 and 7.3, three points are made here.

(1) A small number of outliers can quickly disrupt the cluster form. The poor clustering performance of K-means on fibs' and kddcup based on NMI and Rn lends credence to this claim.

(2) Furthermore, K-means is unable to detect outliers when the cluster size is simply increased. K-means – K-means minimizes the harm that outliers provide to the clusters by outperforming on average while also learning the cluster structure and identifying outliers.

(3) In terms of outliers, K-means performs better than COR. Some Caltech and yeast articles, particularly those on K1B, show an increase over K-means of larger than 30. Unlike the F-measure, K-means is unable to identify any outliers. COR is essentially K-means applied to a binary matrix. The partition space, which enables joint consensus clustering, is responsible for the enormous gains observed in relation to all four criteria (Liu et al., 2017; Lourenco et al., 2013; Fred et al., 2005), develops the concept of clusters,

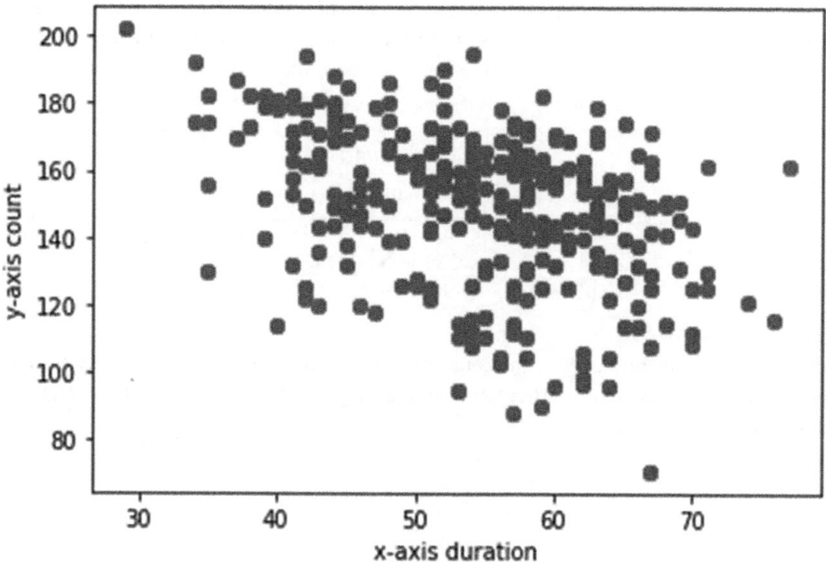

FIGURE 7.2 Range in which data points are present.

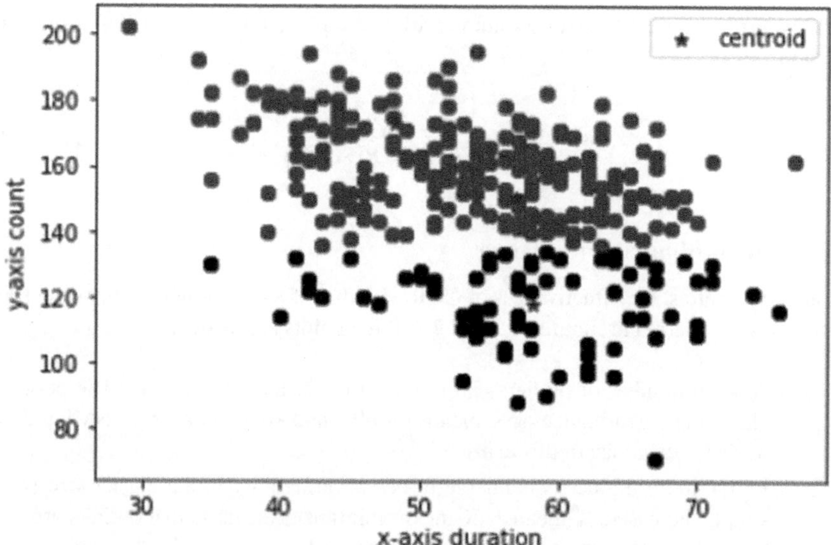

FIGURE 7.3 Assigning cluster and centroids within given range.

and removes outliers; COR performs much better than the two primitive algorithms, as per the score. Since COR functions in the partition space, we also contrast it with Consensus Clustering based on K-means (KCC) (Cao et al., 2013, 2015), which uses the same fundamental partitions but includes an additional cluster to identify outliers.

In addition to these two algorithms, in Figure 7.4, we compare COR to several methods of outlier identification. The efficiency of employing F-measure and Jaccard is to identify outliers. In some situations, these unsupervised outlier identification methods with different underlying assumptions are effective. For example, on shuttle and kddcup, COF and iForest, respectively, perform best. But these rivals usually deliver mediocre outcomes. The causes are numerous and complex, but the initial location and lack of outside supervision may be two of them. The ability of the original space to discern between outliers and inliers is restricted, and it is challenging to set the hyperparameter in an unsupervised manner. The effectiveness of all of the above algorithms will then be evaluated. The cluster-based methods, including TONMF and K-means, are comparatively fast, but angle-based, density-based, and distance-based methods have trouble processing high-dimensional data sets.

The most time-consuming method is FABOD. It is crucial to remember that the density-based, distance-based, and angle-based techniques all need the calculation of the closest neighbour matrix. This requires a significant amount of space complexity and causes a 64GB RAM PC to run out of memory when trying to process large data sets. Furthermore, because COR operates on a binary matrix rather than a complex matrix, its temporal complexity is practically proportional to the number of instances.

7.5.3 Factor Analysis

We offer additional analysis of the factors in this paragraph, the number of fundamental partitions, fundamental partition formation method, and cluster count inside COR. The performance of consensus clustering increases with the number of fundamental partitions. We evaluate COR in a similar way with diverse numbers of

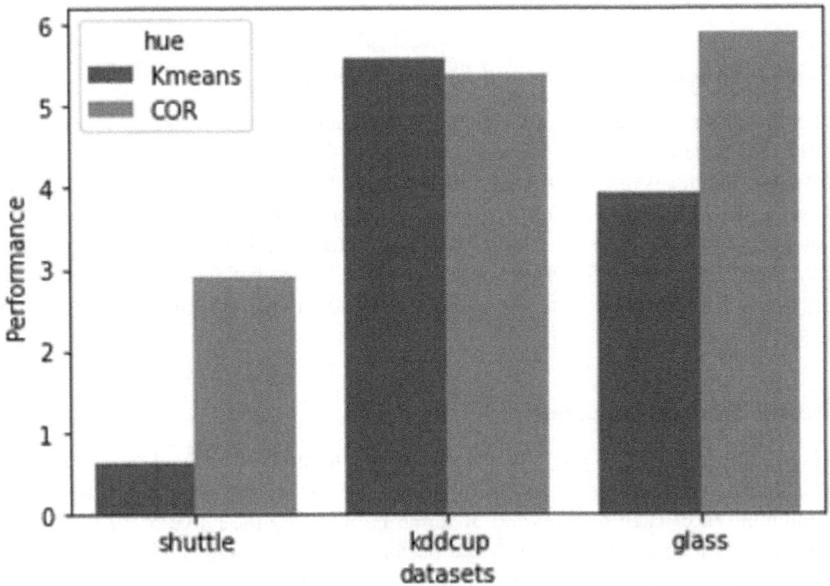

FIGURE 7.4 Performance analysis of K-means and COR with different data sets.

basic partitions. Regarding NMI (Chen et al., 2009) and Jaccard, it is 2. We create 100 sets of basic partitions for a given number of basic partitions, and then we run COR for the boxplot. Even with just 10 fundamental partitions, COR makes high-quality partition strategies for kddcup and shuttle generation. On these two data sets with different measures, RFS outperforms RPS, with the exception of the shuttle in Rn.

As a result, RFS is able to produce fundamental partitions for COR that is of high quality while also effectively decreasing the detrimental effects of noisy features. It is important to remember that the combination of COR and RFS on kddcup yields 21, 18, 34.95 for both the Jaccard and the F-measure, challenging the one with RPS over 5% on iForest. This shows that COR and RFS work together more quickly than iForest and beat their top rival in the KDD Cup.

7.5.4 Application on Healthcare

Clustering is one of the most efficient machine learning techniques. It is used to determine various hidden structures in both the labelled and unlabelled data sets (Pradhan et al., 2022). In our chapter, we are considering the application of clustering in healthcare. We are applying our clustering technique for studying heart disease (Buettner and Schunter, 2019) which is a neurological disease. The role of clustering here is that we are going to partition the people affected by disease based on the similarity in the persons. The same technique is used here since clustering looks for similarities between specific data points, and the outlier is the data point that differs from the other data points. The patients who have heart disease (Ankita and Garg, 2023) are like the similar data points as they have similar symptoms and those who do not have the disease are the outliers as they do not have the symptoms like the disease-affected patients. The clustering algorithm could find similar patterns among the people whereas it is difficult for the medical practitioners to detect.

7.5.4.1 Patient Population and Sample Selection

Patients under the age of 18 were included in the analysis provided they met two criteria: they began at least two HD sessions between 2008 and 2010 and had at least one complete diagnosis of ESRD. They called the first HD claim an "index date". Patients were removed if they had not maintained continuous registration during the index date, which was the "pre-" or "post-" HD period (the index date may have contained data from 2007 or 2011 for the pre- and post-HD periods). Patients who underwent PD or received a transplant were not excluded due to sample size and generalizability concerns.

7.5.4.2 Statistic Evaluation

These analyses aimed to group patients according to the "before" and "after" periods' total expenses for all causes. Values for all-cause costs were normalized by taking the minimum out of each number and dividing the result by the range of all values. On normalized all-cause expenses, CA was performed. Patients with similar cost patterns were "grouped" into a collection of clusters based on their pre- and post-HD period expenses using different CA approaches.

Patterns of comorbidities and demographic data were compared, contrasted, and evaluated within each cluster. Normalized costs from both the pre- and post-HD eras were subjected to hierarchical CA using various linking techniques, as well as K-means (non-hierarchical), which employs a hierarchical CA algorithm, in order to identify clusters. When conducting CA, a number of crucial issues must be taken into consideration, such as which similarity metrics should be used to compare the items in question. How are clusters supposed to form? And how many clusters should there be in total? The most common method for comparing two objects is to employ a distance metric, where larger values (i.e., distances between cases) indicate greater dissimilarity between items. There are several ways to express the similarities and differences between two objects. Euclidean distance, or the straight-line distance between persons in the database, is the most widely used type of similarity measure when analyzing ratio or interval-scaled data, and this is what we used in these analyses. In terms of two variables, x and y, the Euclidean distance between any two objects,

$$\text{Euclidean } (d) = \sqrt{(x_2 - x_1)^2 + (y_2 - y_1)^2} \tag{7.10}$$

According to Figure 7.5, we have taken age on the x-axis and Caltech which is the maximum heart rate beats per minute (bpm) on the y-axis. From the above plot, we can interpret that maximum people in the younger age group have a higher heart rate between the range of 160 and 200 bpm while maximum middle-aged people have a heart rate between the range of 140 and –160 bpm and older people lie between the range of 80 and 130 bpm, however, some exceptions do occur.

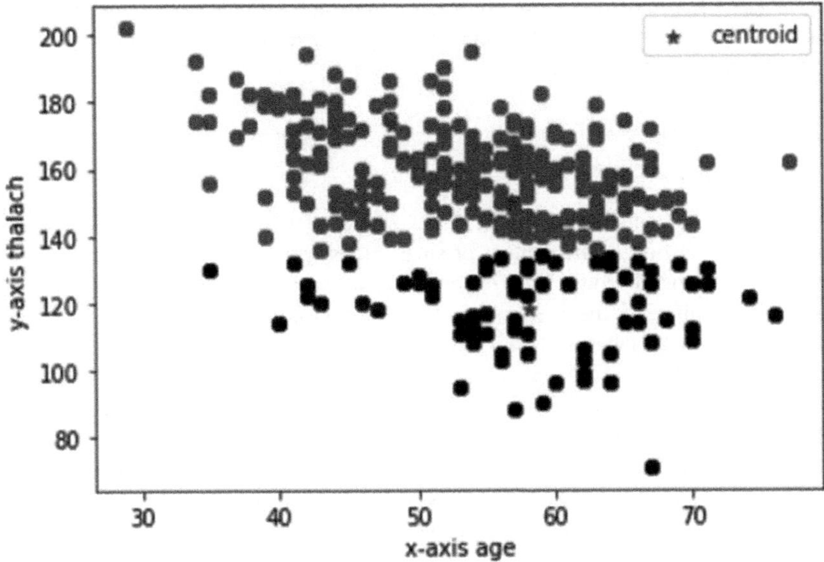

FIGURE 7.5 Clustering with outlier removal on heart disease data set with age and maximum heart rate (bpm).

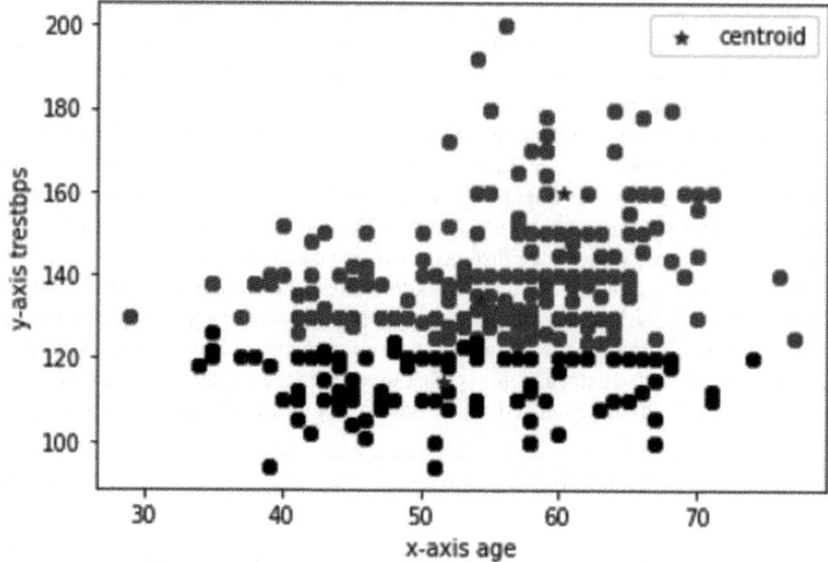

FIGURE 7.6 Clustering with outlier removal on heart disease data set with age and resting blood pressure (mm of Hg).

According to Figure 7.6, resting blood pressure is measured (mm Hg) at hospital admission on the *y*-axis and the age on the *x*-axis. From the above plot, we can interpret that maximum people in the 50–70 age group have a higher blood pressure rate in the range of 160 and 200 mm of Hg while middle-aged people in the range of 35–65 have a resting blood pressure between the range of 100 and 140 mm of Hg, however, some exceptions do occur.

7.6 Conclusion

We used the COR technique to solve the problems of simultaneous clustering and outlier identification in the context of smart cities and healthcare. In this study, we looked at the simultaneous clustering and outlier identification problem and proposed the COR technique for the healthcare industry. We initially divided the original feature space according to the correlation between outliers and clusters, which is different from the prior K-means. Next, we gave the aim function based on the holoentropy utilizing K-means optimization. Moreover, a support binary matrix was made in order for COR to fully address the challenging problem by applying K-means on the concatenated binary matrices. Extensive experimental results showed that COR greatly outperforms competitors, such as K-means and other innovative outlier identification techniques, in terms of cluster strength and outlier identification.

REFERENCES

Ankita, A. S. & Garg, A. (2023). Outlier detection system for cardiovascular disease using time-series data: A comparative analysis. In *IEEE 2nd International Conference on Industrial Electronics: Developments & Applications (ICIDeA).*

Breunig, M. M., Kriegel, H.-P., Ng, R. T., & Sander, J. (2000). Lof: identifying density-based local outliers. In *ACM SIGMOD Record*, *29*(2), 93–104.

Buettner, R., & Schunter, M. (2019). Efficient machine learning based detection of heart disease. In *IEEE International Conference on E-Health Networking*, Applications and Services (Healthcom), Bogota, Colombia, 2019, pp. 1–6, doi: 10.1109/HealthCom46333.2019.9009429

Cao, J., Chen, J., Liu, H., Liu, H., & Xiong, H. (2015). K-means-based consensus clustering: A unified view. *IEEE Transactions on Knowledge and Data Engineering*, *27*(1), 155–169.

Cao, J., Wu, J., Liu, H., & Xiong, H. (2013). A theoretic framework of k-means-based consensus clustering. In *Proceedings of the International Joint Conference on Artificial Intelligence.*

Chen, J., Wu, J., & Xiong, H. (2009). Adapting the right measures for k-means clustering. In *Proceedings of ACM SIGKDD International Conference on Data Mining and Knowledge Discovery.*

Elhamifar, E., & Vidal, R. (2013). Sparse subspace clustering: Algorithm, theory, and applications. *IEEE Transactions on Pattern Analysis and Machine Intelligence*, *35*(11), 2765–2781.

Fahim, A. M., Salem, A. M., & Torkey, F. A. (2006). An efficient enhanced k-means clustering algorithm. *Journal of Zhejiang University Science A*, *10*, 1626–1633.

Fred, A., & Jain, A. (2005). Combining multiple clusterings using evidence accumulation. *IEEE Transactions on Pattern Analysis and Machine Intelligence*, *27*(6), 835–850.

Ghosh, J., & Strehl, A. (2003). Cluster ensembles — a knowledge reuse framework for combining partitions. *Machine Learning Research Journal*, *3*, 583–617.

Guha, S., Rastogi, R., & Shim, K. (1999). ROCK: A robust clustering algorithm for categorical attributes. In *Data Engineering 1999. Proceedings. 15th International Conference on* (pp. 512–521).

Hong, M., Jing, K., & Xiong, L. (2010). Research on clustering algorithms of data streams. In *ICIME the 2nd IEEE International Conference.*

Huang, Z. (1998). Extensions to the k-Means Algorithm for Clustering Large Data Sets with Categorical Values. *Data Mining and Knowledge Discovery*, *2*(3), 283–304.

Hussain, M. W., & Roy, D. S. (2023). Performance Optimization Strategies for Big Data Applications in Distributed Framework. In *Intelligent Technologies: Concepts, Applications, and Future Directions*, Volume 2 (pp. 221–252). Singapore: Springer Nature Singapore.

Hutter, M., Zhang, K., & Jin, H. (2009). A new local distance-based outlier detection approach for scattered real-world data. In *Pacific-Asia Conference Proceedings on Data Mining and Knowledge Discovery.*

Jin, H., Zhang, K., & Hutter, M. (2009). A new local distance-based outlier detection approach for scattered real-world data. In *Pacific-Asia Conference on Data Mining and Knowledge Discovery Proceedings*, Bangkok, Thailand.

Kriegel, H. P., Kroger, P., & Zimek, A. (2010). Outlier detection techniques. In *Tutorial at the 16th ACM International Conference on Knowledge Discovery and Data Mining (SIGKDD)*, Munich, Germany.

Li, W., Mo, W., Zhang, X., Squiers, J. J., Lu, Y., Sellke, E. W., Fan, W., DiMaio, J. M., & Thatcher, J. E. (2015). Outlier detection and removal improves accuracy of machine learning approach to multispectral burn diagnostic imaging. *Journal of Biomedical Optics*, *20*(12), 121305.

Liu, H., Wu, J., Liu, T., Tao, D., & Fu, Y. (2017). Spectral ensemble clustering via weighted k-means: Theoretical and practical evidence. *IEEE Transactions on Data Engineering and Knowledge*, *29*(5), 1129–1143.

Lourenco, A., Bulò, S., Rebagliati, N., Fred, A. L. N., Figueiredo, M., & Pelillo, M. (2013). Probabilistic consensus clustering using evidence accumulation. *Machine Learning*, *98*(1-2), 331–357.

Pagh, R., & Pham, N. (2012). A near-linear time approximation algorithm for angle-based outlier detection in high-dimensional data. In *ACM SIGKDD International Conference Proceedings on Data Mining and Knowledge Discovery*, Beijing, China.

Pang, L., Ramos, F., Chawla, S., & Ott, L. (2014). On integrated clustering and outlier detection. In *Advances in Neural Information Processing Systems*. Cambridge.

Pradhan, B., Hussain, M. W., Srivastava, G., Debbarma, M. K., Barik, R. K., & Lin, J. C. W. (2022). *A Neuro-Evolutionary Approach For Software Defined Wireless Network Traffic Classification*. IET Communications, London.

Reddy, K. H. K., Roy, D. S., Mishra, T. K., & Hussain, M. W. (Eds.). (2023). *Handbook of Research on Network-Enabled IoT Applications for Smart City Services*. IGI Global, USA.

Ting, K. M., Liu, F. T., & Zhou, Z.-H. (2008). Isolation Forest. In *IEEE International Conference Proceedings on Data Mining*.

Wang, Y., Lee, Y., & Yeh, Y. (2013). Anomaly detection via online oversampling principal component analysis. *IEEE Transactions on Knowledge and Data Engineering*, *25*(7), 1460–1470.

Wati, M., Noorlah, M. S., Tejawati, A., Septiarini, A., Jamil, M., & Puspitasari, N. (2022). Implementation of the K-means clustering for the public health center data. In *International Conference on Electrical Engineering, Computer and Information Technology (ICEECIT)*.

Woo, H., Kannan, R., Aggarwal, C. C., & Park, H. (2017). Outlier detection for text data. In *International Conference on Data Mining*, USA.

Wu, J., Liu, H., Liu, T., Tao, D., & Fu, Y. (2017). Spectral ensemble clustering via weighted k-means: Theoretical and practical evidence. *IEEE Transactions on Data Engineering and Knowledge*, *29*(5), 1129–1143.

Wu, S., & Wang, S. (2013). Information-theoretic outlier detection for large-scale categorical data. *IEEE Transactions on Data Engineering and Knowledge*, *25*(3), 589–602.

Xu, R., & Wunch, D. (2005). Survey of clustering algorithms. *IEEE Transactions on Neural Networks*, *16*(3), 645–678.

Yi, J., Jin, R., Jain, S., Yang, T., & Jain, A. (2012). Semi-crowdsourced clustering: Generalizing crowd labeling by robust distance metric learning. In *Advances in Neural Information Processing Systems 25 (NIPS 2012)*.

8

Cluster Weighting—A New Clustering Technique for Outlier Removal and Noise Overlap in Healthcare Diagnosis for Smart City

N. Malathy, J. Grace Sophia, R. Sree Harini, and M. Ramya
Mepco Schlenk Engineering College, Sivakasi, India

8.1 Introduction

A smart city is an evolving urban environment that uses data-driven strategies and technology to improve the prosperity and well-being of its residents. Smart cities create an efficient and sustainable urban environment by fusing advanced technologies such as automation, artificial intelligence, Internet of Things (IoT), sensors, and other infrastructure assets with ease (Reddy et al., 2023). Using a high distance between clusters and a low distance inside each cluster, clustering is an illustration of an unsupervised learning technique used in machine learning (Hussain and Roy, 2023, Pradhan et al., 2022). It extrapolates conclusions from data sets without a target variable. We can examine multivariate data sets using this technique for exploratory data analysis. Gene expression data usually involve a large number of genes, yet there are frequently limited samples available. To solve these problems, various clustering techniques have been proposed (Daxin et al., 2004, Ruskin et al., 2007). The cancer gene data set was clustered using several conventional clustering techniques, but the outcomes of these conventional clustering techniques were frequently erratic and inaccurate. It infers results from the data sets that do not contain a target variable. It is an exploratory data analysis technique through which we can analyze multivariate data sets. Many genes are often involved in gene expression data; however, there are frequently few samples available, thus various clustering techniques have been suggested to overcome the challenges faced with gene expression data (Daxin et al., 2004; Ruskin et al., 2007). The present clustering techniques are ineffective at handling outliers, cluster overlap, and noise dimensions. All of these possible sources of mistakes are frequently present in high-throughput genomic and proteomic data, making it challenging to precisely identify logical grouping patterns (Young et al., 2016;

DOI: 10.1201/9781032631738-8

MacQueen, 1967). Homogeneity—the underlying premise of clustering—must be upheld in the overwhelming majority of tumor gene regulation data. Hierarchical clustering and data partitioning are the two primary types of clustering techniques.

Hierarchical clustering links objects based on a predetermined distance in a tree-like structure. Each object is put into a cluster on its own in hierarchical clustering. The criteria that are used to segregate the items are eased at each level of the analysis to connect the two clusters that are the most similar, and this process continues until all of the objects are joined to form a complete classification tree (Jain and Dubes, 1999). Cluster analysis aims to identify comparable groupings of subjects, where "similarity" refers to a generic assessment of all the attributes of each subject (Rousseeuw, 1987; Arnedo et al., 2013). Clusters have a variety of physical properties, including electrical, magnetic, and optical qualities. The electric characteristics of clusters, such as their conductivity and whether they are metallic or insulating, depend on both the substance and cluster size (Yang et al., 2018). Various industries, including marketing, biology, libraries, and insurance, use clustering. Data on cancer gene expression clustering has several benefits and drawbacks. Although feature weighting has been thoroughly investigated by many scholars, cluster weighting is still a relatively new concept. Many academics are working to develop a useful algorithm for classifying tumor subgroups employing genetic expression data. Researchers require accurate findings when studying cancer. Our technique overcomes the shortcomings and provides accurate results which will be helpful for bioinformaticians. We use a weighting scheme not only for individual objects but also for the cluster itself which tunes the clustering procedure and can result in accurate findings.

8.2 Related Works

To effectively cluster the data, many academics have investigated the issues of cluster overlap, noise dimensions, and outlier detection. Often, improper data clustering results from outliers dominating the data. We require an effective clustering technique that can remove outliers, perform well for data sets with noisy dimensions, and perform well for cluster overlap (Liu et al., 2018; Maderia et al., 2004). Outlier detection is critical in many fields. The concept of an object's outlier factor is broadened in the context of a cluster. This method is used to pinpoint the genes responsible for the development of cancer via recurring chromosomal translocations. Gunawardana et al. created a method to recognize the outlier post-translationally regulated proteins. Gunawardana et al. (2015) provided two methods. The authors established that outliers are trustworthy candidates for post-translational control in a variety of contexts.

To identify outliers and reduce noise, some clustering techniques automatically give feature weights (Makarenkov and Legendre, 2001; De Amorim, 2016; Tseng, 2017). Tseng introduced a brand-new clustering method utilizing a weighted variant of K-means that assigns a weight to each item in the data set (Tseng, 2017). The objects cannot be given weights automatically using Tseng's method (Tseng, 2017). All of the weights must be predefined and remain constant during the clustering procedure. Wei Yang et al. (2020) showed how the shortcomings of poor clustering outcomes caused by the optimal local setting and excessive intra-cluster variance can be significantly reduced by using an adjusted distance volume calculation approach to determine an information set's density throughout the K-means grouping procedure. According to Alexander et al. (2021) and Shen et al. (2010), who recommended a clustering method that assigns weights to each object based on the silhouette, median, and two inter-cluster weighting schemes, the median was determined to be the best weighing system. Each object that is detected is given a weight via an innovative blending technique devised by Gebru et al. (2016) and Kerdprasop et al. (2005). Two expectation–maximization (EM) methods exist. Each object in the first has a constant weight, while each weight in the second is regarded as an unpredictable variable using a gamma distribution. To identify the presence of distributed noise genes, Shen et al. (2010) and Gebru et al. (2016) introduced a weighted clustering method that makes use of functional annotation data. The normalized dispersions of the grouped genes are combined to generate the objective function. Shen et al.'s method (Gebru et al., 2016) utilizes group-specific weights so that each of the genes that make up a part of the same group have the same weights, contrary to Tseng's method (Tseng, 2017), which utilizes individual weights of genes. FeipingNie et al. (2023), by the reweighted approach concept, provided a new weight learning paradigm in the context of multi-view clustering. Zhiqiang Fu et al. proposed a technique to improve the discrimination of the learned affinity matrix, a weighted distance penalty is incorporated into the LatLRR model by leveraging on the weighted distance (2023). This allows the technique to conserve both global and local geometric information. James Lee et al. proposed pixel intensity-weighted K-means clustering (PIKC) to stop biased coordinates from being detected (2023). By assigning touch pixel intensity values as weights during the centroid update procedure of clustering, PIKC can identify unbiased coordinates.

In this chapter, we present a weighting algorithm that takes clusters and individual items into account. The performance of this approach is compared to that of the popular X-means (Pelleg and Moore, 2000), K-means (Tibshirani and Walther, 2005), and feature-weighted K-means algorithms (Jombart et al., 2010).

8.3 Methodology

The conventional K-means algorithm is still the most often used clustering technique. The number of successful clusters produced is a gauge of how well the K-means clustering approach works. The key objective here is to select the appropriate amount of clusters. Although there are various approaches to determining the appropriate number of clusters, the one we present here is the most successful. The elbow approach uses WCSS (within cluster sum of squares) data to estimate the appropriate number of clusters. The total variances found inside a cluster are provided by WCSS using equation 1:

$$\text{WCSS} = \begin{array}{l} \sum\limits_{\text{Li in Cluster1}} \text{distance}\,(L_i, C_1)^2 + \\ \sum\limits_{\text{Li in Cluster2}} \text{distance}\,(L_i \times C_2)^2 + \\ \sum\limits_{\text{Li in CLuster3}} \text{distance}\,(L_i \times C_3)^2 \end{array} \quad (1)$$

The most important changes to the k-means approach have been explored by MacQueen, Hartigan Wong, and Lloyd. It tries to divide n data points into k groups, where each observation belongs to a cluster and the prototype of the cluster is the nearest mean. This vector quantization technique has its roots in signal processing. The technique starts with a random initialization of the centroids. At each iteration, an object x is assigned to the cluster Sk, if its center is nearest to the object. After each iteration, the group's centers are updated. Thus, what comes next is the objective function given in equation 2:

$$\sum_{k=1}^{K}\sum_{x_i \in Sk} wi\left(\sum_{v=1}^{V}(x_{iv} - C_{kv})\right)^2 \tag{2}$$

where $c_k \in C$ is the cluster number and $v = 1, \ldots, V$ are the attributes describing the items in x. To get accurate results, the algorithm has to be run thousands of times, especially when dealing with gene expression data. To overcome this particular limitation, we add weights to each object and thus in the computation equation the weight is also included as follows in equation 3:

$$L(S,C,w) = \sum_{k=1}^{K}\sum_{x_i \in Sk} wi\left(\sum_{v=1}^{V}(x_{iv} - C_{kv})^2\right) \tag{3}$$

where w_i is the calculated object weight for the ith object. However, to obtain reliable findings, we compute weights for each cluster using various weighting algorithms, and each item is given a cluster weight. The fact that all the elements in a specific cluster have the same weights is intriguing. Clustering effectiveness will increase because cluster weights shorten intra-cluster distances while lengthening inter-cluster distances. After adding cluster weights (W), the object's K-means objective function will be as follows in equation 4:

$$L(S,C,w,W) = \sum_{k=1}^{K}\sum_{x_i \in Sk} W(wi(\sum_{v=1}^{V}(x_{iv} - C_{kv})^2 \tag{4}$$

where W is the calculated cluster weight to which the object belongs. The effective clustering properties of the items are strongly supported by the cluster weights. By giving some items low weights and the outliers large weights, the outliers will be punished.

8.3.1 Different Weighting Approaches

Figure 8.1 describes the overall system architecture. This section deals with the different weighting approaches that are used to calculate the weights for each object and cluster. The different approaches used here are the median weighting approach, silhouette weighting approach, the nearest centroid weighting approach, and the sum of distances weighting approach.

In this trade-off approach, the width of an object's silhouette determines its silhouette (Jain and Dubes, 1999). The Euclidean distance that exists between a given object

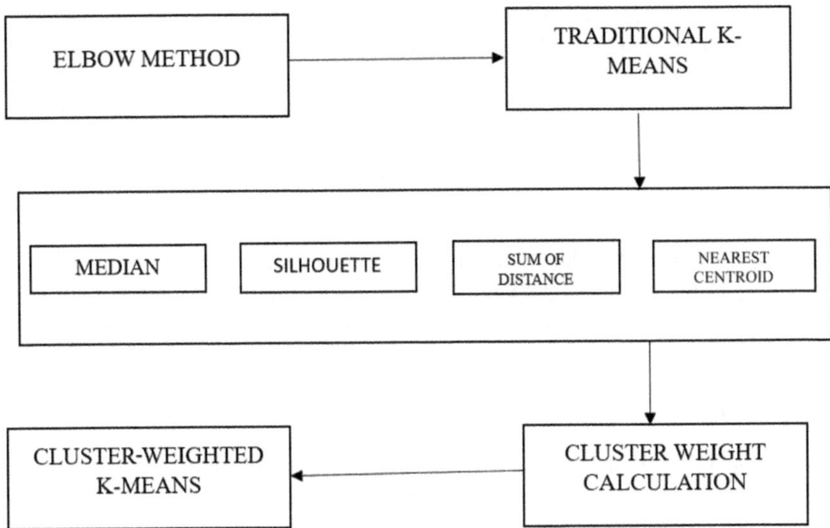

FIGURE 8.1 System architecture.

and the cluster's median serves as the foundation for the median weighting strategy. Based on the item's squared Euclidean distance from the closest centroid of the group to which it does not belong, a nearest-neighbor centroid ranking technique is utilized. The "sum of weights" weighting method is based on the squared Euclidean distance between the centroid of an item group and the center points of all other clusters.

The weight calculation is done using an additional constraint that requires the total weight of objects in a cluster to match the total weight of the objects. Thus, the weight calculation based on the above constraints is calculated as follows using equation 5:

$$\omega_i(\mathrm{n}_\mathrm{k}) = \frac{\omega_i}{\sum_{j \in S_k} \omega j} \times n_k \tag{5}$$

where n_k indicates the total number of objects in the cluster S_k, ω_i is the object's weight x_i calculated using the weighting schemes, and $\sum_{j \in S_k} \omega j$ represents the total weights of all objects in the cluster S_k.

8.3.1.1 Silhouette Weighting Approach

Silhouette is a method that interprets and validates the consistency of data within the clusters. The silhouette is between -1 and +1. The item is appropriately assigned to its group and incorrectly matched to nearby clusters, as indicated by the high value. To determine x_i's weight, begin with the silhouette's width is determined using equation 6.

$$s_i = \frac{zi - yi}{\max(xi, yi)} \tag{6}$$

where z_i is the mean distance between item x_i and all other objects in its group of which x_i is not a member and y_i is the minimal mean separation amongst item x_i and all other objects in its cluster.

The following formula given in equation 7 is used to determine each object's weight:

$$\omega_i = \frac{1 - x_i}{2}, \text{for all i} = 1, \ldots, n \tag{7}$$

where x_i is the object's width of the silhouette. This section provides us with the details pertaining to the myriad of paradigms that exist in the present world to address the application requirements. Also, the merits and limitations of each paradigm have been discussed.

8.3.1.2 Median Weighting Approach

The median is the middle number of an increasingly sorted list of numbers. It describes more about the data set than the mean. Also, compared to the mean, the median is more specific to outliers. Hence, more reliable estimates of the mean can be easily obtained using the median than the mean. But there is a point to be noted that the median is not always better than the mean as given in equation 8.

$$w_i = \sqrt{\sum_{b=1}^{B} \left(x_{ib} - Mdn_{kb}\right)^2} \tag{8}$$

where Mdn_{kvb} is the cluster's median value for feature b.

8.3.1.3 Distance with the Nearest Centroid Weighting Approach

To calculate the squared Euclidean measurement between two objects, this weighting method aims to identify the median of the cluster S_k that is closest to which the item x_i does not belong. In this case, the object's weight will be lower since it is further away from the center of an alternate group, which is closer. This is exactly the weight of the object x_i is calculated using equation 9:

$$\mathrm{Wi} = \frac{1}{\min \mathrm{s}_{\mathrm{k} \neq \mathrm{Sk}'} \sum_{\mathrm{v}=1}^{\mathrm{v}} \left(\mathrm{x}_{\mathrm{i}}\mathrm{b}^{-\mathrm{c}}\mathrm{k}'\mathrm{b}\right)^2}, \tag{9}$$

where $c_{k'}$ is the median of the group $S_{k'}$, which is distinct from S_k, and S_k is the group in which x_i is present, and S_k' is the group in which x_i is absent.

8.3.1.4 Cluster Weights

The sum of distances to the center of another group, the distance to the centroid of the closest cluster, the mean weighing technique, the silhouette balancing method, and other weighting approaches are used to calculate cluster weights. Cluster weights are the name of this inter-cluster weighing system. The cluster weights enhance the clustering quality by giving the object's identity more clarity using equation 10.

$$Wk = \frac{\sum_{v=1}^{V} xi}{nk} \tag{10}$$

where W_k is the weight for cluster k. This cluster weight is identical to the objects present in its cluster. Hence, it is not much variant.

8.4 Cluster Weighted (CW) K-Means

Our cluster balanced K-means approach is next used, which is then followed by the conventional K-means algorithm as reported by Hartigan and Wong (1979). Additionally, it adheres to the object weighting K-means algorithm outlined by Zahia Aouabed et al. and Alexander Gondeau.

8.5 Cluster Weighting on the Iris Data

To illustrate the potency of the group-weighted K-means approach, the data set on the iris (Jain and Dubes, 1988) is combined with several weighting schemes. The Calinski–Harabasz (CH) (Romanski, 2009) cluster validation index suggested the best

ALGORITHM 1. Cluster Weighted K-Means

Input:

- The data set Z with m objects is now incorporated by the data set the object weighting approach (different weighting approach 1–4 defined in Section 8.3.1 cluster weight assignment.

Output:

- effective clustering according to the selected weighting approach.

1. **Setting parameters**
   Select the initial number of clusters L and the weighting approach.
2. **Selecting initial cluster centers**
   Select L objects from Z randomly and assign them as initial cluster centers $c_1, c_2, c_3, c_4, \ldots, c_L$.
3. **Updation of Cluster**
   It is the cluster-weighted Euclidian distance equation used to calculate the distance.
4. **Final Step**
   The iteration should be stopped and the result should be produced if M' = M or the maximum number of iterations has been achieved. Go to step 3 if not.

TABLE 8.1
Summary of the Data Sets Used in Our Study

Cancer Type	Data Set	Objects	Classes
Breast	Kaggle	2147	5
Multi-tissue	Kaggle	4400	10
Brain	Kaggle	2220	5
Lung	Kaggle	2102	7
Blood	Kaggle	3425	5

clustering approach based on the results of several clustering methods after the 100th iteration. Cluster weights with high values inside cluster overlap have been obtained using silhouette-based clustering. Penalties were applied to items with significant levels of instability and cluster overlap from that cause. On the other hand, outlier objects were penalized via median-based grouping. For datasets with outliers, it performs well. Therefore, the median is used to penalize the outliers while the silhouette is used to penalize the objects that cause cluster overlap and excessive instability. Table 8.1 shows the data set used in this chapter.

8.6 Results

To compare the accuracy of our cluster-weighted K-means method with other renowned algorithms for clustering including K-means, X-means, and Feature-weighted K-means, we conducted a detailed simulation study by determining the predicted number of clusters. Figures 8.2–8.6 show the error rate for the given data set.

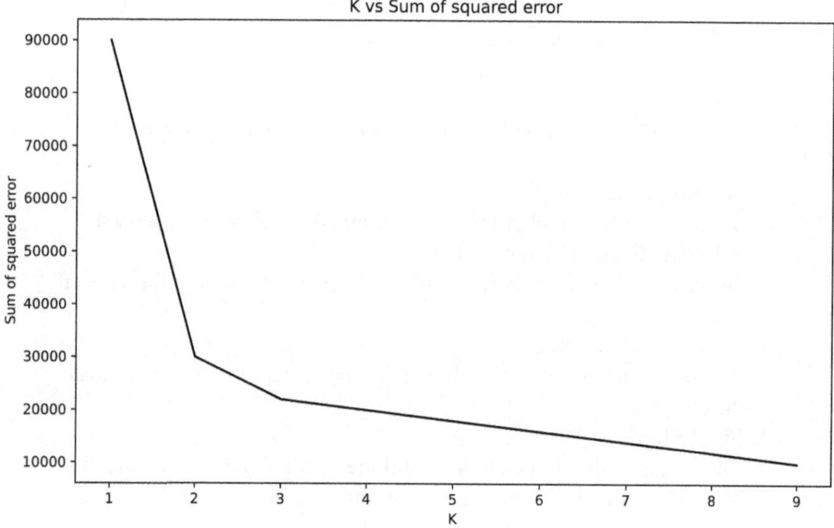

FIGURE 8.2 Elbow method.

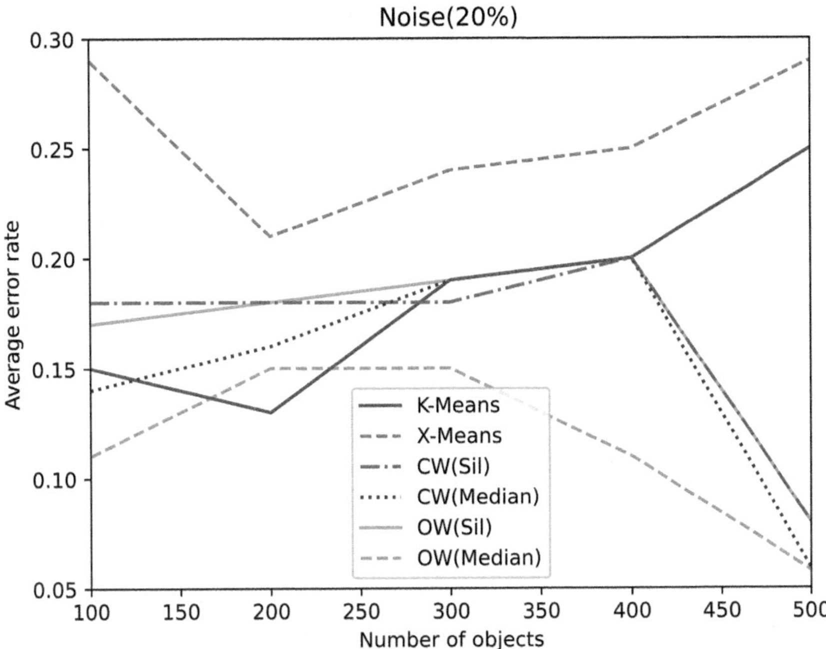

FIGURE 8.3 The data set's normalized error rate with 20% noise.

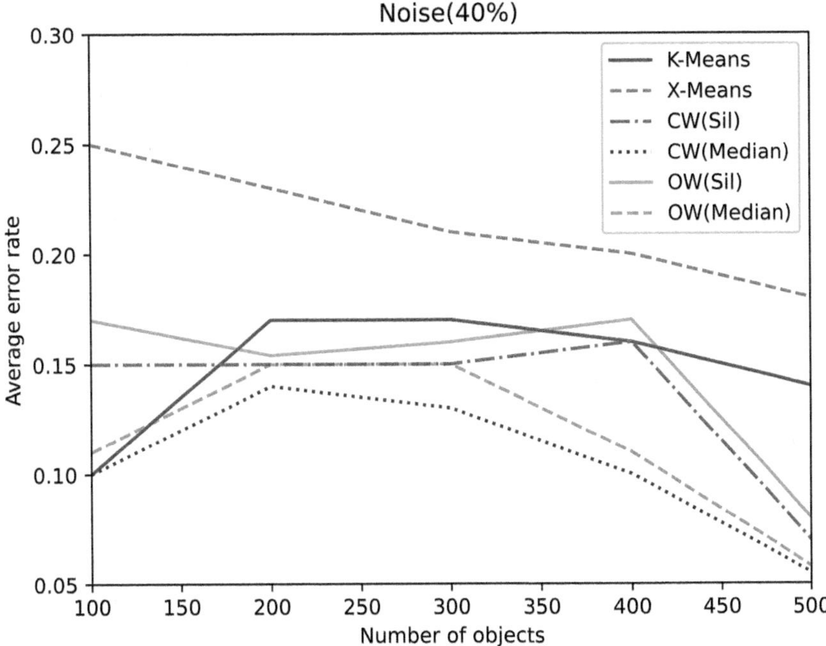

FIGURE 8.4 The data set's normalized error rate with 40% noise.

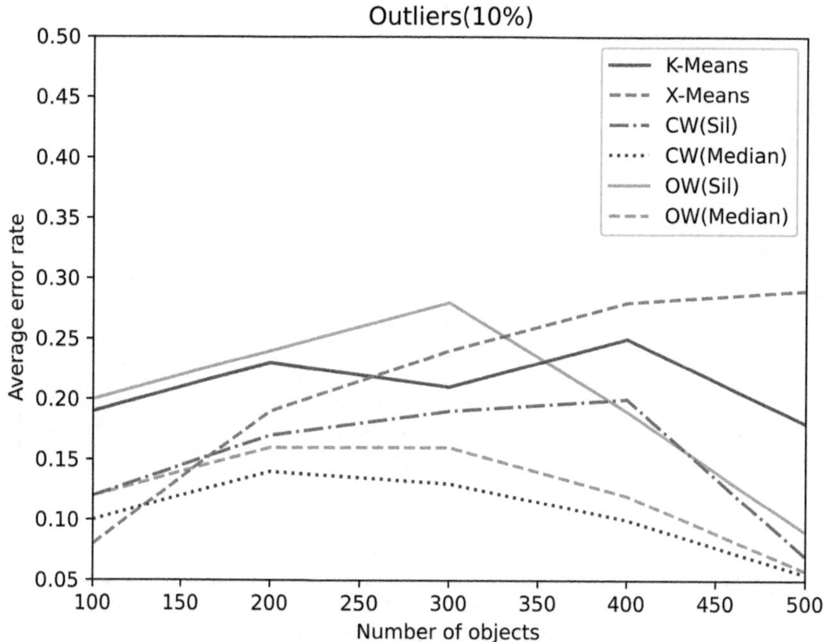

FIGURE 8.5 The average error rate for the data set with 10% outliers.

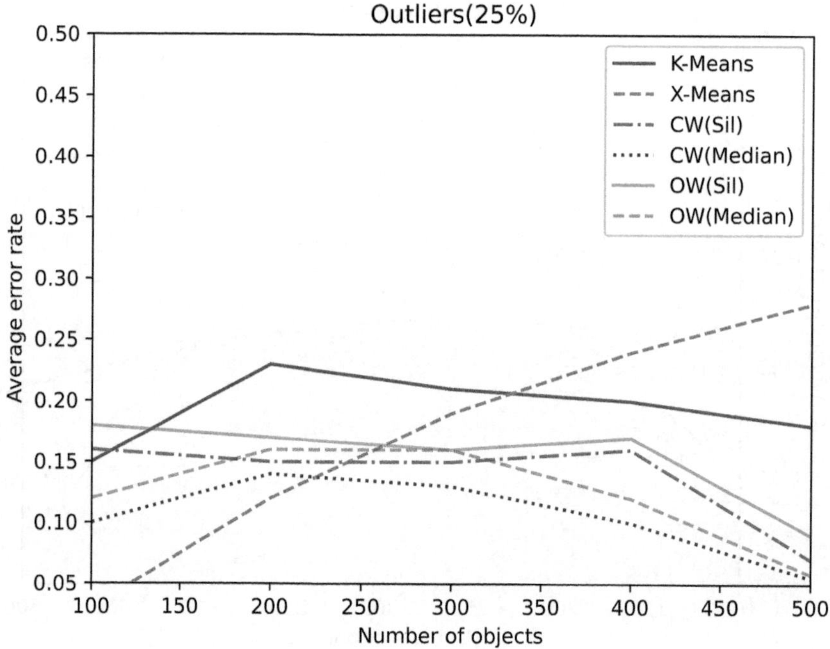

FIGURE 8.6 The average error rate for the data set with 25% Outliers.

8.6.1 Simulation Study

We used the mixSim R package, which replicates distributions of Gaussian shape with various levels of cluster overlap, for comparing and evaluating the best weighting strategy. Second, we used a 20% noise threshold while plotting the data. Third, we created a graphic of data with 10% outliers. By creating the Gaussian groups for 100 randomly assigned data sets, and then standardizing them by the z-score, competition (i.e., mean error rate) was calculated. The mean absolute variance between the total amount of clusters produced and the number provided by competing methods is displayed as competition. To count the clusters, CH or silhouette were utilized.

In the first simulation, we used a silhouette-based CW K-means method and compared the results with those of a traditional K-means approach. Additionally, we compared the CW-K mean values based on the median values. We then ran two other weighted schedules and compared the results with the traditional K-means approach. The true number of clusters was selected using silhouette or CH for each weight-based CW-K mean. Different weighting systems gave very different results for data with 20% noise and 40% noise and with 10% outliers and 25% outliers. For data with outliers, median (nk) produced more accurate results and outperformed alternative weighting schemes such as median WS using silhouette and median WS using CH index. Furthermore, it outperformed OW (median) and OW (silhouette) in terms of superior results. For data affected by cluster overlap, the median WS result based on the CH index performed better than the other results, whereas, for data affected by noise, the silhouette (nk) approach showed better performance. Figures 8.7–8.10 show the silhouette weighting, median weighting, nearest centroid weighting, and sum of distance weighting approaches, respectively. Figures 8.11 and 8.12 show the mean absolute difference and success rate.

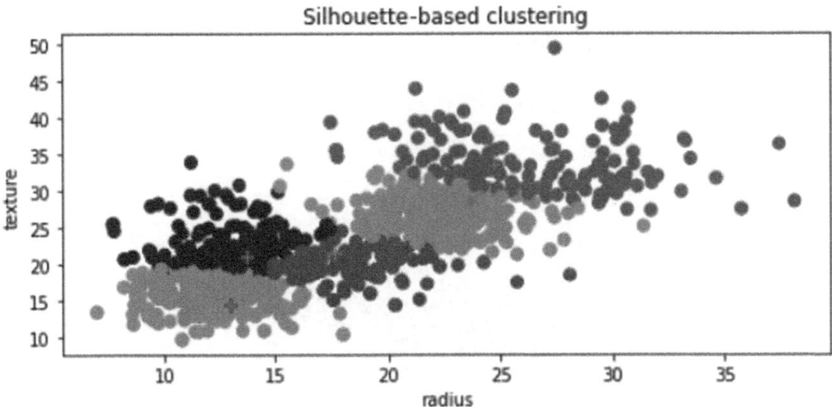

FIGURE 8.7 Silhouette weighting approach.

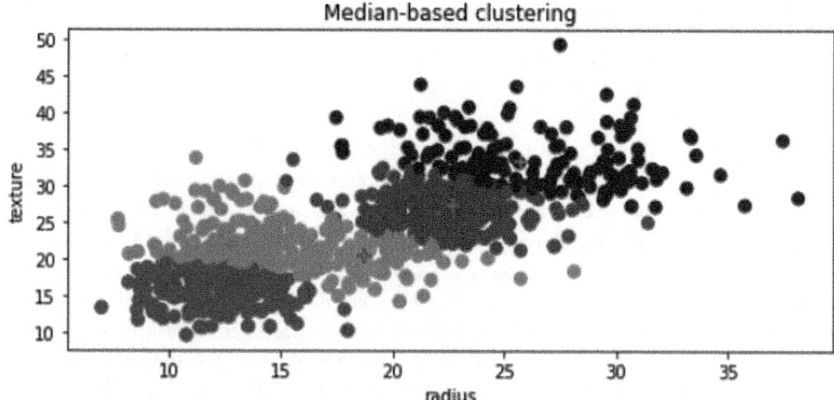

FIGURE 8.8 Median weighting approach.

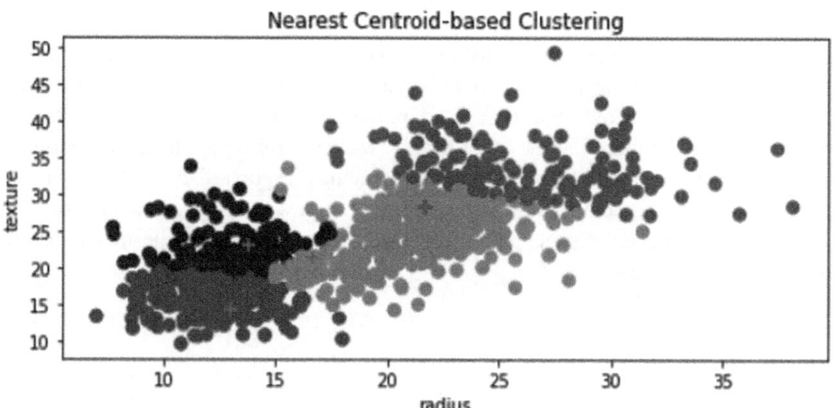

FIGURE 8.9 Nearest centroid weighting approach.

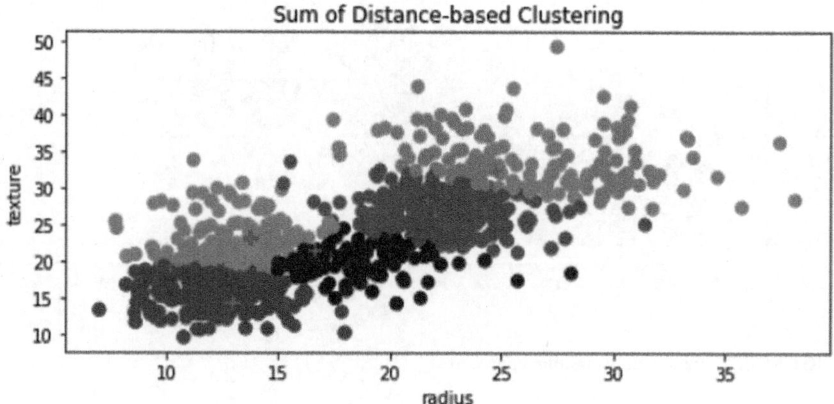

FIGURE 8.10 Sum of distance weighting approach.

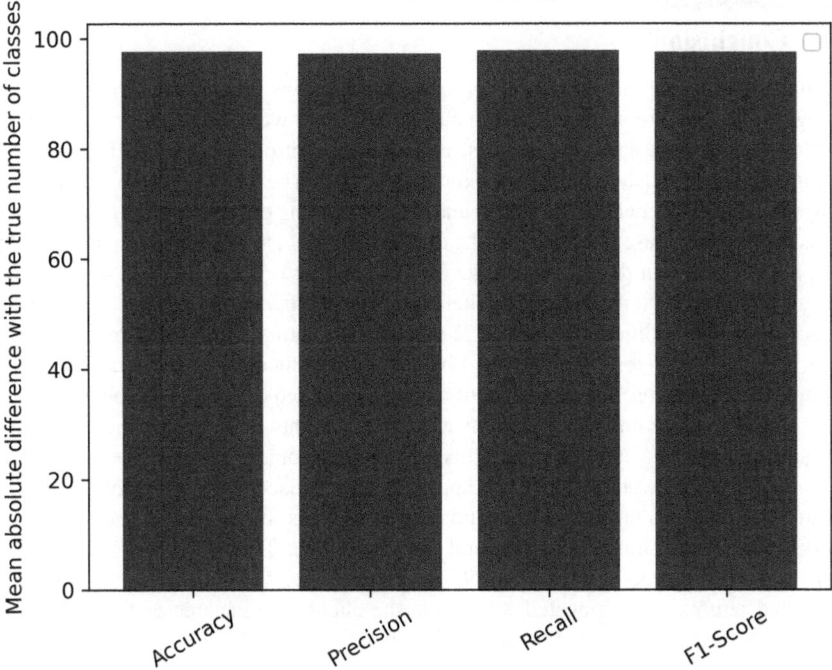

FIGURE 8.11 Mean absolute difference.

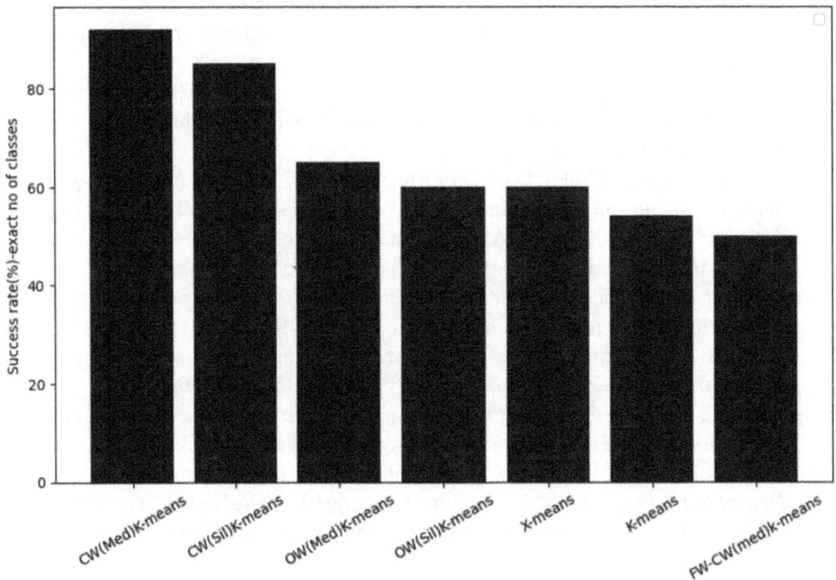

FIGURE 8.12 Success rate.

8.7 Conclusion

In this research, we introduced cluster-weighted K-means, a novel clustering methodology for healthcare applications in smart cities. Four weighting schemes including silhouette, median, sum of distances, and nearest centroid were used. Using these weighting schemes, the cancer gene expression data can be well clustered. The weighting schemes will penalize the outliers and objects causing cluster overlap. Outliers and cluster overlaps cause instability in the clusters. Outliers are the lone data points that are not clustered. In the case of outliers, K-means' performance is quite subpar. The result produced by our algorithm is then compared with various well-known existing algorithms like traditional K-means, X-means, and feature-weighted K-means. Also, we compared our results with the object-weighted-median and object-weighted-silhouette algorithms. The main goal of our work is to detect outliers and objects causing cluster overlap and provide them with high weights to eliminate the clustering instability. Since we add cluster weights in addition to object weights, the outliers are given a very high weight. Thus, our approach can be used to get efficient clustering results for data sets having outliers and cluster overlaps. It can also be used as a preprocessing tool to eliminate outliers and cluster overlaps. The cluster weights could be encrypted and passed to a server where the server collects weights from multiple clients and returns the aggregated weights to the clients. This increases the clustering efficiency further. This could be our future work.

REFERENCES

Alexander G. et al., (2021). Object Weighting: A New Clustering Approach to Deal with Outliers and Cluster Overlap in Computational Biology. *IEEE/ACM Trans. Comput. Biol. Bioinform.*, *18*, 2. https://doi.org/10.1109/TCBB.2019.2921577

Arbelaitz O. et al., (2013). An extensive comparative study of cluster validity indices. *Pattern Recognit.*, *46*, 243–256, https://doi.org/10.1016/j.patcog.2012.07.021

Beaudet D. et al., (2013). Mitochondrial genome rearrangements in Glomus species triggered by homologous recombination between distinct mtDNA haplotypes. *Genome Biol. Evol.*, *5*, 1628–1643.

Bertrand P. and Mufti G. (2006). Loevinger's measures of rule quality for assessing cluster stability. *Comput. Stat. Data Anal.*, *50*, 992–1015. https://doi.org/10.1093/gbe/evt120

Calinski J. and Harabasz T., (1974) A dendrite method for cluster analysis. *Commun. Stat. Theory Methods*, *3*, 1–27. https://doi.org/10.1080/03610927408827101

Daxin J., Chun T. and, Aidong Z. (2004). *Cluster analysis for gene expression data*. Cambridge University Press. https://doi.org/10.4137/BBI.S38316

De Amorim R.C., (2016). A survey on feature weighting based k-means algorithms. *J. Classif.*, *33*, 210–242. https://doi.org/10.1007/s00357-016-9208-4

De Souto M.C. et al., (2008). Clustering cancer gene expression data: a comparative study. *BMC Bioinformatics*, *9*, 497. https://doi.org/10.1186/1471-2105-9-497

Feiping N. et al., (2023). Implicit weight learning for multi-view clustering. *IEEE Trans. Neural Netw. Learn. Syst.*, *34*(I8). https://doi.org/10.1109/TNNLS.2021.3121246

Fisher R.A., (1936). The use of multiple measurements in taxonomic problems. *Ann. Eugen.*, *7* 179–188.

Gebru I.D., Alameda-Pineda X., Forbes F. and Horaud R., (2016). EM algorithms for weighted-data clustering with application to audio-visual scene analysis. *IEEE*

Trans. Pattern Anal. Mach. Intell., *38*(12), 2402–2415. https://doi.org/10.1109/TPAMI.2016.2522425

Gunawardana Y. et al., (2015). Outlier detection at the transcriptome-proteome interface. *Bioinformatics*, *31*, 2530–2536. https://doi.org/10.1093/bioinformatics/btv182

Hartigan J.A. and Wong M.A., (1979). Algorithm AS 136: A k-means clustering algorithm. *J.R. Stat. Soc.*, *28*, 100–108. https://doi.org/10.2307/2346830

Hong L., (2017). BioSeqClass: classification for biological sequences. *R Package*. https://doi.org/10.1093/nar/gkz740

Hubert L. and Arabie P., (1988). Comparing Partitions. *J. Classification*, *2*(4), 193–218. https://doi.org/10.1007/BF01908075

Hussain, M. W. and Roy, D. S. (2023). Performance optimization strategies for big data applications in distributed framework. In *Intelligent Technologies: Concepts, Applications, and Future Directions*, Volume 2 (pp. 221–252). Singapore: Springer Nature Singapore.

Pradhan, B., Hussain, M. W., Srivastava, G., Debbarma, M. K., Barik, R. K., and Lin, J. C. W. (2022). *A Neuro-Evolutionary Approach for Software Defined Wireless Network Traffic Classification*. IET Communications.

Jain A.K. and Dubes R.C. (1988). *Algorithms for clustering data*. Prentice-Hall. https://doi.org/10.5555/46712

Jain A.K. and Dubes R.C. (1999). *Algorithms for clustering data*. Prentice-Hall. https://doi.org/10.5555/46712

Jain A.K. et al., (2012). Data Clustering: A review. *ACM Comput. Surv*. https://doi.org/10.1145/331499.331504

James L. et al., (2023). Classification network-guided weighted k-means clustering for multitouch detection. *IEEE Sensors J.*, *23*(18). https://doi.org/10.1109/JSEN.2023.3292288

Jombart T. et al., (2010). DAPC: A new method for the analysis of genetically structured populations. *BMC Genetics*, *11*(94). https://doi.org/10.1186/1471-2156-11-94

Kerdprasop K., Kerdprasop N. and Sattayatham P., (2005). Weighted K-means for density-biased clustering. In *Data Warehousing and Knowledge Discovery* (pp. 488–497). Berlin Heidelberg: Springer. https://doi.org/10.1007/11546849_48

Liu X. et al., (2018). Analyzing outliers cautiously. *Bioinformatics*, bty793, in press. https://doi.org/10.1093/bioinformatics/btn012

Lloyd S., (1982). Least squares quantization in PCM. *IEEE Trans. Inf. Theory*, *28*, 129–137. https://doi.org/10.1109/TIT.1982.1056489

MacDonald J.W. and Ghosh D., (2006). COPA - cancer outlier profile analysis. *Bioinformatics*, *22*, 2950–2951. https://doi.org/10.1093/bioinformatics/btl433

MacQueen J., (1967). Some methods for classification and analysis of multivariate observations. *Proceedings of the fifth Berkeley symposium on mathematical statistics and probability*, pp. 281–297. https://doi.org/10.1504/ijdmb.2015.067955

Maderia S.D. et al., (2004). Biclustering algorithms for biological data analysis: a survey. *IEEE/ACM Trans. Comput. Biol. Bioinform*. https://doi.org/10.1109/TCBB.2004.2

Makarenkov V. and Legendre, P. (2001). Optimal variable weighting for ultrametric and additive trees and k-means partitioning: Methods and software. *J. Classif.*, *18*, 245–271. https://doi.org/10.1007/s00357-001-0018-x

Manikandan S., (2011). Measures of central tendency: Median and mode. *J. Pharmacol. Pharmacother.*, *2*, 214–215. https://doi.org/10.4103/0976-500X.83300

Melnykov V. et al., (2012). MixSim: An R package for simulating data to study performance of clustering algorithms. *J. Stat. Softw.*, *51*, 1–25. https://doi.org/10.18637/jss.v051.i12

Pelleg D. and Moore A.W. June (2000). X-means: extending k-means withefficient estimation ofthe number of clusters. *Proc. ICML*, pp. 727–734. https://doi.org/10.5555/645529.657808

Reddy, K. H. K., Roy, D. S., Mishra, T. K., and Hussain, M. W. (Eds.). (2023). *Handbook of Research on Network-Enabled IoT Applications for Smart City Services*. IGI Global.

Romanski P., (2009). FSelector: Selecting Attributes, R Foundation for Statistical Computing, Vienna. *Bioinformatics*, *13*, 2247–2255. https://doi.org/10.1093/bioinformatics/bts528

Rousseeuw P.J., (1987). Silhouettes: a graphical aid to the interpretation and validation of cluster analysis. *Comput. Appl. Math.,20*, 53–65. https://doi.org/10.1016/0377-0427(87)90125-7

Ruskin H.J., Crane M. et al., (2007). Techniques for clustering gene expression data. *Curr. Bioinformatics*. https://doi.org/10.5772/intechopen.94069

Shannon P. et al., (2003)Cytoscape: A software environment for integrated models of biomolecular interaction networks. *Genome Res.*, *13*, 2498–2504. https://doi.org/10.1101/gr.1239303

Shen Y.J., Sun W., and Li K.C., (2010). Dynamically weighted clustering with noise set. *Bioinformatics*, *26*(3), 341–347. https://doi.org/10.1093/bioinformatics/btp671

Smith S.E. and Read D.J., (2008). *Mycorrhizal symbiosis*. Academic Press.

Arnedo-Pac C., Mularoni L., Muiños F., Gonzalez-Perez A. and Lopez-Bigas N. (2013). OncodriveCLUSTL: a sequence-based clustering method to identify cancer drivers. *Bioinformatics (Oxford, England)*, *35*(22), 4788–4790. https://doi.org/10.1093/bioinformatics/btz501

Tibshirani R. and Walther R., 2005. Cluster validation by prediction strength. *J. Comput. Graph. Stat.*, *14*, 511–528. https://doi.org/10.1198/106186005X59243

Tseng G.C., (2017). Penalized and weighted k-means for clustering. *Bioinformatics*, *23*, 2237–2245. https://doi.org/10.1093/bioinformatics/btm320

Wei Y. et al., (2020). Weights on clustering based on weighted distance density and k-means. Procedia Computer Center, with scattered objects and prior information in high-throughput biological data. *Bioinformatics*, *23*, 2247–2255. https://doi.org/10.1016/j.procs.2020.02.056

Yang Y. et al., (2018). SAFE-clustering: single-cell aggregated (from ensemble) clustering for single-cell RNA-seq data. *Bioinformatics*, bty793, in press. https://doi.org/10.1093/bioinformatics/bty793

Yang, W. et al. (2020) Research on Clustering Method Based on Weighted Distance Density and K-Means. *Procedia Computer Science*, *166*, 507–511. https://doi.org/10.1016/j.procs.2020.02.056.

Young J.H. et al., (2016). Computational discovery of pathway-level genetic vulnerabilities in non-small-cell lung cancer. *Bioinformatics*, *32*, 1373–1379. https://doi.org/10.1093/bioinformatics/btw010

Zhiqiang F. et al., (2023). Latent low-rank representation with weighted distance penalty for clustering. *IEEE Transactions on Cybernetics*, *53*(11), November. https://doi.org/10.1109/TCYB.2022.3166545

9

Blockchain-Enabled Secured Patient-Centric Data for Smart City Service

V. Sudha
Government Polytechnic College, India

D. Aswini
Kumaraguru College of Technology, India

P. Nancy
SRM Institute of Science and Technology, India

R. Akiladevi
Rajalakshmi Engineering College, Chennai, India

9.1 Introduction

In a growing country like India, cities have a very large effect. It is predicted that by 2030, the cities are going to contribute 75% of our countries' GDP (Ministry, 2015). In this regard, our government has targeted to modernize the cities by introducing the smart city project. The implementation of this project varies from city to city depending upon the individual requirement. This project's major objective is to give people access to environments with reliable electricity, appropriate water supplies, and other amenities that promote good health and education. When considering the health of people, it is important to consider the city because this place is the reason for the outburst of many diseases.

The above facility is achieved using sensors which collect data from various devices and make them automated. Since smartness involves huge data collection, care must be taken to handle the same (Hussain and Roy, 2023). The smart city strives to provide good clinical, mental, social, emotional, physical, and spiritual health (Reddy et al., 2023). If this has to be achieved then data becomes a crucial factor. Patient health record maintenance is a dynamic area that needs to be improved always to sustain the necessity of users.

Telemedicine system is one of the solutions to the above problem. This system helps in identifying the diseases based on the data and patterns (Sahatiya and Singh, 2023). To satisfy user needs, the dynamic field of maintaining PHRs needs to be endlessly improved. The PHR includes the patient's medical history, current treatments,

DOI: 10.1201/9781032631738-9

immunization record, insurance information, and other details. For an effective healthcare system, updating the patient's record every time he/she receives treatment or a vaccination is necessary. This update is significant as it sets the foundation for future treatments. Also, this record needs to be kept securely as it contains sensitive information about a patient.

This chapter covers the basics of blockchain, the importance of health data in smart cities, the different methods that can be used to store health records, as well as the benefits and drawbacks of each.

9.2 Blockchain Fundamentals

9.2.1 Blockchain and Its Features

Blockchain is a distributed database where the contents once stored cannot be removed. Each of the participating nodes in the network broadcasts the data as transaction to every other node using the gossiping protocol. These messages accumulate in the mining pool of the respective node. The node randomly selects a few messages from the pool and forms the block. Only the minor nodes in the network are responsible for block creation. Each of the miner nodes competes to form the block. The block of the miner who wins the race is added to the blockchain. There are various protocols available in the literature for this selection and accordingly the winner is chosen. The hash of the transactions existing in a block is used for linking one block to another. This makes the blocks tamper as the modification of any value within it may lead to a change in the hash value. The tamper-proof nature of the blockchain makes the content not editable.

9.2.2 Blockchain Types

In the literature, there are four distinct varieties of blockchain. They are public, private, consortium, and hybrid blockchain.

- **Public blockchain**

  In this blockchain, anyone can join and leave at anytime. Anyone who is willing to join can join and do transactions. Though the procedure is very simple, there is a lot of security issues. Example: Ethereum.
- **Private Blockchain**

  Permission is needed for joining and creating transactions in the case of private blockchain. This kind of blockchain is mostly used by many enterprises because of the security it provides.
- **Consortium Blockchain**

Consortium blockchains are semi-private in nature where many companies collaborate. Hyperledger is an example of a consortium blockchain.

- **Hybrid Blockchain**

  Blockchain technology that is hybrid combines the advantages of both public and private chains. The program can determine the type of blockchain to use.

9.2.3 Role of Smart Contract in Healthcare

Smart contracts are the pieces of code which get executed when certain conditions are met. This is usually stored in the blockchain. Smart contract finds its application in all the places where certain norms need to be satisfied. In healthcare, smart contracts can be used in the following applications: health insurance claims, patient agreements during medical emergencies, clinical trials, supply chain management, health record management, drug tracing systems, remote monitoring, etc.

9.2.4 Smart Cities and Healthcare

A smart city is an urban area using a variety of sensors, electrical and electronic devices, collects data and analysis, and acts accordingly. By 2050, countries most of the population will be residing in cities. As a result, it is crucial to focus on the health of those who live in cities. The data may be collected from the people residing in the city, buildings, vehicles, electronic equipment, etc., analyzed and used for further action. In smart cities, Internet of Things (IoT) plays a vital role. The following are some of the key aspects of healthcare in smart cities.

1. Smart cities allow their citizen to access the medicinal benefits remotely.
2. Various types of digital health records must be integrated into the healthcare system.
3. IoT devices can be used for tracking the health of the citizens.
4. Analytics applied to the data collected from the city may be used for predicting the place of the outbreak and planning to manage the resources efficiently.
5. It must include a few mobile health access points and IoT-enabled medical facilities.
6. Secured platform must exist for the exchange of patient data between health service providers.

Thus, a smart city must include the features and technologies that improve the health of the residents. In all the above key features, protecting the data collected from the individuals is very much important. Particularly, the health-related details must be safely maintained as they are sensitive.

Healthcare system integrates various entities and provides healthcare services to the target population. Healthcare in smart cities may employ some advanced technologies to provide a smart health service. Few of them are discussed in this section.

- **Remote health monitoring**: Smart city facilities allow the residents to access the medical facilities in online mode through video calls. Also, the user will able to call the ambulance service through SMS and track the location of the service from their location (Poongodi et al., 2021).
- **IoT-enabled health services**: IoT devices help us to collect data very quickly from the end user and indirectly aid in fast prediction. This technology also introduces wearable devices and interaction among different devices (Goyal et al., 2021).

- **Electronic health record (EHR)**: When remote data access needs to be facilitated, then it is necessary to maintain interoperable data records. EHR is one such facility.
- **Smart hospitals**: Smart hospitals include the usage of robots for treatment, automatic operating system, etc.

9.2.5 Novel Use Cases

A smart city and blockchain integration would allow for efficient patient health monitoring. For example, it would be possible to continuously monitor the health of elderly city dwellers so that any unexpected health problems could be treated right away, even in the absence of family members.

A resident of a certain smart city's health information might be transferred outside the city in an emergency by being stored on a blockchain. By doing this, they can receive treatment right away and bring their medical history with them. Likewise, the implementation of Blockchain technology could facilitate the efficient execution of all health-related tracking procedures.

9.3 Existing System and the Issues

Health records are very important to track the patient's treatment and also to ensure that they undergo the proper treatment. Additionally, it helps them to analyze the treatment given and modify the same according to the outcome. Thus, it becomes important to take utmost care in maintaining the health record.

Early health records were maintained physically. Even still in some of the hospitals, this physical record is used. These records make it difficult to search for specific data and also to maintain. In some of the hospitals, they have started to maintain these records electronically in a clear and neat format. When medical records are computerized, it becomes the responsibility of the doctor or the hospital to maintain them securely. Since medical records contain sensitive information about a patient, they should be maintained securely to prevent others from editing and copying the data. Thus, access control over these documents plays a vital role.

In the literature, there are different ways to maintain the health records of patients. They are EHRs, PHRs, hybrid health records (HHRs), regional or national health information exchanges (HIEs), cloud-based health records, biometric health records, and blockchain-based health records.

In the following section, some of the health records in the literature are discussed.

9.3.1 Electronic Health Record (EHR)

EHR is maintained by the health providers. The EHR may be maintained in two ways. Cloud-based and on-premises. The inputs for the patient's records are obtained from the clinics or the hospitals. Since no standard formats are followed, it would be difficult for the patients to maintain the same. To efficiently handle these details, Song et al. (2015) proposed a dynamic health record creation using a mobile device. They have also used medical coding to permit interoperability.

9.3.2 Personal Health Record (PHR)

PHR is maintained by the patient. In PHR, though the patients are able to manage the data by themselves, they don't have the knowledge of where it gets stored and who maintains the same. Roehrs et al. (2017) proposed OmniPHR where the data is divided into different blocks depending upon the nature of the data and stored accordingly. Even it has records to track the location of the data.

9.3.3 Electronic Medical Record (EMR)

The electronic medical record (EMR) is the replacement for EGR or PHR. EMR is an electronic record that collects and maintains the health-related details of a patient. This aids in maintaining the health records up-to-date and facilitates easy maintenance. The EMR also improves the quality of prediction. EMR when implemented with the help of blockchain (Angraal et al., 2017; Mettler, 2016) helps us to maintain easily and impose access control.

9.3.4 Cloud-Based Health Record

Ksibi et al. (2023) proposed an encryption-based system for storing health records in cloud. They have proposed a multi-authority attribute-based encryption for securely safeguarding the details in the cloud. Doukas et al. (2010) and Singh et al. (2020) proposed a mobile-based method for cloud computing to store and access mobile data. Bahga and Madisetti (2013) used a cloud-based health record maintenance system. The Cloud Health Information Systems Technology ARchitecture (CHISTAR) uses a data structure facilitating semantic interoperability among the healthcare records.

Though the above techniques exist for maintaining healthcare data, none of them provide traceable, open, unmodifiable, and secure system. Blockchain is a technology that could overcome the above constraint. Mahajan et al. (2022) used blockchain-based solution to secure health data in the cloud.

9.4 Blockchain and Healthcare in Smart City

Smart cities' management and sharing of healthcare data can be revolutionized by blockchain technology, which offers a safe and patient-focused method of data management. Here's how blockchain can enable secured patient-centric data for smart city services.

9.4.1 Data Security and Integrity

Blockchain uses cryptographic methods to secure healthcare data and maintain the integrity of the same. The tamper-proof nature of the technology makes it difficult to alter the data. Thus, the doctors/patients can view the data but cannot modify the same.

9.4.2 Patient-Centric Data Management Control

When the patient data is stored in a permissioned blockchain then they have control over the data by permitting/deciding the persons accessing the stored data.

9.4.3 Interoperability

Blockchain can facilitate interoperability between different healthcare systems and data sources. In a smart city, where data comes from various sources like hospitals, wearable devices, and health apps, blockchain can act as a standardized platform for aggregating and sharing data seamlessly.

9.4.4 Health Data Exchange

Blockchain can facilitate the secure exchange of health data between different stakeholders, such as hospitals, clinics, pharmacies, and emergency services. This can lead to quicker and more informed decision-making in emergency situations.

9.4.5 Immutable Records

Every transaction in a blockchain needs to be recorded and time-stamped. This process makes all data access and changes as immutable records. This feature is important for regulatory compliance and for guaranteeing transparency in handling data.

Though blockchain technology provides many benefits, it is important to analyze and decide the type of blockchain before getting into the system. The necessity and scalability may be considered as a crucial factor for the above.

9.5 Blockchain-Based Healthcare System

9.5.1 Hyperledger-Based EHR System

The system is designed to adopt a patient-centered approach and uses symmetric key cryptography to provide access control policies. The system is developed using Hyperledger framework which makes use of chaincode concept. It highlights the importance of blockchain in enabling secure and controlled sharing of healthcare data (Tanwar et al., 2020). This approach aims to increase data security and accessibility in the healthcare domain.

The workflow of the system is given below:

User registration: Using a client application or software development kit (SDK), patients and healthcare providers register in the system. The participants ask for the enrollment certificate from the membership service provider (MSP) to access the system. The MSP issues a certificate and a private key, conveying a new credential to the participants. This process guarantees secure access to the system.

Blockchain transactions: All transactions in the systems are done with the help of a Hyperledger Fabric blockchain network. Each user is assigned specific roles, and they access the record based on the privileges given for them.

Patient interaction: Patients interact with the system through the client application. Here, they can add new records. This operation activates the chain code, making it easier to record transactions on the network.

Transaction distribution: After a transaction is committed to the blockchain network, it is distributed across the entire network. This ensures that every participant in the system receives the updated transactions. Importantly, a transaction becomes immutable once it is stored on the blockchain and cannot be changed or removed by unauthorized users.

Security: The network is characterized by a high level of security, where records are regularly updated and visible to all users within the blockchain network. The relevant data can be requested from the network by healthcare professionals such as clinicians and lab workers. The patient is granted access to the EHR ledger network to see and modify their records. Clinicians and laboratory participants can only access and modify records for which they have been given permission by the patient.

9.5.2 EHR Using IPFS

The primary objective of this system is (Shahnaz et al., 2019) to offer a secure, integrated, and scalable solution for EHR systems. The off-chain storage mechanism is employed here. In this system, the blockchain stores essential patient information, while the patients' actual information is stored in offline storage and represented on the blockchain through an inter-planetary file system (IPFS) hash. By conserving the integrity and security of the data on the blockchain, this method permits effective patient data storage and retrieval.

This framework consists of three layers: the user layer with granular access, the blockchain layer enabling user interaction through a Decentralized Application (DApp), and the system implementation layer built using Ethereum and its related components.

User layer: This is the first layer of the system containing various types of users namely, patients, doctors, administrative personnel, and nursing staff. These users are provided with coarse access rights, reflecting their varying levels of authority within the system.

Blockchain layer: This layer takes care of the functionality and processes related to the interaction between blockchain and DApp.

System implementation: The actual implementation of the system is in the third layer where Ethereum and its associated dependencies are built. Ethereum is the fundamental blockchain technology used for creating the structure for the healthcare system.

Thus, this system enables secure and controlled access to healthcare-related data and its functionalities.

9.5.3 Lightweight Blockchain Architecture for Healthcare Data Management

Compared to traditional blockchain networks like Bitcoin, this architecture provides a more effective and secure approach to healthcare data management. It highlights privacy, performance improvements, and the application of a permissioned blockchain for addressing detailed healthcare-related challenges (Ismail et al., 2019). It explains the benefits of a permissioned blockchain network over a permissionless one based on several key issues. These issues include the potential for unauthorized network participation, the exposure of sensitive patient data, limitations in network throughput speed, and the requirement for transaction execution fees. When compared to the Bitcoin network, the blockchain architecture tries to reduce the overhead involved in communication and computation. This is done by grouping network users into clusters and restricting the number of ledger copies retained by each cluster. The system introduces a function called "canal" to allow secure and private transactions between groups of network users. This improves data privacy in a network. This architecture gives a way to overcome forking which is a frequent problem in the Bitcoin network. This aids in maintaining the integrity and consistency of the blockchain. Analyzing different attacks and threats serves as a demonstration of the privacy and security measures implemented within this architecture. The blockchain is simulated using NS3 and from the findings, it is inferred that as the number of blocks rises, the implemented system creates 11 times less network traffic than the Bitcoin network. Additionally, ledger updates are 1.13 times faster.

9.5.4 Patient-Centric Healthcare Framework

To improve interoperability in healthcare systems this system introduces a secure and effective patient-centric healthcare framework (Gohar et al., 2022) by combining blockchain, cloud, and IoT technologies. This method uses blockchain technology for collecting data from various healthcare systems and wearable devices used by patients. This approach is useful for securely storing and managing patients' data by multiple transactions. It also helps access control for a wide range of stakeholders in the healthcare ecosystem. The cloud model is used for reducing cost and managing variations in server capacity usage within the system. This framework uses a five-tiered architecture and facilitates collaboration among the components. An EMR is used as an example to show data handling.

External (public) network tier: This layer acts as the intermediate for the users to communicate with the framework through a variety of platforms, like the web and mobile applications.

Core network tier: This tier is responsible for the location and management of data storage and solution logic. Communication within the blockchain network is done with the help of Hyperledger Fabric client SDK component. This SDK acts as the programming library at the client side by facilitating the selection of Application Programming Interface (APIs) denoted by "methods" and "calls". These APIs help client programs access and use the functionalities and capabilities of the blockchain network proficiently.

Network communication tier: This tier acts as a universal interface for integrating all healthcare applications and smooth communication.

Enterprise network tier: This tier consists of multiple healthcare systems and helps in the internal operations within the framework.

Network governance tier: This tier is responsible for protecting and validating all security and privacy aspects relating to personal and healthcare information.

9.5.5 Patient-Centric Architectural Framework

This system introduces a patient-centric decentralized healthcare management system with blockchain technology. It uses JavaScript-based smart contracts for HER management. It introduces a patient-centric decentralized healthcare management system (Singh et al., 2020). This architecture is built using several modules, assets, and smart contracts for achieving its full functionality. The client interface allows patients to register for appointments, and the chain code speeds up network connectivity. Once a patient commits to an appointment, the transaction is distributed across the network, ensuring data security and resilience against unauthorized tampering. The distributed ledger records these transactions with timestamps and hash values, making it easier to confirm the legitimacy of patients. Authorized parties can access healthcare records and initiate inquiries with fellow authorized participants using the blockchain network. Patients can also raise queries with doctors regarding appointments, medications, reports, clinical diagnoses, and other related matters within this framework.

The implementation of this system was carried out using the Hyperledger platform. Hyperledger Caliper was used to analyze resource utilization and performance evaluation. The experimental results indicate that, on average, the time it takes to write data to the system (write latencies) was approximately 47% higher than the time it takes to read data from the system (read latencies). With a modest drop of roughly 10 transactions per second when switching from a One-org1peer to a Two-org2peer network setup, the maximum throughput of 186 transactions per second was attained. Additionally, it was observed that doubling the block size resulted in a roughly tenfold increase in TPS. Notably, the framework introduced an innovative feature: client communication through a REST server. This capability represents a novel advancement in the healthcare domain, holding the potential to transform next-generation EHR systems.

9.5.6 Permissioned Blockchain

Omar et al. (2019) describes a healthcare data management system that prioritizes patients' needs and uses blockchain technology for data storage. The primary objective of the system is to elevate data privacy and security within the healthcare domain. To protect patient data, elliptic curve cryptography (ECC) functions are applied for encryption and pseudonymity. The system makes use of permissioned blockchain which restricts the user to gain access only by validating their credentials. The system has analyzed the transaction and execution costs with the help of a smart contract.

9.5.7 Integrity and Privacy-Aware Framework

The primary goal of the system is to improve the integrity and privacy of patient data. It also provides access control by restricting access to health information (Abutaleb et al., 2023). This framework combines blockchain technology and usage control (UCON) principles, allowing patients to revoke access as needed. The blockchain caches the access control details when finalized by the user. The UCON monitor module continuously implements real-time access control by leveraging the blockchain, while also tracking the records. The dynamic access control within the system is implemented using the UCON model. It actively monitors and manages runtime access to PHRs, ensuring that access adheres to predefined time constraints and other relevant policies. Additionally, patients could view the history of the access made with their data. Unauthorized access attempts are logged in an immutable ledger secured by blockchain technology.

The following illustrates how the framework utilizes Hyperledger Fabric and employs blockchain technology to safeguard the privacy of PHR access.

User request: The process initiates when a patient makes a request through a subscriber node, which is responsible for overseeing access control. This node verifies user credentials to manage access control effectively.

Access verification: Once the user credentials are validated, the subscriber node issues a digital certificate and transfers the same to the endorsement node through a smart contract for further processing.

Enhanced security: The access control mechanism implemented in the system ensures security by preventing unauthorized access to the private blockchain. It ensures that only authenticated and authorized users can interact with the blockchain.

Transaction validation: Following the request's processing, the endorsement node proceeds to execute a chaincode. This chaincode facilitates ledger access and assesses the validity of a transaction based on predefined criteria.

Response: Following an assessment of the transaction, the endorsement node encourages its validity by signing the proposal. Subsequently, it conveys the response to the patient using a smart contract application.

Blockchain commit: The validated transaction is broadcasted to the ordering node. The ordering node creates a block containing the transaction data. Next, the created block is sent to the committing peer which acts as the consensus node. The committing peer ensures that the transaction is added to the blockchain ledger. Thus it ensures consensus across the network regarding the state of the blockchain.

Ledger update: Once the transaction is validated, the committing peer makes the transaction as part of the ledger's history. The invalid transactions are identified and removed as part of the consensus mechanism.

Patient oversight: Upon completion of each transaction, the patient plays a vital role in managing all information logs and getting feedback responses. This process assures transparency and authorizes the patient by allowing them control over their health records, raising trust and responsibility in the system.

9.5.8 Secure and Fast Emergency Road Healthcare Service

This system (Ksibi et al., 2023) concentrates on the issues of the increasing number of road accidents and casualties. It talks about the importance of quick response from the emergency vehicles and doctors. The growth in the IoT technologies provides solution for the above issues.

The integration of the healthcare industry and IoT technology helps improve the speed and effectiveness of emergency services. This integration introduces two essential concepts: the Internet of Vehicles (IoV) and the Internet of Medical Things (IoMT).

In the IoV model, sensors kept within the vehicles are for collecting medical data from patients involved in emergencies. This data is transported in real-time to healthcare professionals, aiding them in prompt assessment and response to medical needs in critical situations.

As the data involved in the above process are sensitive in nature, secure management becomes crucial. To address these needs, a comprehensive system is proposed by integrating the following three concepts: Blockchain technology, IoV and IoMT. The system is organized using three core components: a list of hospitals, an EMR for patients, and a network of interconnected ambulances. This integrated system enables the persons involved in accidents to quickly report their location to nearby hospital and ambulances. Thus, this system improves the emergency response times and helps to overcome the critical situations positively.

In this proposed system, emergency vehicles, connected vehicles, and hospital emergency services are the three main components. Its primary goal is to augment road safety and streamline emergency response rules on the account of a road accident.

The work flow of the system is given below:

Broadcasting information: When a road accident occurs, details about the incident are sent to nearby vehicles. This detail aids other drivers to give way or adjust their routes.

Locating emergency vehicles: The system searches for the availability of nearby emergency vehicles and transmits the exact location of the accident to them.

Data collection: When the ambulance arrives at the accident location, with the help of sensors vital factors about a patient are collected. This collected data is processed for immediate assessment and treatment of injured individuals.

Prompt emergency response: The processed data is further sent to the hospital helping them to prepare in advance for the arrival of the patients. This advanced process increases the probability of saving lives.

To achieve these goals, the system is divided into three sub-systems, all of which are automated using blockchain technology and smart contracts. This automation ensures efficient and timely processing of data in emergency situations. This system was implemented using the Ethereum platform.

9.6 Conclusion

Nowadays healthcare has become an important keyword among people. With the enhancement of cities into smart cities, it becomes necessary to revolutionize healthcare methods and technologies. One such technique is the integration of blockchain and healthcare. This integration may ensure security, privacy, and patient-centricity of healthcare data. This also improves transparency and helps the system to be more beneficial for the customer. In this chapter, various techniques existing in the literature are discussed. However, it is important to note that various challenges need to be faced when implementing this technology in the real-life. It needs the collaboration of all the stakeholders involved in the system.

REFERENCES

Abutaleb, R. A., Alqahtany, S. S., & Syed, T. A. (2023). Integrity and Privacy-Aware, Patient-Centric Health Record Access Control Framework Using a Blockchain. *Applied Sciences*, *13*(2), 1028. https://doi.org/10.3390/app13021028

Angraal, S., Krumholz, H. M., & Schulz, W. L. (2017). Blockchain Technology Applications in Health Care. *Circulation: Cardiovascular Quality and Outcomes*, *10*(9), e003800.

Bahga, A., & Madisetti, V. K. (2013). A Cloud-based Approach for Interoperable Electronic Health Records (EHRs). *IEEE Journal of Biomedical and Health Informatics*, *17*(5), 894–906. https://doi.org/10.1109/jbhi.2013.2257818

Doukas, C., Pliakas, T., & Maglogiannis, I. (2010, August 1). *Mobile healthcare information management utilizing Cloud Computing and Android OS*. IEEE Xplore. https://doi.org/10.1109/IEMBS.2010.5628061

Gohar, A., AbdelGaber, S., & Salah, M. (2022). A Patient-Centric Healthcare Framework Reference Architecture for Better Semantic Interoperability Based on Blockchain, Cloud, and IoT. *IEEE Access*, 1. https://doi.org/10.1109/access.2022.3202902

Goyal, S., Sharma, N., Bhushan, B., Shankar, A., & Sagayam, M. (2021). IoT Enabled Technology in Secured Healthcare: Applications, Challenges and Future Directions. In: Hassanien, A.E., Khamparia, A., Gupta, D., Shankar, K., Slowik, A. (Eds) *Cognitive Internet of Medical Things for Smart Healthcare. Studies in Systems, Decision and Control*, 311.

Hussain, M. W., & Roy, D. S. (2023). Performance Optimization Strategies for Big Data Applications in Distributed Framework. In *Intelligent Technologies: Concepts, Applications, and Future Directions*, Volume *2* (pp. 221–252). Singapore: Springer Nature Singapore.

Ismail, L., Materwala, H., & Zeadally, S. (2019). Lightweight Blockchain for Healthcare. *IEEE Access*, *7*, 149935–149951. https://doi.org/10.1109/access.2019.2947613

Ksibi, A., Mhamdi, H., Ayadi, M., Almuqren, L., Alqahtani, M. S., Ansari, M. D., Sharma, A., & Hedi, S. (2023). Secure and Fast Emergency Road Healthcare Service Based on Blockchain Technology for Smart Cities. *Sustainability*, *15*(7), 5748. https://doi.org/10.3390/su15075748

Mahajan, H. B., Rashid, A. S., Junnarkar, A. A., Uke, N., Deshpande, S. D., Futane, P. R., Alkhayyat, A., & Alhayani, B. (2022). Integration of Healthcare 4.0 and Blockchain into Secure Cloud-Based Electronic Health Records Systems, *Applied Nanoscience*. https://doi.org/10.1007/s13204-021-02164-0

Mettler, M. (2016). Blockchain Technology in Healthcare the Revolution Starts Here. In *Proceedings of the 2016 IEEE 18th International Conference on E-Health Networking, Applications and Services (Healthcom)*, Munich, Germany, 14–17 September, 520–522.

Ministry of Urban Development Government of India. (2015). https://smartcities.gov.in/sites/default/files/SmartCityGuidelines.pdf

Omar, A. A., Bhuiyan, M. Z. A., Basu, A., Kiyomoto, S., & Rahman, M. S. (2019). Privacy-friendly Platform for Healthcare Data in Cloud Based on Blockchain Environment. *Future Generation Computer Systems*, *95*, 511–521. https://doi.org/10.1016/j.future.2018.12.044

Poongodi, M., Sharma, A., & Hamdi, M. (2021). Smart Healthcare in Smart Cities: Wireless Patient Monitoring System Using IoT. *The Journal of Supercomputing*, *77*, 12230–12255.

Roehrs, A., da Costa, C. A., & da Rosa Righi, R. (2017). OmniPHR: A Distributed Architecture Model to Integrate Personal Health Records. *Journal of Biomedical Informatics*, *71*, 70–81. https://doi.org/10.1016/j.jbi.2017.05.012

Reddy, K. H. K., Roy, D. S., Mishra, T. K., & Hussain, M. W. (Eds.). (2023). *Handbook of Research on Network-Enabled IoT Applications for Smart City Services*. IGI Global.

Sahatiya, P., & Singh, D. K. (2023). Role of Telemedicine in Healthcare Sector for Betterment of Smart City. *Soft Computing: Theories and Applications*, 925–935. https://doi.org/10.1007/978-981-19-9858-4_79

Shahnaz, A., Qamar, U., & Khalid, A. (2019). Using Blockchain for Electronic Health Records. *IEEE Access*, *7*(1), 147782–147795. https://doi.org/10.1109/access.2019.2946373

Singh, A. P., Pradhan, N. R., Luhach, A. K. K., Agnihotri, S., Jhanjhi, N., Verma, S., Kavita, Ghosh, U., & Roy, D. (2020). A Novel Patient-Centric Architectural Framework for Blockchain-Enabled Healthcare Applications. *IEEE Transactions on Industrial Informatics*, 1. https://doi.org/10.1109/TII.2020.3037889

Song, Y. T., Hong, S., & Pak, J. (2015). Empowering patients using cloud based personal health record system. *2015 IEEE/ACIS 16th International Conference on Software Engineering, Artificial Intelligence, Networking and Parallel/Distributed Computing (SNPD)*, Takamatsu, Japan, 1–6.

Tanwar, S., Parekh, K., & Evans, R. (2020). Blockchain-based Electronic Healthcare Record System for Healthcare 4.0 Applications. *Journal of Information Security and Applications*, *50*(1), 102407. https://doi.org/10.1016/j.jisa.2019.102407

10

Pneumonia Classification in Chest X-Ray Images Using Fusion of Deep Features and Light GBM

A. Beena Godbin and S. Graceline Jasmine
Vellore Institute of Technology, Chennai, India

10.1 Introduction

In the case of pneumonia, there is a bacterial infection or fungus in one or both lungs, causing an acute respiratory illness. A number of people of all ages suffer from this disease, which is one of the most important life-threatening diseases. As reported by the World Health Organization (WHO) in their latest report, under-five mortality rates are expected to increase to 808,000 by 2017. As a matter of fact, even people over the age of 65 are at a high risk of dying. Approximately 18% of all deaths caused by this disease occur every year as a result of this disease. The use of tobacco and being overweight are two of the main causes of these diseases. There is a WHO report that suggests that a reduction of at least 8% in heart diseases, diabetes, and 40% in cancer can be achieved through the avoidance of tobacco use. The most popular technique for diagnosing this disease, known as the chest X-ray, is one of the common methods of identifying this disease. As well as being used to diagnose heart problems, collapsed lungs, broken ribs, emphysema, and lung cancer, chest X-ray imaging can also be used for diagnosing different heart problems. Pneumonia specifically can be detected on X-rays of the chest based on the area of increased opacity that is present. As a result, imaging reviews of chest X-rays are often complicated because there are many factors, such as the position of the patient and the depth of inspiration when the patient is breathing, that can alter the appearance of a chest X-ray (Labhane et al., 2020). The expert radiologist still makes mistakes sometimes because observing X-ray images is still regarded as subjective according to the institution, even though he or she has a lot of experience. With the growing use of computer advancements in diagnosis and image acquisition devices, as well as medical image sets, the possibility of diagnosing patients has increased exponentially in recent years. As a result of the advanced digital processing and content storage system, both clinical science and medical treatments benefit from innovation in the field of medical treatment. Many hospitals and diagnostic centers in the country have access to a great deal of data (Chaudhary et al., 2019).

DOI: 10.1201/9781032631738-10

There have been several algorithms proposed to analyze these data in order to make sense of them. A significant advancement in the classification of medical images has been the use of convolutional neural networks (CNNs). A network that is very popular among security practitioners is one that learns based on the extraction of discriminating features from images in order to classify them. The light gradient boosting machine (LGBM), a machine learning (ML) classifier, is used in this study in order to classify the features extracted from MobileNet and DenseNet architectures with the use of ML algorithms. In the future, this application will be able to assist radiologists and medical experts in making more accurate diagnoses.

In the smart city context, in the field of disease diagnosis, ML, deep learning (DL), and statistical methods have shown great promise (Sirazitdinov et al., 2019; Sharma et al., 2021a; Reddy et al., 2023; Hussain and Roy, 2023). By tackling intricate vision tasks within the healthcare imaging field, tasks like classifying lung diseases and segmenting lungs represent key areas of focus, they can achieve a high degree of sophistication. Recent advances in the field of DL have contributed, in many cases, to the attainment or even the surpassing of human performance in many activities. As well as finding out the outcome of treatments, there are also a number of other ways in which DL can be applied in order to make predictions, such as chevalier methods as well as cancer treatments. In this study, X-ray images were used with labeled data and ML algorithms to locate and categorize a wide range of thoracic illnesses with encouraging results (Stephen et al., 2019). Traditionally, deep neural networks (DNNs) were developed and validated through a laborious and resource-intensive trial-and-error process conducted by humans, demanding significant time and expertise. This chapter presents a new model that uses DNN architecture to address the issue of efficiently executing ideal classifications. CXR radiographs are used exclusively in the proposed model for categorizing and predicting pneumonia based on CXR images. The technique is based on structural features of neural networks (NNs), which are used to determine the significance of images by concatenating, identifying, and extracting significant features from a set of images, based on an artificial NN architecture. In spite of the state-of-the-art models, NN offers a similar network architecture oriented toward training and testing, which was also the primary premise on which they developed their prototypes. The utilization of the NN model enhances the precision of predicting and classifying healthcare-based image data sets. This has spurred the adoption of DL-based algorithms that are the best choice for making predictions and classifications in the context of healthcare-based image data sets. The results of classification can be predicted by using DL (Saravagi et al., 2022). Similar to that, there are a number of models in the domain of DL which are used in the healthcare sector in order to predict diseases (Hasan et al., 2021). DL models are, however, only useful for a certain type of data, depending on how they are used that has been collected. In the chapter, the data set used for the experiment is in the form of images, which is an indication that the NN model is a good fit for the data set type used for the procedure. There is a method called the NN that uses a uniform grid to analyze information, such as radiography in the healthcare industry, and it is based on the structure of the human vision model when analyzing radiographs (Gayathri et al., 2022; Sharma et al., 2021b). Employing autonomous and adaptable techniques, the system gathers spatial stratifications of features, encompassing structures from the lowest to the highest levels. The NN architecture is structured with three hierarchical levels: convolution, pooling, and fully connected layers. The initial two layers extract information from the nodes, and the third layer interconnects all nodes, transmitting these features to the output layer, where the classification outputs are presented. Various NN models are available for classification tasks, each with distinct applications. In order to predict accurate results in various sectors, there have been a growing number of architectures including Visual Geometry Group, GoogleNet, ResNet, etc. The reason for utilizing the VGG16 transfer learning method for feature extraction is its applicability to a wide range of strides and window sizes, and due to its application to smaller strides and window sizes, we present it here as an example. As it has the capability of inserting 16 deep layers, it will do a better job on large data sets since it can insert 16 layers deep. By leveraging one of the NN architecture named VGG16, the DL-based model is presented in this work that can detect pneumonia in humans rapidly and early. The total number of layers is limited to 16, which reduces computational time.

There are three main sections in this chapter: Section 10.1 presents a review of related methods, Section 10.2 shows a review of the original study. The proposed method for CNN classification as well as the existing CNN models is presented in Section 10.3. A description of the pneumonia classification measures of the proposed method can be found in the fourth section. Furthermore, the conclusion of Section 10.5 provides a framework for future research and development.

10.2 Literature Survey

Rahamn et al. proposed a new model for focusing attention on disease-specific regions was proposed. The lung portion of the image is erased and designated as a non-pneumonia sample in this manner. To reduce background interference, transfer learning is used to segment the lung area of interest. A data set was utilized to train a convolutional neural network (CNN) using SE-ResNet (Varshni et al., 2019). The aim of this chapter is to generate medical images by utilizing convolutional data augmentation (CDA) and generative adversarial networks (GANs) (Bhagat and Bhaumik, 2019). As a result of this GANs technology, unprecedented images of chest X-rays of patients were produced using the DCNN model to classify the images. Using synthetic data produced by the GAN model increased the accuracy of the analysis.

Ozturk et al. employed the DarkNetwork for their research in 2020 (Ozturk et al., 2020). Seventeen convolution layers make up the training model. During three-way classification, they obtained an accuracy performance of 88.03% and during two-way classification methods, they obtained an accuracy of 98.8%. For their research, they used a data set consisting of 1126 images, including 520 pictures from normal group people, 500 pictures from patients with pneumonia, and 125 pictures from patients with COVID-19 disease. The accuracy of 93.1% was achieved by Abbas et al. by using the DeTraC deep convolutional NN (DCNN architecture) (Abbas et al., 2021). Their study involved 128 people with COVID-19 and 82 normal persons and their chest images. In order to address the issue of both classes, Minaee et al. (2020) developed four models with CNN architecture. There are ResNet18, ResNet50, SqueezeNet, and DenseNet121. Alavi and Nasiri described a framework combining DL and ANOVA (Nasiri and Alavi, 2022). To classify, they used XGBoost. A study by Gunraj and colleagues (2020) using COVID-Net achieved 93.3% accuracy. According to Hemdan and colleagues (2020), 90% accuracy was achieved using VGG19 and DenseNet201 networks. On three different data sets, we tested five pre-trained NNs, Nasiri and Hasani (2022) selected the ResNet50 NN, which obtained an average accuracy performance of 97.6%. To classify the images, Barstuvˇgan et al. (2021) extracted features from four other data sets. Based on the results of the research, 99.88% accuracy was achieved in two classes. The DenseNet169 DNN was applied by Nasiri and Hasani (2022) in order to retrieve image characteristics from the image and classify them using the XGBoost algorithm. Three classes scored 98.70% accuracy, while two classes scored 98.244% accuracy, and three classes scored 98.244% accuracy. Using COVID-19 detection system COV-ADSX, Hasani and Nasiri proposed a system for automatically detecting COVID-19 (Hasani and Nasiri, 2022). COV-ADSX is implemented using Django, a Python-based programming language. Using chest X-ray images from three different classes (COVID-19, healthy, and pneumonia) of X-ray images, a data set of a DL model was trained. In order to classify the data, SVM was applied. The overall accuracy for this study was 99.27% (Toğaçar et al., 2020). Based on chest X-rays, Ucar and Korkmaz (2020) reported that the Bayes deep SqueezeNet was 76.37% accurate in detecting COVID-19 when using the Bayes deep SqueezeNet algorithm. In his study, Asnaoui classified COVID-19 pneumonia using chest X-ray images and eight transfer learning methods employed by MobileNet-V2 and Inception-V3 (El Asnaoui et al., 2021). The accuracy score achieved using X-ray chest images and seven transfer learning techniques was 96% in the classification of COVID-19 pneumonia based on X-ray chest images. Using DenseNet169 and ANOVA feature selection, Ezzodding et al. extracted and selected chest X-ray features. Classifying COVID-19 cases with LGBM (Ezzoddin et al., 2022). Thejeshwar proposed a KE Sieve NN architecture using X-ray images (Thejeshwar et al., 2020). This model achieves 98% accuracy. The classification of pneumonia was done by Godbin and Jasmine (2022; Godbin and Jasmine, 2023). Revathi et al. explained ML classifiers (Revathi et al., 2022).

10.3 Materials and Methods

10.3.1 Data Set

There is an X-ray chest data set available on the Kaggle site.[1] There is no error in the distribution of data in this case. A representative image from the data collection is shown in Figure 10.1. Approximately 20% of the data set is earmarked for testing, while the remaining 80% is designated for training. A total of 2000 images of bacterial pneumonia, 2370 normal lung images, and 1345 viral pneumonia photos are included in this set of data.

10.3.2 Model Architecture

Figure 10.2 illustrates the process of extracting features from chest X-ray images using two different DL architectures, DenseNet and MobileNet. An X-ray image is analyzed by using these extracted feature sets as input to an LGBM. The following is a step-by-step explanation.

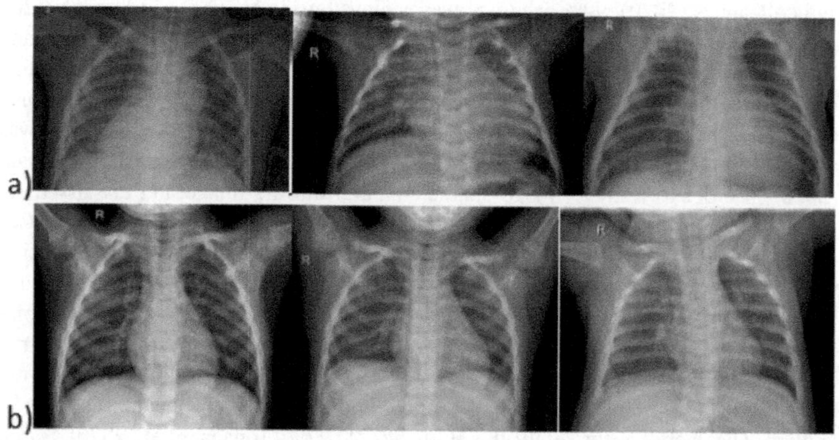

FIGURE 10.1 Example images from the data set (a) images of pneumonia and (b) healthy lung images.

Input data: A chest X-ray image is the input data. On the basis of these images, determine whether that patient has pneumonia or not based on his/her lung X-ray scan.

10.3.2.1 Feature Extraction with DenseNet and MobileNet

DenseNet: Pre-trained DenseNet models are used to process a part of the input data. High-level features are retrieved from the images by DenseNet. Patterns, shapes, and textures are represented in a features vector for each X-ray image. The architecture of the DenseNet model is illustrated in Figure 10.3. DenseNet is an architecture for computer vision methods involving image identification and densely connected convolutional networks. The method was developed by Gao Huang et al. (2017). The paper titled "Densely Connected Convolutional Networks" by Weinberger published in 2016 has gained popularity for its ability to improve training efficiency, parameter utilization, and overall performance when compared to traditional convolutional NNs.

DenseNet has the following key concepts and features:

The dense block is at the heart of DenseNet. Traditional CNNs connect each layer only to its predecessor. DenseNet, on the other hand, connects every layer within the same block to every other layer within the same block. In the network, this dense connectivity promotes information flow and gradients.

Bottleneck layers: In dense blocks, bottleneck layers are typically followed by convolutional layers to reduce computational complexity. Convolutional layers take accept feature maps and reduce them in number before passing them through the bottleneck layer. In this design, important features are preserved while parameters are reduced.

Transition layers: Transition layers are mainly used to control the spatial vector dimensions (width and height) of feature maps of the image. The process usually consists of batch normalization, convolutional layer 1×1, and

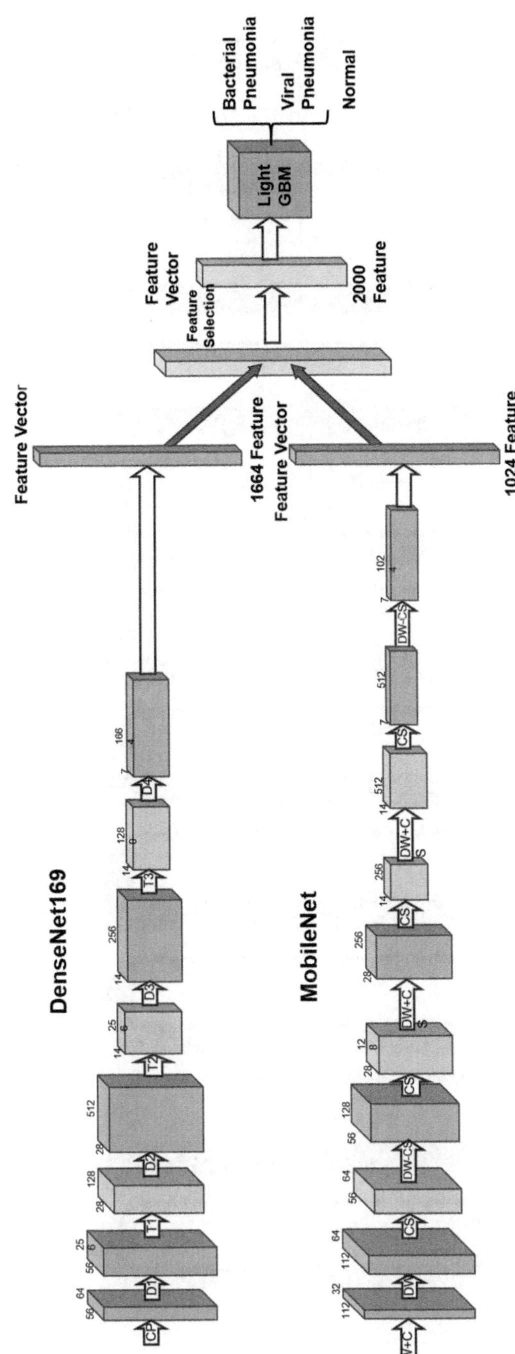

FIGURE 10.2 Workflow of the proposed model.

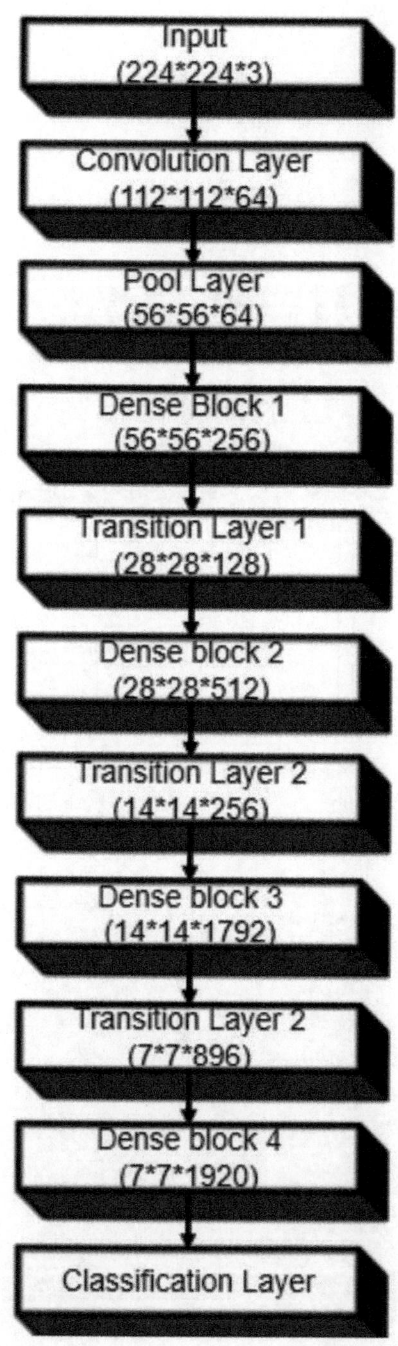

FIGURE 10.3 Densenet model.

downsampling (usually average pooling). As a result of transition layers, feature maps are smaller and parameters are fewer.

Growth rate: This hyperparameter determines how many new feature maps each level layer produces in a separate dense block. The capacity of the model is directly influenced by it. Larger growth rates can retrieve more difficult patterns but need more computing resources, whereas small growth rates result in smaller, more computationally efficient models.

Feature reuse: The densely featured connections in DenseNet enable characteristics from previous layering to be reused efficiently, reducing the risk of vanishing gradients during training.

Global average pooling: In DenseNet, global average pooling (GAP) is typically used instead of completely connected layers at the bottom of the networks. The GAP generates a fixed-size representation for each class by averaging the feature maps spatially. It reduces overfitting and parameterization.

Skip connections: DenseNet is a skip connection architecture where every layer is connected to every other layer. When training deep networks, skip connections facilitate gradient flow.

The densely connected architecture of DenseNet allows it to train deeper networks with fewer parameters, improve feature reuse, and provide strong regularization. In addition to image classification, it can also detect objects and segment images using computer vision techniques.

MobileNet: Data is also passed through a pre-trained MobileNet model, MobileNet, a lightweight NN architecture, also extracts features from images, although with fewer parameters than DenseNet. Each image also contains a feature vector containing the features extracted by MobileNet.

Designed specifically for computer vision and DL applications on mobile devices, MobileNet is one type of NN architectures. Google researchers developed it to use effectively on mobile devices and embedded systems with restricted computing resources. Known for its lightweight and fast inference, MobileNet is suitable for real time image classification, object identification, and other vision tasks on smartphones, IoT devices, and embedded systems.

Key features and concepts of MobileNet include the following:

Depthwise separable convolution: MobileNet's convolutional layers are based on depthwise separable convolution, which is computationally effective compared to previous convolutional layers. A depthwise separable convolution consists of two steps:

Depthwise convolution: A convolutional filter independently processes each input channel.

Utilizing 1x1 convolutional filters diminishes the computational expenses by reducing the total calculations.

Pointwise convolution: On the output channels, a 1x1 convolution (pointwise convolution) is applied after depthwise convolution.

"Width Multiplier": MobileNet introduces a hyperparameter known as the "width multiplier" (usually indicated by an "α"). The width multiplier determines how many channels (i.e., the width of a model) are present in each layer. Using fewer parameters and thinner models can make them more computationally efficient because they can be made thinner and thinner. Choosing a model size and accuracy compromise allows you to find the right balance for your needs.

Resolution multiplier: This hyperparameter (often denoted by "ρ") can be used to reduce the input image resolution. Using this method will reduce both the computational requirements and the memory footprint of the model, but it may have an adverse effect on its performance. A lower ρ value corresponds to a lower resolution of the input image.

Inverted residuals: The concept of "inverted residuals" is introduced in MobileNetV2, an improvement over MobileNet. A layer is expanded using 1x1 convolutions before depthwise separable convolutions are applied. While maintaining efficiency, it enhances the model's representation power.

Bottleneck blocks: Using bottleneck blocks, MobileNetV2 further reduces computation. There are a variety of components in these blocks, such as 1x1 convolutions to reduce dimensionality, and 3x3 depthwise separable convolutions to reduce size. In addition to capturing features efficiently, these blocks also help to decrease the model size.

Efficient design: MobileNet architectures maintain competitive accuracy while being efficient and lightweight. In mobile and embedded devices, where memory and computation resources are limited, they are optimized for deployment.

Variants: MobileNet comes in different versions, such as MobileNetV1, MobileNetV2, and MobileNetV3, each with incremental improvements. Speed and accuracy can be traded off with these variants. Mobilenet model is shown in Figure 10.4.

Feature combination: X-ray images are analyzed using both DenseNet and MobileNet to extract features. Concatenation or element-wise addition can be used to combine these elements. By combining both models, complementary information can be captured (Huang et al., 2017). On the contrary, a classification model is the output provided by your classifier through ML. The process of categorizing data is governed by an algorithm, sometimes called a set of rules. You train a classifier, which then categorizes your data using the classifier (Howard et al., 2017). It is possible to use a supervised or an unsupervised classifier. It is used to classify unlabeled data sets using patterns, anomalies, and structures. In both supervised and semi-supervised learning, classifiers utilize training data sets to improve their performance and make predictions. Sentiment analysis relies on classifiers to identify and categorize the polarity of opinions. ML classifiers analyze content from various sources such as social media, online reviews, and emails to gain insights into customer sentiments about a company (Pradhan et al., 2022).

LGBM model: In an LGBM model, the combined feature vectors are used as input. As the combined features are treated as tabular data, LGBM is an efficient and effective gradient boosting framework. Lavanya and Subbulakshmi (2023) explained ML methods for non-communicable diseases. (In LGBM, a histogram-based method is used to calculate the volume. As a result of making continuous variables discrete, the cost of calculating those variables is reduced. The training's duration of decision tree is inversely proportional to the number of computations and division methods involved. As a result, fewer resources are used, and training time is reduced (Muratlar, 2020). It is possible to learn from a decision tree in a leaf-wise manner or in a depth-wise manner. By expanding the tree level-by-level,

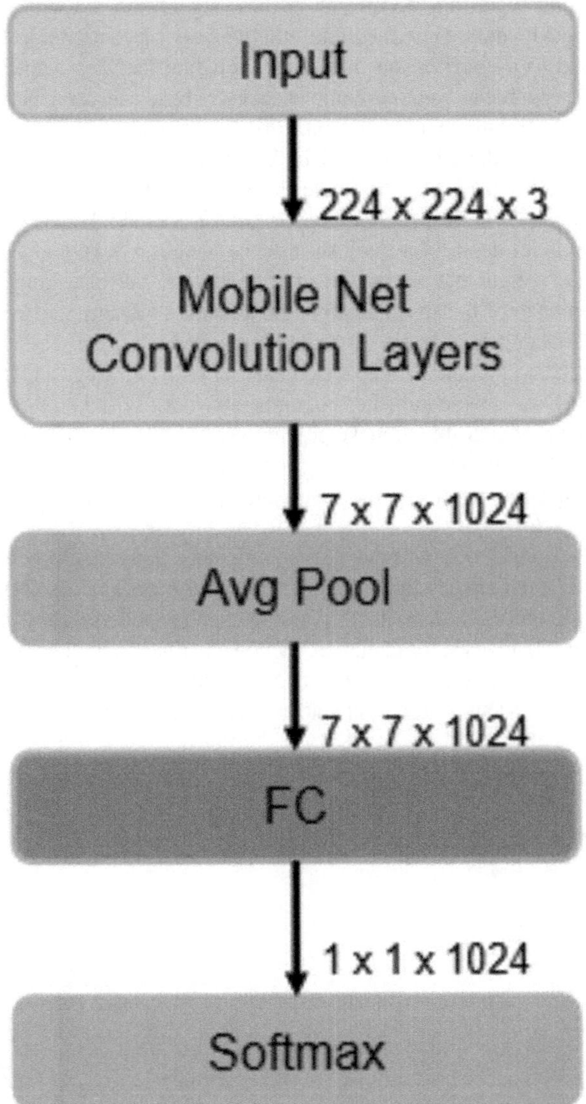

FIGURE 10.4 Mobilenet model.

the balance within the tree remains as the tree grows. LGBM differs from other boosting algorithms since it starts splitting leaves from the top, which lowers the loss, and continues splitting leaves from the bottom, thereby reducing the loss even further. Leaf-oriented methods facilitate the model in achieving quicker and more precise learning. Whenever the amount of data is low, the leaf focused growth strategy is vulnerable to being overtrained. It is, therefore, more suitable for the application of the technique when dealing with huge data sets. In addition, it is possible to tune factors such as leaf count and depth in order to avoid over learning the algorithm. As a result of these algorithms, you will be able to train them quickly and they will require little memory of your computer. This can be attributed to a combination of factors, including leafwise splitting, which can result in significantly more complex trees, which can contribute to improved accuracy (Minastireanu and Mesnita, 2019). A boosting decision tree is one that is based on gradient boosting, which is a type of boosting tree. With LGBM, a learning rate of 0.1 is used and there are 100 boosted trees. It is assumed that each tree contains 31 leaves, so a learning rate of 0.1 is used. There is no upper limit to the maximum depth of a tree. An instance weight of 0.001 pounds is the least amount of weight that can be needed in a leaf. Generally speaking, 21 data points are deemed to be the absolute minimum amount of data needed in a leaf. LGBM and XGBost differences are shown in Figure 10.5.

Training: LGBM is trained on a labeled data set with known ground truth (whether an chest X-ray image indicates pneumonia or not). Based on the combined features, the model is able to make predictions.

Prediction: Once trained, LGBM can predict new, unseen X-ray images. Using an X-ray image as input, the model predicts pneumonia likelihood based on the feature vector.

Evaluation: Considering accuracy, sensitivity, specificity, and other relevant metrics, the model's predictions can be evaluated for pneumonia detection in chest X-rays. In this method, both DL (DenseNet and MobileNet) and gradient boosting (LGBM) are used for feature extraction and final prediction. An image model that combines features from different NNs could be made more accurate by capturing a wider range of image characteristics by combining the extracted features.

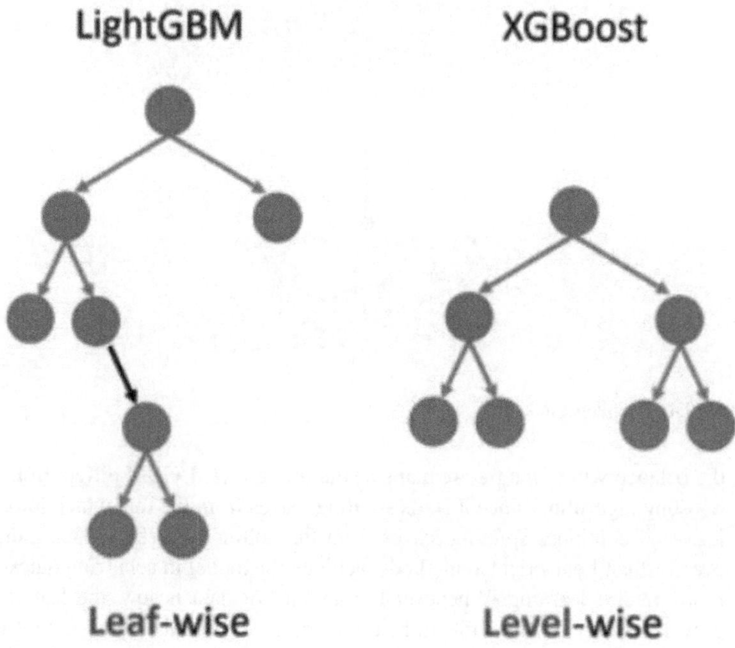

FIGURE 10.5 LightGBM vs XGBoost.

10.4 Implementation and Result Analysis

Training and test results were compiled on a Windows 10 machine using CXT pictures for pneumonia classification. 8GB of RAM and an Intel Core i5 processor were used. Scikit-learn 0.23.1 was used as well as Python 3.7.10. An LGBM classifier was used to classify images. To control classifier learning, hyperparameters are used. Each categorization method was controlled by several variables. Grid searching with a 10-fold CV (cross validation) was used to develop the model hyperparameters for each classification method. Using the 10-fold cross-validation method, this study generated more accurate and realistic results. Model accuracy was based on its precision, sensitivity, and accuracy as well as its F1 support. Predictions that are accurate are proportional to all other hypotheses. Precision can be determined by comparing the rate of correct positive class predictions with the rate of correct negative class predictions. An accurate positive class prediction is equal to a correct negative class guess, and that is what is known as sensitivity. The harmonic mean provides a balanced measure that considers both precision and recall, making it a useful metric for evaluating the overall performance of a classification model.

In the LGBM data set classifier, Figure 10.6 displays a confusion matrix. Figure 10.7 shows LGBM model performance. Positive class labels that are classified accurately are termed "true positives" (TP). Negative class examples that are incorrectly predicted are referred to as TN. A false positive rate (FP) refers to the overall number of negative class samples that were misclassified as positive. Negative cases are

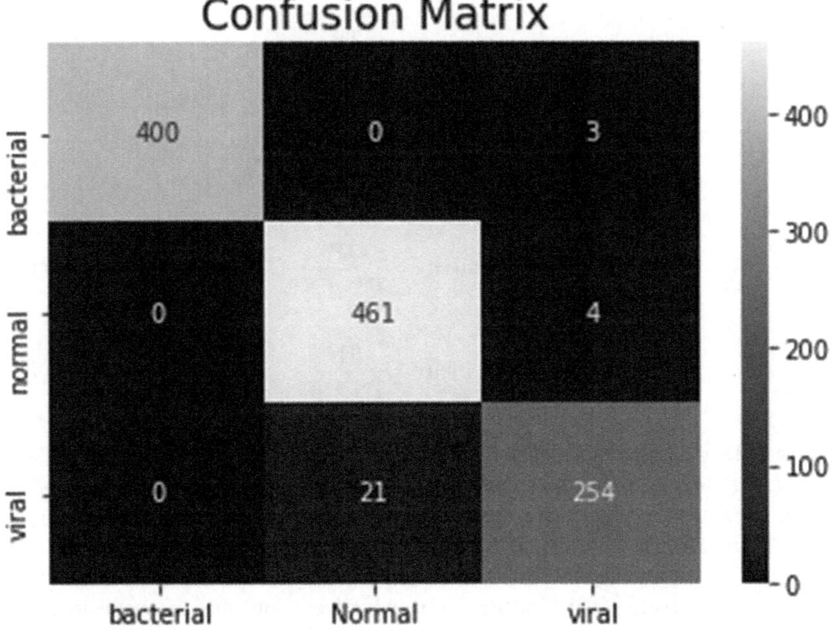

FIGURE 10.6 Confusion matrix.

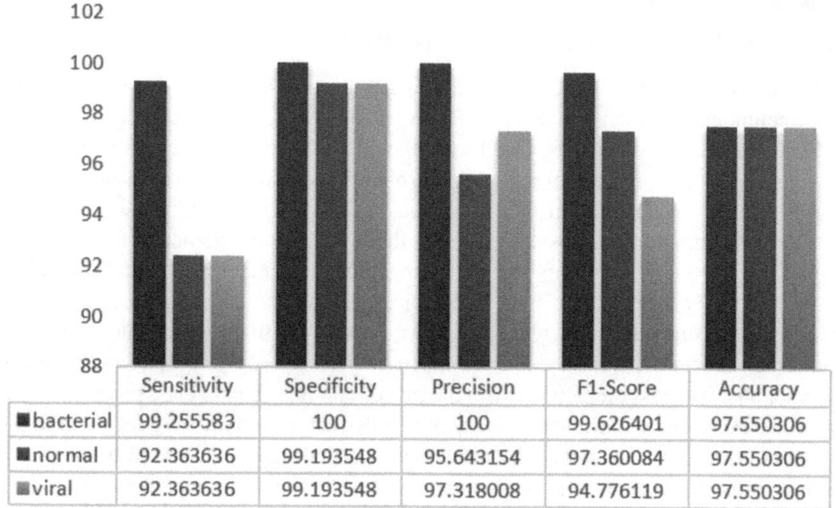

	Sensitivity	Specificity	Precision	F1-Score	Accuracy
bacterial	99.255583	100	100	99.626401	97.550306
normal	92.363636	99.193548	95.643154	97.360084	97.550306
viral	92.363636	99.193548	97.318008	94.776119	97.550306

FIGURE 10.7 Performance measure of LGBM model.

mistakenly labeled as positive cases in false negatives. The calculation metrics are shown in equations 10.1–10.5.

$$\text{Accuracy} = \frac{\text{TP} + \text{TN}}{\text{TP} + \text{FP} + \text{TN} + \text{FN}} \tag{10.1}$$

$$\text{Precision} = \frac{\text{TP}}{\text{TP} + \text{FP}} \tag{10.2}$$

$$\text{F1} - \text{score} = 2 * \frac{\text{Precision} * \text{sensitivity}}{\text{Precision} + \text{sensitivity}} \tag{10.3}$$

$$\text{Sensitivity} = \frac{\text{TP}}{\text{TP} + \text{FN}} \tag{10.4}$$

$$\text{Specificity} = \frac{\text{TN}}{\text{TN} + \text{FP}} \tag{10.5}$$

The accuracy number is calculated by dividing the portions of the method that accurately identified the data set as a whole by the number of predictions. A true positive, a true negative, a false positive, and a false negative are denoted by the symbols TP, TN, FP, and FN. Those values of the event that were correctly predicted are shown by true positives. A true negative is used for event values that were false positives due to inaccurate forecasting. A true positive is used for event outcomes that were accurately guessed as no-events. An incorrectly anticipated non-event value is displayed by a false negative. To assess performance, expressions based on the confusion matrix are crucial. Performance metrics encompass precision, accuracy, specificity, F1-score, log loss, sensitivity, and error rate. These metrics collectively provide a comprehensive evaluation of the model's effectiveness in classification tasks.

10.5 Discussion and Conclusion

An early prediction of COVID-19 is presented using a DL-based model built on lung X-ray images of patients. DenseNet169 and MobileNet models are used to retrieve features of the image, after the feature selection method is used to select some of the most essential feature properties, and the LGBM method is used to identify the images. We achieved a 98.54% accuracy rate with our proposed algorithm. For this study, readers will use the LBGM classifier to categorize pneumonia. In the future, we will test our technique against various data sets in order to improve its performance for diagnosing pneumonia more efficiently and accurately. In the realm of smart cities, it has been demonstrated that a variety of models can be utilized in the identification of various diseases using the findings of this research.

NOTE

1 https://www.kaggle.com/datasets/paultimothymooney/chest-xray-pneumonia.

REFERENCES

Abbas, A., Abdelsamea, M. M. and Gaber, M. M. "Classification of covid-19 in chest x-ray images using detrac deep convolutional neural network," *Applied Intelligence*, vol. *51*, no. 2, pp. 854–864, 2021.

Barstuv̌gan, M., Özkaya, U., and S. Öztürk, "Coronavirus (covid-19) classification using ct images by machine learning methods," in *CEUR Workshop Proceedings*, vol. *2872*, 2021.

Bhagat, V. and Bhaumik, S. "Data Augmentation using Generative Adversarial Networks for Pneumonia classification in chest Xrays," *Proceedings of the IEEE International Conference on Image Processing*, vol. *2019*, pp. 574–579, 2019.

Chaudhary, A., Hazra, A., and Chaudhary, P., "Diagnosis of Chest Diseases in X-Ray images using Deep Convolutional Neural Network," *2019 10th Int. Conf. Comput. Commun.Netw.Technol.ICCCNT2019*, pp. 6–11, 2019.

El Asnaoui, K., Chawki, Y., and Idri, A. "Automated methods for detection and classification pneumonia based on x-ray images using deep learning," in *Artif. Intell. Blockchain Fut. Cybersecurity Appl.*, Springer, 2021, pp. 257–284.

Ezzoddin, M., Nasiri, H., and Dorrigiv, M. "Diagnosis of COVID-19 Cases from Chest X-ray Images Using Deep Neural Network and LightGBM," in *2022 Int. Conf. Mach. Vis. Image Proc. (MVIP)*. IEEE, 2022, pp. 1–7.

Gayathri, J.L., Abraham, B., Sujarani, M.S., and Nair, M.S. A computer-aided diagnosis system for the classification of COVID-19 and non-COVID-19 pneumonia on chest X-ray images by integrating CNN with sparse autoencoder and feed forward neural network. *Computers in Biology and Medicine*, vol. *141*, p. 105134, 2022.

Godbin, A.B. and Jasmine, S. G. "Analysis of pneumonia detection systems using deep learning-based approach," *2022 Int. Conf. Innov. Comp., Intel. Commun. Smart*

Electr. Syst. (ICSES), Chennai, India, 2022, pp. 1–8, doi: 10.1109/ICSES55317.2022.9914321.

Godbin, A.B. and Jasmine, S.G. Screening of COVID-19 based on GLCM features from CT images using machine learning classifiers. *SN Computer Science*, vol. *4*, p. 133, 2023. https://doi.org/10.1007/s42979-022-01583-2

Gunraj, H., Wang, L., and Wong, A. "Covidnet-ct: A tailored deep convolutional neural network design for detection of covid-19 cases from chest ct images," *Frontiers in Medicine*, p. 1025, 2020.

Hasan, M.D., Ahmed, S., Abdullah, Z.M., Monirujjaman Khan, M., Anand, D., Singh, A., AlZain, M., and Masud, M. "Deep learning approaches for detecting pneumonia in COVID-19 patients by analyzing chest X-ray images," *Mathematical Problems in Engineering*, vol. *2021*, p. 9929274, 2021.

Hasani, S. and Nasiri, H. "COV-ADSX: An Automated Detection System using X-ray images, deep learning, and XGBoost for COVID-19," *Software Impacts*, vol. *11*, 2022.

Hemdan, E. E.-D., Shouman, M. A., and Karar, M. E. "Covidx-net: A framework of deep learning classifiers to diagnose covid-19 in x-ray images," *arXiv preprint arXiv:2003.11055*, 2020.

Howard, A. G., Zhu, M., Chen, B., Kalenichenko, D., Wang, W., Weyand, T., Andreetto, M., and Adam, H. "Mobilenets: Efficient convolutional neural networks for mobile vision applications," *arXiv preprint arXiv:1704.04861*, 2017.

Huang, Z., Liu, L., Van Der Maaten, and Weinberger, K. Q. "Densely connected convolutional networks," in *Proc. IEEE Conf. Comp. Vision and Pattern Recog.*, 2017, pp. 4700–4708.

Hussain, M. W., & Roy, D. S. (2023). Performance Optimization Strategies for Big Data Applications in Distributed Framework. In *Intelligent Technologies: Concepts, Applications, and Future Directions*, Volume *2* (pp. 221–252). Singapore: Springer Nature Singapore.

Labhane, G., Pansare, R., Maheshwari, S., Tiwari, R., and Shukla, A., "Detection of Pediatric Pneumonia from Chest X-Ray Images using CNN and Transfer Learning," *Proc. 3rd Int. Conf. Emerg. Technol. Comput. Eng. Mach. Learn. Internet Things, ICETCE2020*, no. February, pp. 85–92, 2020.

Lavanya, J. S., & Subbulakshmi, P. (2023, January). Machine Learning Techniques for the Prediction of Non-Communicable Diseases. In *2023 Int. Conf. Artif. Intel. Knowledge Disc. Concurrent Eng. (ICECONF)* (pp. 1–8). IEEE.

Minaee, S., Kafieh, R., Sonka, M., Yazdani, S., and Soufi, G. J. "Deepcovid: Predicting covid-19 from chest x-ray images using deep transfer learning," *Medical Image Analysis*, vol. *65*, p. 101794, 2020.

Minastireanu, E. and Mesnita, G. 2019 Light GBM machine learning algorithm to online click fraud detection. *Journal of Information Assurance & Cybersecurity*, vol. *2019*, pp. 1–12.

Muratlar, E. R., LightGBM. [Internet].[cited 06.12.2020]. Available from: https://www.veribilimiokulu.com/lightgbm/

Nasiri, H. and Alavi, S. A. "A Novel Framework Based on Deep Learning and ANOVA Feature Selection Method for Diagnosis of COVID-19 Cases from Chest X-Ray Images," *Computational Intelligence and Neuroscience*, vol. *2022*, p. 4694567, 2022.

Nasiri, H. and Hasani, S. "Automated detection of COVID-19 cases from chest X-ray images using deep neural network and XGBoost," *Radiography*, vol. *28*(3), pp. 732–738, 2022.

Ozturk, T., Talo, M., Yildirim, E. A., Baloglu, U. B., Yildirim, O., and Acharya, U. R. "Automated detection of covid-19 cases using deep neural networks with x-ray images," *Computers in Biology and Medicine*, vol. *121*, p. 103792, 2020.

Pradhan, B., Hussain, M. W., Srivastava, G., Debbarma, M. K., Barik, R. K., & Lin, J. C. W. (2022). *A Neuro-Evolutionary Approach for Software Defined Wireless Network Traffic Classification*. IET Communications.

Reddy, K. H. K., Roy, D. S., Mishra, T. K., & Hussain, M. W. (Eds.). (2023). *Handbook of Research on Network-Enabled IoT Applications for Smart City Services*. IGI Global.

Revathi, M., Godbin, A. B., Bushra, S. N. and Anslam Sibi, S. "Application of ANN, SVM and KNN in the Prediction of Diabetes Mellitus." *2022 Int. Conf. Elect. Syst. Int. Comp. (ICESIC)*, Chennai, India, 2022, pp. 179–184, doi: 10.1109/ICESIC53714.2022.9783577.

Saravagi, D., Agrawal, S., Saravagi, M., and Rahman, M.H. Diagnosis of Lumbar spondylolisthesis using a pruned CNN model. *Computational and Mathematical Methods in Medicine*, vol. *1*, p. 2722315, 2022.

Sharma, A., Guleria, K., and Goyal, N. Prediction of Diabetes Disease Using Machine Learning Model. In: *Int. Conf. Commun., Comp. Electro. Sys.*, Springer, Singapore, 2021a, pp 683–692.

Sharma, S., Khanra, P., and Ramkumar, K.R. Performance analysis of biomass energy using machine and deep learning approaches. *Journal of Physics: Conference Series*, vol. *2089*(1), p. 012003, 2021b.

Sirazitdinov, I., Kholiavchenko, M., Mustafaev, T., Yixuan, Y., Kuleev, R., and Ibragimov, B. (2019) Deep neural network ensemble for pneumonia localization from a large-scale chest x-ray database. *Computers & Electrical Engineering*, vol. *78*, 388–99.

Stephen, O., Sain, M., Maduh, U. J., Jeong, D. U. An efficient deep learning approach to pneumonia classification in healthcare. *Journal of Healthcare Engineering*, vol. *1*, p. 4180949, 2019.

Thejeshwar, S. S., Chokkareddy, C., and Eswaran, K. "Precise prediction of covid-19 in chest x-ray images using ke sieve algorithm," *medRxiv*, 2020.

Toğaçar, M., Ergen, B. and Cömert, Z. "Covid-19 detection using deep learning models to exploit social mimic optimization and structured chest x-ray images using fuzzy color and stacking approaches," *Computers in Biology and Medicine*, vol. *121*, p. 103805, 2020.

Ucar, F. and Korkmaz, D. "Covidiagnosis-net: Deep bayes-squeezenet based diagnosis of the coronavirus disease 2019 (covid-19) from x-ray images," *Medical Hypotheses*, vol. *140*, p. 109761, 2020.

Varshni, D., Thakral, K., Agarwal, L., Nijhawan, R. and Mittal, A. "Pneumonia Detection Using CNN based Feature Extraction," *Proc. 2019 3rd IEEE Int. Conf. Electr. Comput. Commun. Technol. ICECCT 2019*, pp. 1–7, 2019.

11

AI-Driven Prioritization and Detection of COVID-19 Cases in Smart City: An Integration of X-Ray Imaging and ResNet-18 Machine Learning Model

Deepa Parasar, Naufil Arif Kazi, Lachiket Narendra Warule, and Vaibhav Guru
Amity University Maharashtra, Mumbai, India

11.1 Introduction

During the COVID-19 pandemic, global healthcare infrastructures have experienced unprecedented stress, necessitating immediate and precise diagnostic procedures to manage and mitigate viral transmission. Traditional diagnostic methodologies, such as reverse transcription polymerase chain reaction (RT-PCR), although considered the gold standard, exhibit inherent limitations including extended processing time and substantial resource allocation. The most current research on endoscopic otolaryngology procedures and data assessment was done during the COVID-19 pandemic and was presented. In this context, computational technologies present a viable alternative for expediting diagnostic procedures.

Machine learning, a specialized branch of artificial intelligence (AI), offers capabilities for data analysis at a scale and speed unattainable by human intervention (Hussain and Roy, 2023; Pradhan et al., 2022). Within the medical domain, machine learning algorithms applied to radiological imaging, specifically chest X-rays, have demonstrated potential for enhancing the speed and efficiency of COVID-19 diagnosis (Oishee et al., 2021). COVID-19 exposes limitations in healthcare preparedness for emerging infectious diseases, necessitating the exploration of diagnostic tools. This review examines cell culture, indirect fluorescent antibody, radiologic imaging, reverse transcriptase PCR, isothermal amplification, CRISPR-Cas, microfluidics, immunoassays, and advancements in NGS for early detection and viral analysis in the global challenge. Utilizing the widespread availability and operational simplicity of X-ray imaging devices, this computational approach emerges as a particularly effective solution in healthcare environments constrained by limited resources.

DOI: 10.1201/9781032631738-11

The focal point of this chapter is to use an advanced machine learning model, that is implemented to diagnose X-ray images of the chest and subsequently rank patients for testing of RT-PCR. This model is summarized within a web platform-based application developed using the Django framework, aiming to facilitate rapid and automated diagnostic procedures for COVID-19.

While the machine learning model does not serve as a substitute for RT-PCR testing, it functions as an essential triage mechanism. It aids healthcare practitioners in the rapid identification of individuals at elevated risk, thereby streamlining the allocation of medical resources and potentially reducing mortality rates. Highly lethal respiratory disease COVID-19 has led to the adoption of CT and chest X-ray modalities in radiological imaging for non-invasive screening has been stated (Lasker et al., 2022). For computer-assisted COVID-19 identification, researchers have created AI/ML algorithms in response to the lack of medical specialists. This thorough study discusses the uniqueness and limitations of the published research while summarizing and contrasting various ML/DL algorithms, datasets, and outcomes in employing CT and X-ray imaging for diagnostic prediction.

11.1.1 The Global Crisis

In December 2019, the emergence of the coronavirus disease (COVID-19) in Wuhan, China, marked the inception of a global health crisis. Initially perceived as a localized outbreak, the situation rapidly escalated into a pandemic of international proportions. Data from the World Health Organization, as of April 25, 2021, indicates that the virus has infected in excess of 147 million individuals globally and has been responsible for more than 3.1 million deaths (Sanyaolu et al., 2021). The COVID-19 pandemic, which was caused by the rapid global spread of SARS-CoV-2, has resulted in a significant number of cases and fatalities, especially in the elderly and those with comorbidities. It is vital to identify, test, and isolate affected people in order to avoid overloading healthcare facilities (Sanyaolu et al., 2021). This chapter looks at the topographical possibility of the virus's spread, the effects it had on the distressed nations, and the successful countermeasures some of them took to lessen the pandemic and flatten the COVID-19 spread curve. This widespread transmission and high mortality rate have exerted immense pressure on healthcare infrastructures worldwide, leading to a crisis that is unparalleled in its scope and complexity. The pandemic has not only overcome healthcare systems but has also posed significant challenges in terms of allocation of medical resources, improving diagnostic capabilities, and treatment protocols. The condition of the worldwide healthcare landscape was presented which is grappling with an exigent situation that demands immediate and effective interventions to lessen the spread of the virus and manage its impact (Nanaiah et al., 2022).

11.1.1.1 The Diagnostic Challenge

A crucial element in the proper management of the COVID-19 pandemic is the capability for rapid and accurate diagnostic procedures. The RT-PCR test, widely considered an important standard for COVID-19 diagnosis is fraught with limitations that complicate its utility. Among these boundaries related to diagnosis others, are extended processing times, which can vary significantly, ranging between 1 and 2 days. Moreover, the availability of testing of RT-PCR is often constrained, particularly in healthcare centre settings that are limited in terms of resources like financial and logistical resources. These challenges create a diagnostic bottleneck, which has a flowing effect on multiple facets of managing healthcare issues. Specifically, the delays and limitations associated with RT-PCR testing obstruct the required allocation of medical resources and compromise the efficacy of strategies aimed at containing the spread of the virus. Consequently, the inadequacies of the RT-PCR testing methodology underscore the crucial need for alternative diagnostic approaches that can address these constraints while maintaining a high level of accuracy (Valent et al., 2021; Torres et al., 2021; Lanzilao et al., 2023; Kunac et al., 2021).

11.1.1.2 The Urgency for Alternate Solutions

By considering the limitations related to pandemic and healthcare management, there is an immediate need for substitute diagnostic strategies that can deliver quick and reliable results. One such alternate method lies in leveraging existing medical imaging technologies, specifically X-rays of chest images. Radiography of the chest has been widely available, even in low-resource availabilities, and can produce diagnosis in a much quicker manner than RT-PCR tests. This speed is vital for effective patient triage, a crucial step in managing healthcare resources during any pandemic (Augustine et al., 2020; Yin et al., 2021; Mehta et al., 2022).

11.1.2 Purpose of This Work

The core aim of this research work is to improve the diagnosis by applying different machine learning methods to X-ray images of the chest for the rapid identification of COVID-19 infections. A deep learning model based on ResNet-18 architecture aims to differentiate COVID-19 cases from other types of pneumonia, viral, and normal cases. The model is trained on a dataset comprising 3,896 X-ray images of the chest, achieving an accuracy rate of 95.56%. The sample images of the dataset are shown in Figure 11.1.

The outcome of the proposed work highlights the enduring relevance of the proposed model in post-pandemic healthcare scenarios, underscoring its vital role in fortifying the healthcare infrastructure of smart cities. This model, with its adaptable and predictive capabilities, stands as a testament to our commitment to long-term healthcare resilience.

11.2 Literature Review

11.2.1 Review of Existing Literature

Artificial intelligence (AI) encompasses computer science as a kind of machine-driven technological advancement. The phrase "artificial intelligence" often refers to computer systems that replicate the cognitive abilities associated with human intelligence,

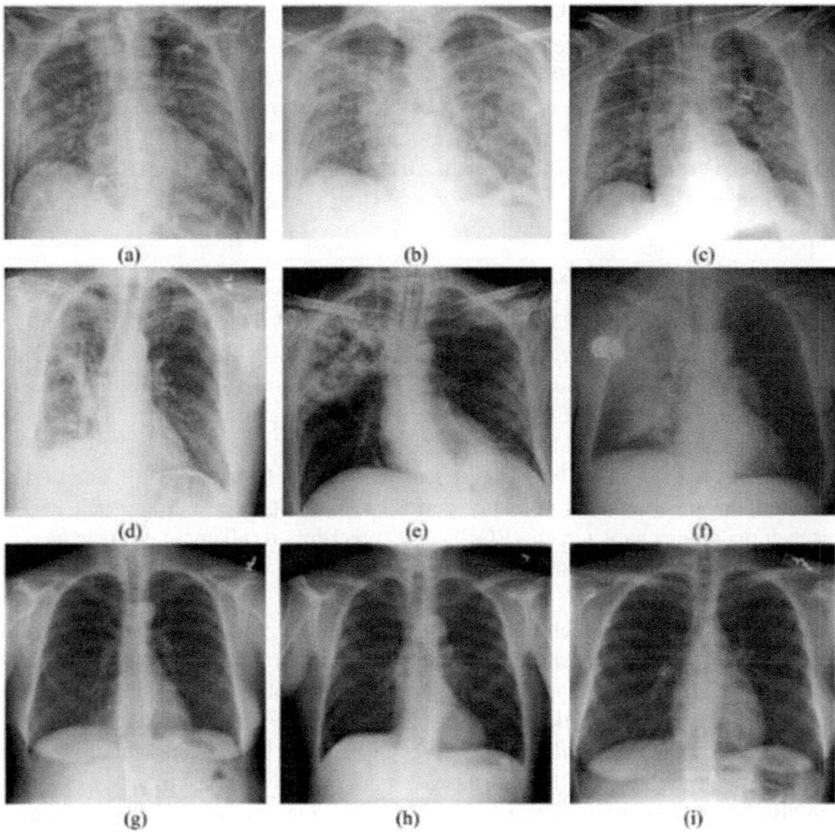

FIGURE 11.1 (a–c) COVID-19-infected chest X-ray images, (d–f) pneumonia-infected chest X-ray, and (h–i) normal chest X-ray images.

such as learning and problem-solving, as opposed to the innate intelligence shown by humans (Reddy et al., 2023).

The convolutional neural networks (CNNs) algorithm is a very advanced technique in deep learning that surpasses previous models, hence qualifying as a kind of "artificial intelligence." CNN is expected to be the predominant method for computer vision processing applications. The objective of this research is to examine the feasibility of using CLAHE and CNN in various deployment scenarios and transfer learning experiments.

Researchers use contrast limited histogram equalization (CLAHE) to improve the quality of X-ray chest images when they have established an appropriate method for detecting COVID-19. This entails implementing a histogram equalization technique on the X-ray datasets and assessing the effectiveness of combining CNN with CLAHE (Mehta et al., 2022; Khasawneh et al., 2021; Gupta et al., 2023).

Pneumonia is one of the worst lung diseases. A radiologist examines a sequence of chest radiographs to detect pneumonia. However, human-assisted diagnosis is constrained by factors such as the availability of experts, associated expenses, and other related issues. In order to achieve the utmost precision in terms of dataset quantity, the researchers have included the non-COVID-19 pneumonia dataset in the existing X-ray chest imaging of COVID-19 patients. To consider it through another approach, the dataset included in this work comprises both regular X-ray chest images and X-ray chest images of COVID-19 (Suganyadevi and Seethalakshmi, 2022; Farhat et al., 2022; Taresh et al., 2021; Solaiman et al., 2021; El-Kenawy et al., 2021; Takara et al., 2022; Shadin et al., 2021).

11.2.1.1 Existing Models/Architectures

In their study, Saheb et al. (2022) introduced a deep-COVID model that utilizes deep transfer learning. Four renowned CNNs, including ResNet-18, ResNet-50, SqueezeNet, and DenseNet-121, underwent transfer learning on a subset of 2000 radiograms to accurately identify cases of COVID-19 in the analyzed chest X-ray pictures. Upon assessing these models with the remaining 3000 pictures, most of these networks had a specificity rate of about 90% and a sensitivity rate of 98% (± 3%). The design included the incorporation of many performance evaluation metrics such as the receiver operating characteristic (ROC) curve, precision–recall curve, average prediction, and confusion matrix for each model. Additionally, the sensitivity and specificity rates were also considered.

A system suggested which will compile the COVID-19 statistics database that is accessible on official websites, making it easier for travellers to plan their trips (N. Kazi et al., 2021). The application will provide a list of locations, and upon selecting a location, various statistics will be displayed. All cases, all active cases, all deaths, all recovered, chances of infection, chances of recovery if infected, and chances of dying if infected are among the statistics given. An individual's past travel experiences can also be used to predict travel safety. Travellers and anyone in social touch with them will find this feature useful.

Relative convolution network: ResNet-18 and ResNet-50 Pre-trained ResNet-18, which was trained on the ImageNet dataset, is one of the models utilized in the study described by Polat et al. (2021).

SqueezeNet is a concise CNN design that employs much fewer parameters, around 50 times less, while yet achieving accuracy comparable to that of AlexNet on the ImageNet dataset. By using model compression methods, the authors successfully decreased the size of SqueezeNet to around 0.5 MB. This achievement has greatly enhanced its appeal for applications requiring compact models. To compress the incoming data vertically, a layer of size 1 x 1 is being used, while two parallel 1x1 and 3x3 convolutional layers are considered to restore the input's depth.

One of the prominent models is DenseNet which is described by Patel (2021) and is also known as the dense convolutional network, which also achieved the top position in the 2017 ImageNet competition. Every layer of DenseNet gets added inputs from all previous layers and transmissions its own feature maps to all subsequent levels. Each layer acquires all the information from the preceding ones. The network may achieve a reduced size and increased density by having a less number of channels since each layer gets feature maps from all preceding levels which leads to the enhancement of the computational and memory efficiency of the network.

11.2.2 Theoretical Framework

ResNet-18 is a CNN with a depth of 18 layers. The network has undergone pretraining using a version that was trained on more than one million photographs from the ImageNet database. The pretrained network has the capability to classify images of 1000 distinct item categories, such as a keyboard, mouse, pencil, and various animals. As a result, the network has been trained to generate a wide range of feature representations that include a large amount of visual information. The network has the capability to process pictures with an input size of 224 × 224.

ResNets effectively address one of the prominent issues known as the vanishing gradient problem. This phenomenon occurs when gradients originating from the point where the loss function is computed rapidly diminish to zero after numerous iterations of the chain rule, particularly when the network is too deep. Consequently, the absence of learning occurs due to the weights failing to update their values.

ResNets allow for direct propagation of gradients from subsequent layers to initial filters via the skip connections. The many ResNet architectures for ImageNet, categorized by the number of layers and parameters, are shown in Table 11.1.

It is well acknowledged that increasing the number of layers in a deep neural network leads to a reduction in the error rate. This phenomenon, known as the Vanishing/Exploding gradient, is often seen in deep learning as the network grows in size and complexity. This results in the gradient either being zero or too huge. Therefore, when the number of layers is raised, both the training and test error rates similarly rise.

Figure 11.2 demonstrates that a 56-layer CNN design yields higher error rates on both the training and testing datasets in comparison to a 20-layer CNN architecture. If overfitting was the cause, the 56-layer CNN should have a smaller training error. However, it paradoxically demonstrates a larger training error as well. Additional examination of the error rate revealed that the vanishing/exploding gradient is the cause. To address this problem, the concept of leftover blocks is used.

11.2.2.1 Residual Blocks

The residual blocks network has been used to address the issue of the vanishing/exploding gradient. This network operates using a technique known as skip connections. A skip connection bypasses the training process of some layers and immediately links to the output.

TABLE 11.1

ResNets Architectures for ImageNet

Number of Layers	Number of Parameters
ResNet-18	11.174M
ResNet-34	21.282M
ResNet-50	23.521M
ResNet-101	42.513M
ResNet-152	58.157M

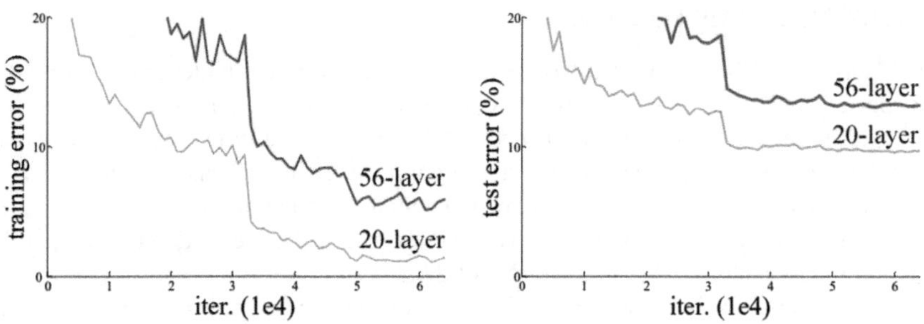

FIGURE 11.2 Increasing network depth leads to an increase in error.

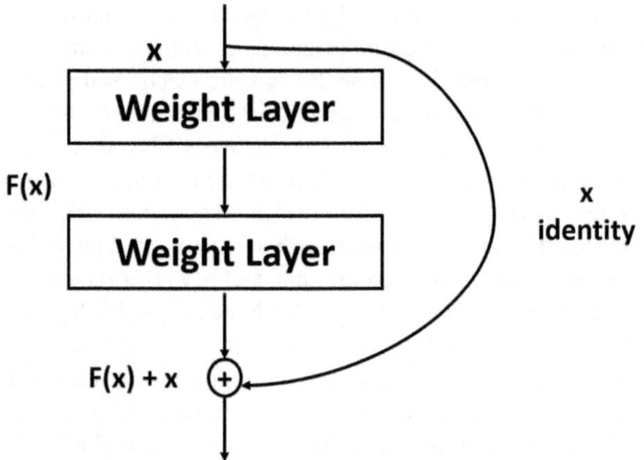

FIGURE 11.3 Logical scheme of base building block for ResNet.

The approach of this network is to allow the network to adapt to the residual mapping instead of having layers learn the fundamental mapping.

Instead of using the initial mapping H(x), we may use the network fit as shown in Figure 11.3. In this case, the function F(x) is defined as H(x) minus x, which implies that H(x) is equal to F(x) plus x.

11.2.2.2 ResNet Layers

The layers of a ResNet consist of several blocks. This phenomenon occurs because when ResNets increase in depth, they often do this by including more processes into a block, while maintaining the same total number of layers. Except for the last action in a block, which excludes the ReLU activation, an operation in this sense pertains to a convolution, batch normalization, and ReLU activation.

Consequently, throughout the implementation, they differentiate between the Basic Block, which consists of two operations, and the Bottleneck Block, which consists of three actions. Typically, each of these operations is called a layer. However, the proposed system already designates a layer as a group of blocks.

Layer Name	Output Size	ResNet-18
conv1	$112 \times 112 \times 64$	7×7, 64, stride 2
conv2_x	$56 \times 56 \times 64$	3×3 max pool, stride 2 $\begin{bmatrix} 3 \times 3, 64 \\ 3 \times 3, 64 \end{bmatrix} \times 2$
conv3_x	$28 \times 28 \times 128$	$\begin{bmatrix} 3 \times 3, 128 \\ 3 \times 3, 128 \end{bmatrix} \times 2$
conv4_x	$14 \times 14 \times 256$	$\begin{bmatrix} 3 \times 3, 256 \\ 3 \times 3, 256 \end{bmatrix} \times 2$
conv5_x	$7 \times 7 \times 512$	$\begin{bmatrix} 3 \times 3, 512 \\ 3 \times 3, 512 \end{bmatrix} \times 2$
average pool	$1 \times 1 \times 512$	7×7 average pool
fully connected	1000	512×1000 fully connections
softmax	1000	

FIGURE 11.4 ResNet-18 architecture.

The literature review has elucidated the distinctive aspects of the study in the context of COVID-19 X-ray image analysis within smart city frameworks. By leveraging the ResNet-18 machine learning model as shown in Figure 11.4, the technical frontier not only has been advanced but also tailored our approach to the unique dynamics of urban healthcare systems. This juxtaposition of advanced computational techniques with the practical realities of urban healthcare distinguishes our work from existing literature. The comparative analysis presented herein underscores the novelty and potential impact of our approach, particularly in how it harnesses technology for more efficient and effective pandemic response in smart cities.

11.3 Methodology

The overall illustration of our proposed architecture consists of two distinct stages. In the first stage, the one pre-trained CNN that is well-known for its performance in image classification tasks is used. In the second stage, Web Application has been developed for classifying the X-ray images. A rapid, non-invasive, and reasonably priced way to discover anomalies in the chest is through X-ray imaging. Suitable for COVID-19 identification, the ResNet-18 model is a deep CNN that excels in extracting subtle patterns from medical pictures. The flow diagram of the proposed system is shown in Figure 11.5. ResNet-18 retains computing efficiency while extracting complex information for precise diagnosis from X-rays. In the complex circumstances,

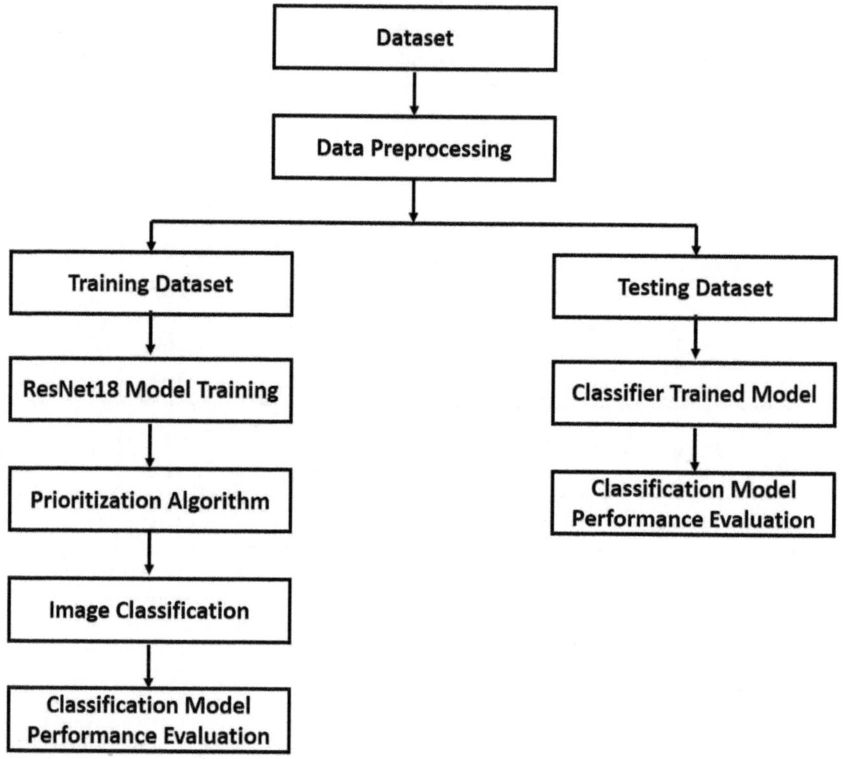

FIGURE 11.5 Flow diagram of the proposed system.

minor irregularities are detected that are frequently missed by human sight simplifying treatment planning and diagnostics for better patient outcomes.

11.3.1 Dataset

The Kaggle repository provided the dataset used for this study, which included chest X-ray scans of pneumonia patients, normal individuals, and COVID-19-afflicted individuals. The purpose of this dataset collection is not to validate the diagnostic performance of any deep learning model, but rather to investigate potential methods for effectively identifying coronavirus infections through computer vision techniques (Chandra et al., 2021; Yang et al., 2023). There are 3886 chest X-ray pictures in the entire dataset. The training (i.e., 3796) and test (i.e., 90) sets of normal, COVID-19, and pneumonia are further separated from this dataset. Around 1341 is normal, 1200 is COVID-19, and 1345 is pneumonia in the training set. Thirty samples each of a normal case, COVID-19, and pneumonia were taken into consideration for this analysis throughout the test phase. Also, approximately 200 posteroanterior (PA) view scans of COVID-19-affected patients from another dataset 150 of which were randomly selected and added to the existing dataset to reduce class imbalance. The scans were scaled down to 224 × 224 (another option was 227 x 227) to help our model train quickly. It was determined that the PA view scans were compatible with our COVID-19 dataset.

11.3.2 Data Preprocessing

The model's weights have been utilized. The model offered us two options for each image: 224 x 224 or 227 x 227. The former has been selected to expedite training times. Random horizontal flip has been used to enhance the data. For example, an image that has been inverted and normalized should both be in the same class. Images are normalized to a specified range, which was utilized to train the ImageNet dataset for our ResNet-18 Model. Data loaders are used as an iterator to loop through the dataset and retrieve the batch size samples and labels. In the test set, no data augmentation will be necessary.

11.3.3 Model Formulation

When necessary, the data that was taken from the repositories was cleansed. A substantial dataset is needed to apply a deep learning algorithm and produce trustworthy findings. However, it's conceivable that not all problems have enough data, particularly when it comes to medical difficulties. Medical data collection can occasionally be costly and time-consuming. Augmentation can be used to address these kinds of issues. Through augmentation, the overfitting issue can be resolved and the suggested model's accuracy raised. In order to avoid over-fitting, augmentation is also applied to this gathered dataset. Zoom, rotation, and picture sharing were among the enhancements. Next, to lessen over-fitting and help the model become broader, the data was shuffled. Subsequently, the suggested model was trained using the prepared dataset.

11.3.4 Model Creation: ResNet-18

The ResNet-18 architecture was strategically selected for this research initiative due to several technical merits. The ResNet-18 architecture mainly focuses on implementing a resolution of the vanishing gradient problem, a well-known obstacle in deep learning. It does this by using residual or skip connections, which facilitate the backpropagation of gradients in deeper layers, enhancing the model's capabilities in learning complex features. Furthermore, the architecture is known for efficiency in image classification, both computationally and temporally; thus, the architecture serves as a suitable base model for this study (Wang, 2023).

11.3.5 Hyperparameter Selection

To balance the speed of convergence and model performance the learning rate is set to 3e-5. For its adaptive learning rate capabilities, the Adam optimizer was chosen.

11.3.6 Challenges Faced

1. **Computational constraints**: The initial training phase was computationally expensive, demanding hardware advancements.

2. **Data scarcity**: The shortage of publicly available medical imaging data played limitations on the training phase.
3. **Model interpretability**: Ensuring that the model's predictions could be interpreted by healthcare professionals was a significant challenge, as explaining the model's findings is especially difficult when dealing with neural networks with multiple layers and dense networks, which both enable in-depth automated feature selection.

11.4 Experimental Results and Discussion

The model has been trained using a medical imaging dataset consisting of chest X-ray images. The training was conducted on a Google Colab GPU to leverage its processing capabilities. The dataset was pre-processed and carefully curated to guarantee consistent and high-quality photographs. The initial learning rate was set to 0.00003 and the training was conducted over the course of 160 epochs. The Adam optimizer is used to facilitate convergence by using a learning rate that gradually decreases over time. The fetching and displaying of a batch of datasets by using data loaders is shown in Figure 11.6.

The dataset consists of 3886 chest X-ray pictures, divided into a training set of 3796 photos and a test set of 90 images. The dataset includes instances of normal, COVID-19, and pneumonia. The training set comprises 1341 photos classified as normal, 1200 images classified as COVID-19, and 1345 images classified as pneumonia. The test set included 30 samples each of normal, COVID-19, and pneumonia cases, which were used for analysis. To mitigate class imbalance, an additional dataset including 150 randomly sampled PA view scans of COVID-19-affected individuals was included, resulting in a total of around 200 scans. In order to expedite the training process of our model, the scans were downsized to dimensions of 224 × 224 (alternatively, there was

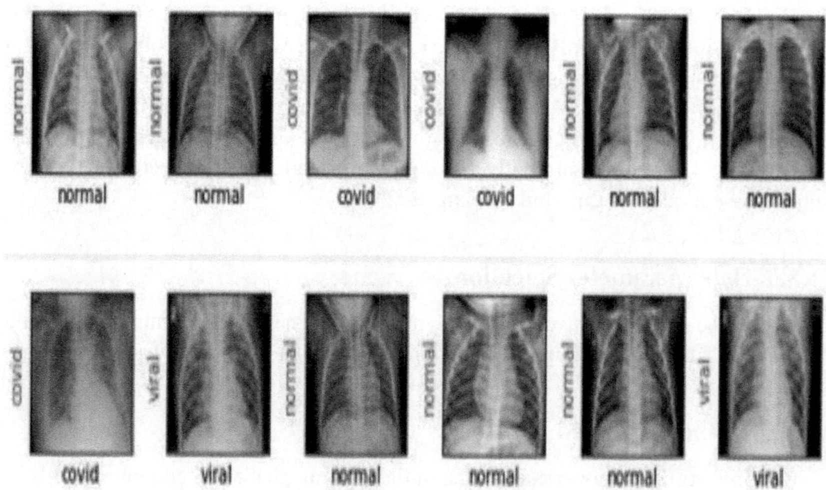

FIGURE 11.6 Fetching and displaying a batch using data loaders.

the choice to use dimensions of 227 x 227). According to the given information, the PA view scans were determined to be consistent with the COVID-19 dataset. The data distribution for training and testing the data is shown in Table 11.2.

11.4.1 Model Performance Metrics

Validation loss and accuracy were computed at different epoch levels that were used to evaluate the performance of the model.

Validation loss: A key indicator of how successfully a model generalizes to new data is validation loss. It displays the discrepancy between the validation set's actual values and the values predicted by the model. Better model generalization and an increased capacity for precise prediction on fresh data are shown by a decreased validation loss.

Accuracy: The percentage of accurate predictions the model made on the validation set is known as validation accuracy. It provides a clear indicator of how well the model can categorize or forecast results. A model that performs better is usually indicated by a higher validation accuracy.

Collaborating for the best possible model evaluation: Accuracy and validation loss offer complementary perspectives on the performance of the model. The model's performance on real-world data can be ensured by adjusting model architecture, fine-tuning hyperparameters, and preventing overfitting by keeping an eye on these two measures throughout training. Figure 11.7 shows that the suggested model appears to have performed well on the validation dataset following 160 epochs of training, based on the reported validation loss of 0.1898 and accuracy of 95.56% at the 160th epoch.

TABLE 11.2

Dataset Distribution in Training and Testing

	Train	Test
Normal	1341	30
COVID-19	1350	30
Pneumonia	1345	30

```
Evaluating at step 160
Validation Loss: 0.1898, Accuracy: 0.9556
```

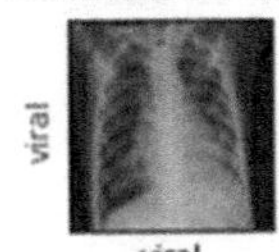

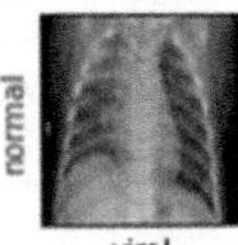

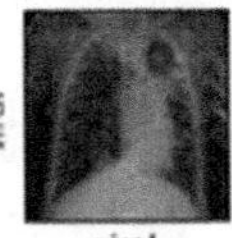

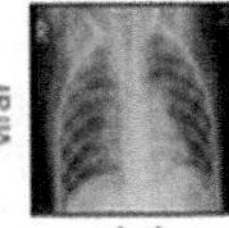

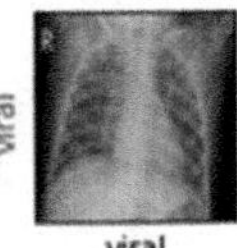

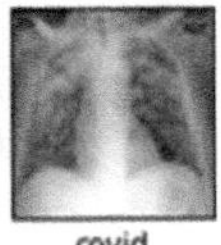


```
Performance condition satisfied, stopping..
CPU times: user 6min 17s, sys: 5.28 s, total: 6min 22s
Wall time: 9min 48s
```

FIGURE 11.7 Epoch 160 when the performance condition was satisfied.

Loop visualizing predictions refers to a dynamic, ongoing process that creates visual representations of model predictions over time in order to track and assess and may be to improve the model's performance. When models must adjust to shifting data distributions or when ongoing monitoring is essential for making decisions, this iterative technique is useful. By using loop visualization, it classification of X-ray images into normal, viral, and COVID-19 is shown in Figure 11.8.

Table 11.3 shows the achieved validation loss and accuracy by the proposed model at different levels of epoch between 1 and 160.

Table 11.4 displays the accuracy, validation loss, and training time of different deep learning models: ResNet-18, ResNet-50, SqueezeNet, and DenseNet121. It gives insights of their performance.

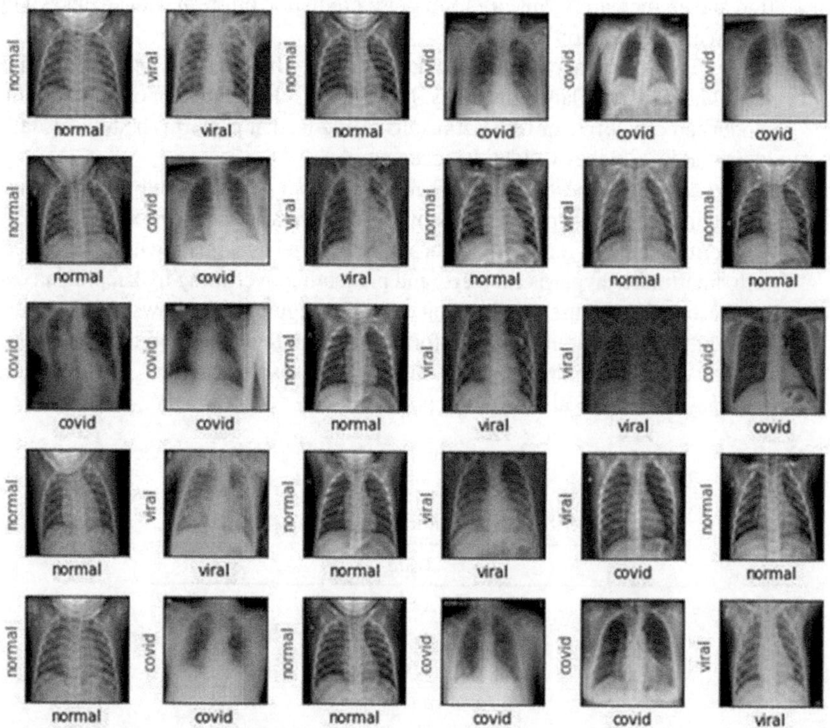

FIGURE 11.8 Loop visualizing predictions.

TABLE 11.3

Epoch, Accuracy, and Loss

Epoch	Accuracy (%)	Loss
1	91.2	0.25
...	...	...
160	95.56	0.1898

TABLE 11.4

Model Accuracy, Loss, and Training Time

Model	Accuracy (%)	Loss	Training Time
ResNet-18	95.56	0.1898	9m 48s
ResNet-50	94.1	0.21	15m 30s
SqueezeNet	92.3	0.25	8m 20s
DenseNet-121	93.7	0.23	14m 15s

11.4.2 Significance of Accuracy and Loss Rates

The model's diagnostic accuracy, quantified at 95.56%, is of significant relevance given the exigent circumstances surrounding COVID-19 diagnosis. This high accuracy rate indicates a substantial degree of reliability in the model's predictive capabilities. However, it is crucial to consider the accompanying validation loss, which is recorded at 0.1898. This metric serves as an indicator that the model's performance is not yet fully optimized. Specifically, the validation loss points to the necessity for further refinement in the model's ability to minimize both Type I and Type II errors, commonly referred to as false positives and false negatives, respectively. The presence of these errors could have serious implications in a clinical setting, where the stakes are elevated due to the life-threatening nature of the virus. Therefore, while the high accuracy rate is indicative of the model's potential utility, the non-negligible validation loss underscores the imperative for additional tuning and validation to enhance its diagnostic precision.

11.4.3 Hypothetical Scenarios

Imagine a remote village where healthcare facilities are minimal, and the nearest city with comprehensive medical facilities is hundreds of miles away. A sudden outbreak of respiratory illnesses, suspected to be COVID-19, has the local health workers worried. In such a scenario, the proposed system can be very useful. When multiple patients come in with symptoms of respiratory distress, Health workers can take chest X-rays and can use the proposed application to quickly categorize the cases. During the peak of the COVID-19 pandemic, even well-equipped hospitals in cities are overwhelmed. The application could play a crucial role in speeding up the diagnostic process. A backlog of untested patients and long waiting times for RT-PCR tests can be handled well. This can lead to efficient utilization of RT-PCR tests, quicker isolation of confirmed cases, and effective patient management.

11.5 Conclusion

The model implemented in this work performs well on the dataset, with an accuracy of 95.56% at the 160th epoch with a validation loss of 0.1898. In the context of an ongoing global pandemic, the integration of AI, specifically machine learning algorithms, into healthcare diagnostics has become increasingly critical. This chapter provides a comprehensive analysis of the deployment of machine learning techniques for the expedited and accurate diagnosis of COVID-19 via chest X-ray imaging. This type of initiative serves dual purposes: it acts as a compound for technological advancement in healthcare and it aims to mitigate the escalating straining on global healthcare infrastructures.

The work has yielded a high degree of diagnostic accuracy, thereby establishing a healthy foundation for further work and real-time world applications. However, there are a range of limitations, including but not restricted to insufficient data and ethical quandaries. Despite the presence of these constraints, the technological implications are significant. The model has the capability to accelerate diagnosis procedures, which can lead to expedite the treatment process and reduce mortality rates. Moreover, the efficacy of machine learning-based models, such as the one elaborated in this chapter, is not confined to COVID-19 diagnostics; it has wider pertinence to other forms of medical imaging, thereby expanding the scope of AI integration into global healthcare systems. Ethical considerations, however, will always remain a paramount concern.

The proposed research work has been extended as a web application for the development of a city as smart city that will let patients upload X-ray images of the chest, self-screening for COVID-19, and offer useful medical diagnosis at a preliminary level for enhancing the test's accuracy over time. The application is made up with a special importance on data privacy, guaranteeing that user information is secure and anonymized. After processing of provided chest X-ray images, the images are divided into three categories: normal, viral, and COVID-19. After the model delivers a categorized class index, the web application's frontend user interface displays the chest X-ray image, name of image, location, and calculated probabilities for each class. The performance gives an accuracy of 95.56%.

11.6 Future Scope

Subsequent similar research work may concentrate on improving the existing dataset by integrating a wider range of image samples, hence potentially improving the model's resilience and precision. Adding more classes of different categories can improve the model's comprehensiveness and can also lower the possibility of inaccurate classifications. With subsequent updates, the application might be able to operate independently, receiving X-ray images of the chest and giving outcomes without the need of human intervention. More advanced optimization methods such as Bayesian optimization or grid search could be used for more precise adjustment of the hyperparameters. Thorough experimental trials might confirm the safety and efficacy of the approach in real-time practical situations. The development of such kind of healthcare systems can lead to smart cities with well-equipped healthcare systems.

REFERENCES

Augustine, R., et al. (2020). Loop-mediated isothermal amplification (LAMP): A rapid, sensitive, specific, and cost-effective point-of-care test for coronaviruses in the context of COVID-19 pandemic. *Biology*, *9*(8), 182.

Chandra, T. B., Verma, K., Singh, B. K., Jain, D., & Netam, S. S. (2021). Coronavirus disease (COVID-19) detection in chest X-ray images using majority voting-based classifier ensemble. *Expert Systems with Applications*, *165*, 113909.

El-Kenawy, E.-S. M., et al. (2021). Advanced meta-heuristics, convolutional neural networks, and feature selectors for efficient COVID-19 X-ray chest image classification. *IEEE Access, 9*, 36019–36037.

Farhat, H. J., Sakr, G. E., & Kilany, R. (2022). Pneumonia and COVID-19 detection in chest X-rays using faster region-based convolutional neural networks (Faster R-CNN). *IEEE-EMBS International Conference on Biomedical and Health Informatics (BHI)*. IEEE.

Gupta, H., et al. (2023). A hybrid convolutional neural network model to detect COVID-19 and pneumonia using chest X-ray images. *International Journal of Imaging Systems and Technology*, *33*(1), 39–52.

Hussain, M. W., & Roy, D. S. (2023). Performance optimization strategies for big data applications in distributed framework. In *Intelligent Technologies: Concepts, Applications, and Future Directions*, Volume *2* (pp. 221–252). Singapore: Springer Nature Singapore.

Kazi, N., Parasar, D., & Jadhav, Y. (2021). Predictive risk analysis by using machine learning during COVID-19. In N. Mohanty, S. K. Saxena, S. Satpathy, & J. M. Chatterjee (Eds.), *Applications of artificial intelligence in COVID-19*. Medical Virology: From Pathogenesis to Disease Control. Springer, Singapore.

Khasawneh, N., et al. (2021). Detection of COVID-19 from chest x-ray images using deep convolutional neural networks. *Sensors*, *21*(17), 5940.

Kunac, N., et al. (2021). Building the COVID-19 testing capacities in Croatia: Establishing the interdepartmental COVID-19 unit at the Split University Hospital Centre. **Acta Clinica Croatica*, *60*(2), 254.

Lanzilao, L., et al. (2023). A computational approach in the diagnostic process of COVID-19: The missing link between the laboratory and emergency department. **Frontiers in Bioscience-Landmark*, *28*(2), 31.

Lasker, A., et al. (2022). Application of machine learning and deep learning techniques for COVID-19 screening using radiological imaging: A comprehensive review. *SN Computer *Science*, *4*(1), 65.

Mehta, V., et al. (2022). Correlation between chest CT and RT-PCR testing in India's second COVID-19 wave: A retrospective cohort study. *BMJ Evidence-Based Medicine*, *27*(5), 305–312.

Nanaiah, A., et al. (2022). Managing COVID-19 through collaboration: Applying a novel patient care model in a rural Indian community. *Journal of Global Health Reports*, *6*, e2022044.

Oishee, M. J., Ali, T., Jahan, N., Khandker, S. S., Haq, M. A., Khondoker, M. U., … & Adnan, N. (2021). COVID-19 pandemic: Review of contemporary and forthcoming detection tools. *Infection and Drug Resistance*, 1049–1082.

Patel, S. (2021). Classification of COVID-19 from chest X-ray images using a deep convolutional neural network. *Turkish Journal of Computer and Mathematics Education (TURCOMAT)*, *12*(9), 2643–2651.

Polat, Ç., et al. (2021). COVID-19 diagnosis from chest X-ray images using transfer learning: Enhanced performance by debiasing dataloader. *Journal of X-ray Science and Technology*, *29*(1), 19–36.

Pradhan, B., Hussain, M. W., Srivastava, G., Debbarma, M. K., Barik, R. K., & Lin, J. C. W. (2022). *A Neuro-Evolutionary Approach for Software Defined Wireless Network Traffic Classification*. IET Communications.

Reddy, K. H. K., Roy, D. S., Mishra, T. K., & Hussain, M. W. (Eds.). (2023). *Handbook of Research on Network-Enabled IoT Applications for Smart City Services*. IGI Global.

Saheb, S. K., Narayanan, B., & Rao, T. V. N. (2022). Prediction of COVID-19 through chest X-ray images employing various machine learning techniques. *International Conference on Intelligent Controller and Computing for Smart Power (ICICCSP)*. IEEE.

Sanyaolu, A., et al. (2021). *Global pandemicity of COVID-19: Situation report as of June 9, 2020*. Infectious Diseases: Research and Treatment, 14.

Shadin, N. S., Sanjana, S., & Farzana, M. (2021). Automated detection of COVID-19 pneumonia and non-COVID-19 pneumonia from chest X-ray images using convolutional neural network (CNN). *International Conference on Innovative and Creative Information Technology (ICITech)*. IEEE.

Solaiman, I. A., et al. (2021). *X-Ray classification to detect COVID-19 using an ensemble model*. Brac University.

Suganyadevi, S., & Seethalakshmi, V. (2022). Cvd-hnet: Classifying pneumonia and COVID-19 in chest x-ray images using a deep network. *Wireless Personal Communications, 126*(4), 3279–3303.

Takara, B., et al. (2022). Artificial intelligence to evaluate diagnosed COVID-19 chest radiographs. *Brazilian Journal of Radiation Sciences, 10*(3), 1–16.

Taresh, M. M., et al. (2021). Transfer learning to detect COVID-19 automatically from x-ray images using convolutional neural networks. *International Journal of Biomedical Imaging, 2021*(1), 1–9, 8828404.

Torres, I., Sippy, R., & Sacoto, F. (2021). Assessing critical gaps in COVID-19 testing capacity: The case of delayed results in Ecuador. *BMC Public Health, 21*, 1–8.

Valent, F., et al. (2021). RT-PCR tests for SARS-CoV-2 processed at a large Italian Hospital and false-negative results among confirmed COVID-19 cases. *Infection Control & Hospital Epidemiology, 42*(4), 498–499.

Wang, C. (2023). Federated learning with ResNet-18 for medical image diagnosis. *Proceedings of the 2023 8th International Conference on Multimedia Systems and Signal Processing*.

Yang, C., Gan, X., Peng, A., & Yuan, X. (2023). ResNet Based on Multi-Feature Attention Mechanism for Sound Classification in Noisy Environments. *Sustainability, 15*(14), 10762.

Yin, G., et al. (2021). An efficient primary screening of COVID-19 by serum Raman spectroscopy. *Journal of Raman Spectroscopy, 52*(5), 949–958.

12

Depression Detection in Social Media Text Using Machine Learning Techniques

Thirumoorthy Karpagalingam
Mepco Schlenk Engineering College, Sivakasi, India

J. Jerold John Britto
Ramco Institute of Technology, Rajapalayam, India

S. K. Manasa
Mepco Schlenk Engineering College, Sivakasi, India

12.1 Introduction

In this modern healthcare era, which is the focal point of smart cities, various machine learning (ML) techniques have been employed to detect depression (Reddy et al., 2023). Depression is a significant psychiatric condition characterized by persistent feelings of sadness, yet it can be effectively treated. In simple terms, it is related to our mood or state of mind. Depressive disorder affects our daily routine, inner peace, and how we feel and react. Experiencing this condition may result in a range of negative emotional and behavioral issues, which can ultimately impair one's ability to perform effectively both in their personal and professional life. Depression symptoms may vary in adults, teens, and children which include being sad, loss of interest in daily and usual activities, sudden weight loss or gain, excess amount of sleep or inadequate sleep, feeling guilty, thoughts of being worthless, or suicide. As per stats, 1 in 15 adults gets affected by depression per year. On average, depression appears during the teens to 20s. In today's world, teens and adults are involved in social media like Facebook, Twitter, Instagram, etc. Hence, some people express their emotions and thoughts in their social media texts and posts. They share all their emotions through social media which they feel comfortable with. Therefore, we will utilize ML classifiers to forecast whether an individual is experiencing depression based on their social media writings. The social media texts are unstructured; hence ML classifiers can be used which is good for handling unstructured data and non-linearity (Hussain and Roy, 2023; Pradhan et al., 2022). A classifier can be defined as an ML scheme that helps to categorize the data into classes. An unsupervised classifier uses unlabelled datasets and separates the data according to pattern or structure. Supervised classifiers

DOI: 10.1201/9781032631738-12

use a labelled dataset and it classifies data according to predetermined categories. We would be using the supervised classifiers. There are lots of classification algorithms available to categorize the data into classes.

In our work, we have used the Twitter-labelled dataset, Eye. Even though this study utilized Twitter tweets to train its machine-learning models, the findings could potentially be extended to other forms of text-based communication. The models were initially trained and tested on a publicly available Twitter dataset, which included and excluded specific phrases "depression" and "diagnosis." Subsequently, the Twitter-labelled dataset was employed to further train and test the models. We have employed supervised ML classifiers that include single and ensemble models, which are commonly used for prediction tasks due to their high prediction accuracy. However, the efficacy of the models is highly dependent on the type of data and features that are used for training purposes. Furthermore, the features utilized for training are retrieved and preprocessed utilizing a variety of techniques. More precisely, part-of-speech (POS), lemmatization, and text preprocessing techniques such as tokenization, stop word removal, correction of elongation words, and tokenization are used. To extract features from the input, we employ the Bag of Words (BoW) feature extraction approach. The models that are trained are primarily preprocessed and feature extraction is done. After features are extracted, the feature selection method is performed (Duric and Song, 2012) on the data using mutual information (MI), chi-square test (Chi2), and ReliefF. Although our objective is to develop a generalized method for detecting distress in social media, the dataset contains only the text and does not contain any of the frequently included emoticons, emojis, images, videos, or web links. We concentrate our efforts on resolving the imbalanced data sample issue, which has the possibility of affecting the effectiveness of classification models. The following provides an overview of this chapter's major contributions:

1. Constructing a framework for depression detection using text-based features for social media messages.
2. Incorporating feature selection techniques using MI, Chi2, and ReliefF.
3. Achieving greater accuracy for various ML classifiers.

The layout of this chapter is as follows: Section 12.2 represents the literature review of social media text using ML techniques, and Section 12.3 represents the dataset description. Section 12.4 represents the proposed methods. Section 12.5 encompasses the findings and analysis, while Section 12.6 provides the last remarks and conclusions of the work.

12.2 Related Works

There is a lot of automatic detection available for depression and these have been carried out using ML techniques which is one of the artificial intelligence methods. Researchers have utilized ML methods, including logistic regression, support vector machine (SVM), multilayer perceptron, and decision tree (DT), to detect and predict depression and stress. Chiong, et al. (2021) used a dataset from Twitter and other social media sites like Reddit and Facebook, a total of five datasets. They have used these six classifiers for depression prediction and trained the Twitter-labelled dataset. The researchers performed the testing after removing the keywords "depression" and "diagnosis" and compared the accuracy of each classifier. They have an accuracy of measuring around 80–93% on each classifier and dataset, respectively. In the work, William and Suhartono (2021) have undertaken a systematic literature review and found that it indeed is possible to detect depression earlier on social media because of the existence of characteristics that are used in the social media text. It is found that most of the studies on detecting depression using text, use deep learning techniques like Recurrent Neural Network (RNN) for early detection. Based on the research, the authors have found that the Bidirectional Long Short-Term Memory (BiLSTM) + Attention methods yield the best result compared to other classifiers and methods and it is also noted that the detection models being utilized require optimization, such as hyperparameter tuning, in order to enhance the performance of any given model. Many researchers have focused on the early detection of depression through social media posts. Yang et al. (2022) employ the Knowledge-aware and Contrastive Network (KC-Net). The authors initially retrieved mental state knowledge by utilizing a commonsense knowledge base called COMET. Subsequently, they included this knowledge into their model using gated recurrent units (GRUs) and employed dot-product attention. The work uses a depression detection dataset, a stress detection dataset, and a stress factors recognition dataset for testing the model and has acquired an F1 score of 95.4% with a 2.07% of average improvement. The model includes Convolutional Neural Network (CNN), GRU, BiLSTM, KC Net, Concatenation of multiple Networks (C-Net), and Bidirectional Encoder Representations from Transformers (BERT) for the comparison of performance metrics. Chatterjee et al. (2022) worked on suicide detection from online social media using a multi-modal feature-based technique. They used a labelled dataset from Reddit and Twitter and identified six groups of clinical behaviours on social media. They used a classification model such as logistic regression, random forest (RF) classifier, linear SVC, and gradient boosting classifier and got an accuracy of 0.86, 0.83, 0.87, and 0.77, respectively. The authors also analyzed the dataset based on time slots as suicidal and non-suicidal. In order to build a model for predicting and recognizing public opinion from the pandemic Twitter data, the author Mahdikhani (2022) utilized feature extraction methods like BOW, TF-IDF and topic analysis, document embedding, and supervised learning algorithms. Sewnet Amare et al. (2022) worked on detecting depression and associated factors in the pregnant stage. They used the logistic regression model and got an accuracy of 95% confidence interval. The participant count was about 422 and based on the study and interview, the prediction was done. Ghosh et al. (2023) used attention-based bidirectional LSTM- and CNN-based models for detecting mental health. The dataset used by the authors was Bangla social media texts. They followed and employed different preprocessing and embedding methods and got an overall accuracy of 96.02%. The embedding methods include fast text, word2vec, and GloVe, and among these, the word2Vec produces greater accuracy of 94.325%. Using the Shapley value, Jothi et al. (2021) were able to forecast that women will suffer from generalized anxiety disorder. In their work, the Shapley value is implemented as a feature extraction selection method of the data mining classifier. Knowledge discovery database (KDD) has been utilized. It has five stages: data collecting, pre-processing, feature selection, classification, and assessment. The classification model here includes Naive Bayes, RF, and J48 and has an accuracy of 61.40%, 70.65%, and 91.20%, respectively. The Shapley value contains the evaluation criteria such as sensitivity and specificity. Thus, the J48 classifier works well in their study when compared with other classifiers. Tao et al. (2021) detected depression using an ensemble binary classifier. This ensemble classifier tries to improve the performance of the ML model. Kim et al. (2020) collected posts from Reddit, analyzed the posting information that is written by the users and identified whether a person has a mental disorder. They have employed a synthetic minority over-sampling technique (SMOTE) to overcome the imbalance issue of the data they have collected. The CNN-based classification model was proposed along with the XGBoost classifier for the prediction of depression, anxiety, bipolar disorder, BPD, schizophrenia, and autism and has acquired an accuracy of 75.13%, 77.81%,9 0.20%, 90.49%, 94.33%, 96.96%, respectively. Thus, it is clear that the deep learning method with appropriate NLP processing could provide great performance in mental illness detection. Kaur et al. (2021) proposed a sentiment analysis using deep learning scheme for analyzing the COVID-19 Tweets. The authors have used the R programming language for analyzing the Tweets. The data were collected from Twitter keywords that include COVID-19, new cases, and recovered. The contributors have employed their algorithm named hybrid heterogenous SVM (H-SVM) and classified the data as positive, negative, and neutral based on the sentimental scores in addition to this, a comparison has also been done between their proposed algorithm and with models such as RNN and SVM. Islam et al. (2018) and Ahmed et al. (2022) employed the ML schemes to devise the depression detection model. The author provided the review study about the healthcare system in Edo-Osagie et al. (2020). In Vandana and Chaudhary (2023), the author devised the deep learning-based depression model using textual features and audio features.

12.3 Proposed Work

In this chapter, we describe the framework designed for detecting a person's depression using textual data. Before the removal of the words "Depression" and "Diagnosis" from the datasets, it is first trained and tested using various classifiers. Following the conclusion of the aforementioned process, the terms "depression" and "diagnostic" are eliminated from the datasets, and feature selection techniques are applied. Subsequently, the data is subjected to training and testing procedures employing diverse classifiers. The system design is represented in Figure 12.1.

Data pre-processing: Data pre-processing is the initial and most important stage in any ML model. The data has to be in the usable form before training the model using the dataset. To gain an accurate result the data must be free of noise. The fundamental problem with social media tweet is that it has an erratic text format that includes acronyms, special characters, numbers, and other symbols. To preprocess data, the Natural Language Toolkit (NLTK) is utilized. This procedure entails the following:

1) Removing URLs: Eliminating URLs, such as "https.//" or "http.//," as well as special characters like the #hashtag, @mentions, punctuation, and numbers.
2) Removing elongated words: People may employ text embellishment in informal writing to emphasize or change the meanings of words. For example: "whyyyyyyyyyyyyyyyy" and "missssssssss" to "why" and "miss."

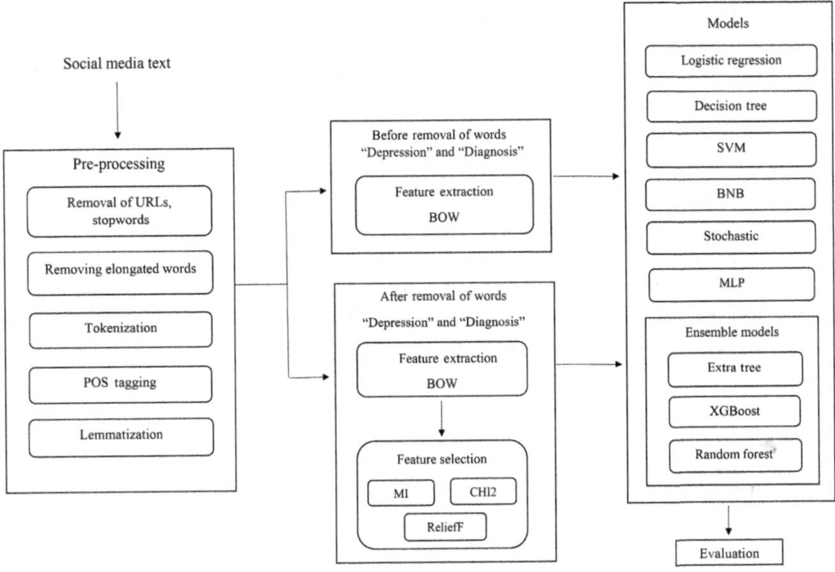

FIGURE 12.1 System design of proposed depression prediction model.

3) Removing stopwords and punctuations: Stopwords, which are the most prevalent words in any language and have no effect on the classification of data, include "a," "in," "will," and similar words. Punctuation (',',":", etc.) is also viewed as superfluous for jobs involving natural language processing.
4) Tokenization: Breaking the text into smaller chunks. For example: "It is hot" is tokenized into "It," "is," "hot."
5) POS tagging: The act of assigning appropriate parts of speech to words in a text (e.g., noun, verb, adjective).
6) Lemmatization: The lemmatization procedure entails discovering a word's root form. For instance, "Listen" is used in place of words like "Listens," "Listened," "Listening," etc. As a result, cleaning of data has been done to remove the incorrect or duplicate data in the dataset.

Feature extraction: Here, the features are extracted using BoW for the Twitter dataset. For the process of non-removal of keywords, the extracted features are directly fed into ML models to evaluate the performance of each classifier used and for the process of after removal, the extracted features are selected using feature selection techniques. To represent a corpus of texts using the BoW method, a vocabulary of all the distinct words must be created. Each word in the vocabulary is assigned a unique index, which is then used to represent the word in a vector. The vocabulary size is the same length as the vector. As a result, it produces a sparse matrix of unique words and it can be calculated as follows:

$$\text{Bag of Words}\left(\text{Document}\right) = \frac{\left(\text{Count of each unique word in the document}\right) /}{(\text{Total number of unique words in the document}).}$$

Feature Selection: The Twitter Labeled dataset – EYE contains a huge number of "depression" and "diagnosis" words in it. So, the words are removed from the datasets and used for further processing. Here, the extracted features from both datasets are selected using feature subset selection schemes such as Chi2, MI, and ReliefF.

a) Mutual information (MI): It is the measure of interdependence among two variables. MI is used in feature selection to evaluate how much knowledge a feature contributes to the target variable. Features with higher MI scores are chosen for the final model because they are thought to be more relevant to the target variable. MI is based on the concept of entropy, which measures the level of uncertainty in a variable. The variable is considered to be more uncertain when the entropy is higher.

$$(feature;target) = Entr(feature) - Entropy(feature \mid target) \tag{12.1}$$

b) Chi-squared (Chi2): It assesses the degree of categorical variables' dependence on one another. The Chi2 statistic is to assess the significance of the link between each feature and the target variable. Features with higher Chi2 scores are chosen for the final model because they are thought to be more relevant to the target variable. Chi2 is based on the discrepancy between the frequency of a variable that is observed and the frequency that would be predicted under the null hypothesis.

$$x_c^2 = \frac{\Sigma\left(O_i - E_i\right)^2}{E_i} \tag{12.2}$$

where c represent the degrees of freedom, O represents the observed value, and E represents the expected value.

c) ReliefF: It is a feature selection technique for locating important features in high-dimensional datasets, and it has been used in some fields, including text classification, image processing, and bioinformatics. Each feature is taken into account individually by the ReliefF method, which determines its significance by comparing the feature values of two randomly chosen examples that are close to one another.

The average difference in feature values between the closest instance with the same class label (i.e., the closest hit) and the closest instance with a different class label is calculated by ReliefF specifically for each feature (i.e., the nearest miss).

$$\text{ReliefF}(\text{i}) = \text{sum\_\{j=1\}\^{}\{k\}}\left(\text{w\_\{j\}}/\text{k}\right)^{*} \text{diff\_\{j\}}(\text{i}) \tag{12.3}$$

The weight is calculated as,

$$w\_\{j\} = 1/\left(d\_\{j\} + \text{eps}\right) \tag{12.4}$$

where $w\_\{j\}$ is the weight assigned to jth instance. k is a number of nearest neighbours. diff_{j}(i) is the difference in feature i and jth instance.

By averaging the difference values across all instances in the dataset, the final feature scores are produced. The features with the highest values will be chosen for the final model because they are thought to be more relevant to the target variable.

The features selected are based on target variables "0" and "1" and it is stored as a CSV file to know how the selected features play an important role after the keywords have been removed in detecting the depression of an individual and to prove that this model performs well even after the removal of keywords in the dataset and the features got selected using these feature selection techniques are shown in Table 12.1.

Class Imbalance: Synthetic minority oversampling technique (SMOTE), a popular oversampling technique, is used in this study to address the issue of class imbalance (Padurariu and Breaban, 2019; Turlapati and Prusty, 2020; Srinivasan and Subalalitha, 2023). An expanding minority class, it aims to balance out the distribution of class. Synthetic data is produced by SMOTE using the KNN algorithm. Between the random data and the randomly selected K-nearest neighbour, synthetic data is produced. Until the minority class is proportionate to the majority class, this process is perpetuated. In this study, the datasets are balanced using SMOTE technique.

Classifier model: Before the removal of the words "Depression" and "Diagnosis," the data are trained and tested using various ML classifiers to detect higher accuracy. After the removal of the words "Depression" and "Diagnosis," the selected features from the Chi2, MI, and ReliefF are fed into the models and it is trained and tested which provides excellent detection performance on models. Those classifiers are

a. Logistic regression: It is one of the supervised ML algorithms. A statistical technique known as logistic regression is used in ML to investigate the relationship between a binary-dependent variable and one or more independent variables, which can be of nominal, ordinal, or period types. This approach is appropriate for exploring data and assessing the correlation between variables.
b. Linear SVM (LSVM): It is one of the supervised learning models. It uses data for training to categorize user input. It functions by

TABLE 12.1

Features Selected Using Chi2, MI, and ReliefF

Chi2	MI	ReliefF
Accounting	Bulk	Dysphoria
Acoustic	Burst	Entirety
Agitated	Desire	Simple
Artist	Illness	Inevitable
Bully	Loneliness	Usual
Celebrate	Plenty	Royalty
Captive	Protect	Apologize
Confidence	Rid	Competitive
Illness	Sad	Brutal

establishing a hyperplane to split classes and then aims to increase the separation from the hyperplane. The SVM algorithm identifies the support vectors, which are the closest points from the classes to the line. By maximizing the margins between these support vectors, the algorithm determines the optimal hyperplane.

c. Bernoulli Naive Bayes: Bernoulli Naive Bayes is a type of algorithm that serves as an alternative to the Naive Bayes (NB) algorithm. It is also a binary algorithm which is very useful to find whether the feature is present or not otherwise when the dataset is in the binary distribution.
d. XGBoost classifier: Extreme gradient boosting (XGBoost) is an ML library that employs a gradient descent algorithm and DTs. It is distributed in nature and belongs to the class of supervised learning algorithms.
e. Stochastic gradient descent: It is an efficient way to fit linear classifiers and regressors in SVM and logistic regression. Here, one can calculate the gradient using a little part of the observations instead of using all the observations.
f. DT classifier: The DT (Geurts, et al., 2006) classifier is a model that classifies data by constructing a tree structure, where each node represents a feature, and each branch indicates a possible outcome. The DT is based on Hunt's algorithm and was developed by Quinlan. This allows the DT to effectively classify new data based on the patterns and relationships identified in the training set.
g. Extra trees classifier: A DT-based ensemble approach, extra trees classifier (Geurts et al., 2006). To provide the categorization result, it combines the output from various DTs. It creates several trees and divides nodes according to a randomly chosen subset of attributes.
h. RF classifier: The RF uses an ensemble of DTs, each trained on a random subset of data and features. The model's generalization and robustness to outliers depend on the strength and correlation of the trees. Randomness reduces overfitting, while diversity improves accuracy. However, the model's performance can be affected by various factors, such as data quality, the complexity of relationships, and hyperparameters.
i. Multi-layer perceptron (MLP): The MLP classifier is a frequently used neural network for supervised learning tasks such as classification and regression. The MLP is composed of several layers of nodes, where each node is a straightforward computational unit that accepts input values, transforms the input, and then transfers the result to the following layer. Here, all ML algorithms are trained and tested and the best model and best feature selection technique will be predicted based on the highest accuracy rate obtained.

Performance Evaluation: The dataset used here is Twitter labelled – EYE. The dataset at hand must be divided into separate training and testing datasets in order to evaluate the performance of the model trained on the training dataset. The dataset is divided into a 70:30 ratio, with 70% allocated for training data and 30% for testing data. The dataset is then fitted and trained using various classifiers like LR, DT, RF, etc.

Before the removal of the words "Depression" and "Diagnosis," the data are trained and tested using various ML classifiers to detect higher accuracy. After the removal of the words "Depression" and "Diagnosis," the selected features from the Chi2, MI, and ReliefF are fed into the model and it is trained and tested which provides excellent detection performance on models.

Here, the performance of each classifier is evaluated before and after the removal of keywords, and the evaluation of the feature selection techniques is also done based on the accuracy score of the classifiers. Each classifier is evaluated using evaluation metrics and it is defined as follows:

i. Accuracy: The ratio of accurately predicted observations to all observations.
ii. Recall: The ratio of positively observed observations that were accurately predicted to all observations in the actual class that was in the yes/positive/1 category.
iii. Precision: Measure how often positive observations are successfully anticipated compared to all positive observations that were forecasted.
iv. F1-score: The harmonic mean of recall and precision. Calculating the average of precision and recall for the F1 score.

The formula for calculating evaluation metrics is

$$\text{Accuracy} = \text{TP} + \text{TN} / \text{TP} + \text{TN} + \text{FP} + \text{FN}, \text{recall} = \text{TP} / \text{TP} + \text{FN}, \text{precision} = \text{TP} / \text{TP} + \text{FP}, \text{F1 score} = \left(2^{*}\text{precision}^{*}\text{recall}\right) / \left(\text{precision} + \text{recall}\right)$$

where TP, true positive; TN, true negative; FP, false positive; FN, false negative.

12.4 Results and Discussion

The dataset is preprocessed and then fed into the feature extraction module without removing the keywords "depression" and "diagnosis." The strings will be in the form of a sparse matrix which is the output of feature extraction using BOW. Then the result of feature extraction is trained and tested using various classifiers. Table 12.2 shows the obtained result before the removal of keywords. The highest accuracy obtained is 99.11% by the XGBoost classifier whose precision, recall, and f1-score are 99.72%, 96.26%, and 97.96%, respectively. The accuracy, precision, recall, and f1-score of each classifier are represented in Table 12.1. After the implementation of the eye dataset before the removal of keywords, the implementation is performed by removing the keywords "depression" and "diagnosis." The feature selection technique is employed. The techniques include Chi2, MI, and ReliefF.

The selected features are then trained and tested using the classifier models and the performance evaluation is carried out to predict the model of those models. The visualization of these techniques along with the accuracy score on each classifier is represented in Figure 12.2 and their accuracy is tabulated in Table 12.3. From the table, it is clear that the MI performs well on the models with an accuracy of 80% and above whereas the Chi2 and ReliefF perform well only on some of the models. Chi2

TABLE 12.2

The Results of the Eye Dataset Before the Removal of the Keywords "Depression" and "Diagnosis"

Model Name	Accuracy (%)	Precision (%)	Recall (%)	F1-score (%)
LR	99.08	99.86	95.94	97.88
DT	91.15	72.17	97.32	82.88
SVM	98.50	97.54	95.59	96.56
RF	94.97	83.44	96.26	89.39
ET	95.12	84.66	95.06	89.55
BNN	98.70	98.35	95.72	97.02
XG	99.11	99.72	96.26	97.96
Stochastic	99.00	99.03	96.39	97.69
MLP	95.82	92.09	88.65	90.34

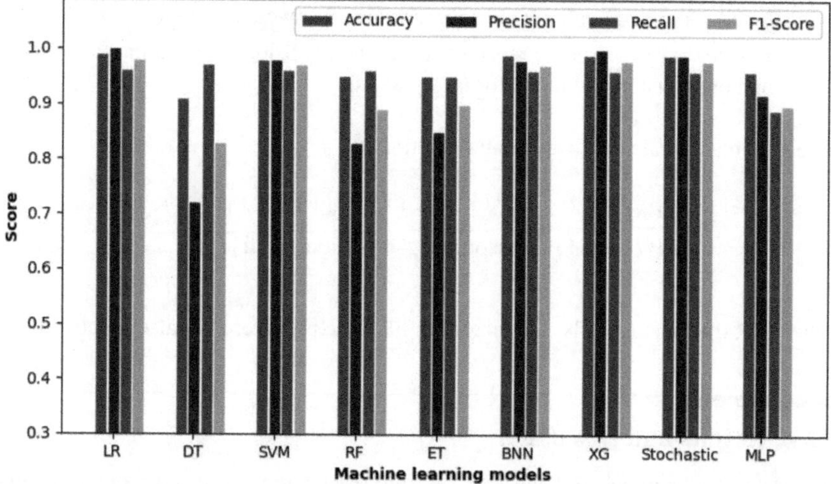

FIGURE 12.2 The performance of various classifiers before removing the keywords "depression" and "diagnosis."

TABLE 12.3

Accuracy of Models, When Implemented with Feature Selection Techniques

Model Name	Chi2 (%)	MI (%)	ReliefF (%)
LR	68.33	84.34	78.17
DT	83.57	82.99	76.73
SVM	68.74	83.93	77.84
RF	84.40	83.04	78.23
ET	84.63	83.02	78.64
BNN	88.68	85.54	79.34
XG	66.98	84.34	74.35
stochastic	68.50	83.96	77.20
MLP	86.72	82.22	80.14

performs well on BNN with an accuracy of 88.68% and ReliefF has the highest accuracy of 80.14% on MLP. Though MI has better accuracy, it best performs on the model BNN with an accuracy of 85.54%. The Receiver Operating Characteristic (ROC), Area Under the Curve (AUC) score measures the ability of a binary classifier to distinguish between positive and negative classes, where a higher score is indicative of better performance. While a model with an AUC value of 1.0 generates excellent predictions, one with a value of 0.5 does no better than random guessing. The AUC-based performance comparisons are as follows: among the various classifiers, the ones with the highest scores are BNB and RF, with ROC AUC scores of 99.18% and 98.75%, respectively. The remaining classifiers, namely, logistic regression, SVM, stochastic, and XGBoost, demonstrate strong performance with scores above 98%. Although the DT and extra tree classifiers display slightly lower scores, they still perform well. The MLP classifier has the lowest score; however, it is crucial to note that its performance might be impacted by the specific dataset and problem it was trained on. Overall, the high scores achieved by these classifiers indicate their potential for binary classification tasks and their capability to accurately classify new, unseen data.

12.5 Validity Threats

This section addresses the validity difficulties associated with our proposed scheme. Although the suggested depression detection method outperforms the alternative scheme, it necessitates a longer computational time. The suggested work utilizes three filter-based approaches to identify the most suitable features. It results in increased processing expenses.

12.6 Conclusion

Among children and young adults, social media use is linked to mental health symptoms like anxiety and depression. An increase in signs and symptoms of depression, anxiety, and stress were shown to be moderately and significantly correlated with youth while using social media in a 2022 meta-analysis. In this study, Twitter tweets help to detect depression in individuals. We proposed our healthcare system to detect whether a person is depressed or not before and after the removal of the keywords "depression" and "diagnosis." ML classifiers have performed well before and after the removal of keywords and helped in gaining better performance results. The feature selection techniques do perform well in this study along with those ML classifiers. This project which attempts to develop a technique for identifying depression in people using social media has shown encouraging results while employing feature selection techniques. In the future, we plan to use more features with more data, including sentiment scores (VADER), BING, Afinn, and NRC lexicons to predict the magnitude of the depression, LIWC characteristics, emoticons, and other linguistic features. Given that our research treats depression as a unified category, we suggest investigating many subcategories of depression and criteria that can indicate the extent of the condition. This study might be viewed as an initial phase in the creation of a social media-driven system that assesses, predicts, and provides suggestions on psychological issues.

REFERENCES

Ahmed, A., Aziz, S., Toro, C. T., Alzubaidi, M., Irshaidat, S., Serhan, H. A., ... Househ, M. (2022). Machine learning models to detect anxiety and depression through social media: A scoping review. *Computer Methods and Programs in Biomedicine Update*, *2*(100066), 100066. doi:10.1016/j.cmpbup.2022.100066

Chatterjee, M., Kumar, P., Samanta, P., & Sarkar, D. (2022). Suicide ideation detection from online social media: A multi-modal feature based technique. *International Journal of Information Management Data Insights*, *2*(2), 100103. doi:10.1016/j.jjimei.2022.100103

Chiong, R., Budhi, G. S., Dhakal, S., & Chiong, F. (2021). A textual-based featuring approach for depression detection using machine learning classifiers and social media texts. *Computers in Biology and Medicine*, *135*(104499), 104499. doi:10.1016/j.compbiomed.2021.104499

Duric, A., & Song, F. (2012). Feature selection for sentiment analysis based on content and syntax models. *Decision Support Systems*, *53*(4), 704–711. doi:10.1016/j.dss.2012.05.023

Edo-Osagie, O., De La Iglesia, B., Lake, I., & Edeghere, O. (2020). A scoping review of the use of Twitter for public health research. *Computers in Biology and Medicine*, *122*(103770), 103770. doi:10.1016/j.compbiomed.2020.103770

Geurts, P., Ernst, D., & Wehenkel, L. (2006). Extremely randomized trees. *Machine Learning*, *63*(1), 3–42. doi:10.1007/s10994-006-6226-1

Ghosh, T., Banna, M. H. A., Nahian, M. J. A., Uddin, M. N., Kaiser, M. S., & Mahmud, M. (2023). An attention-based hybrid architecture with explainability for depressive social media text detection in Bangla. *Expert Systems with Applications*, *213*(119007), 119007. doi:10.1016/j.eswa.2022.119007

Hussain, M. W., & Roy, D. S. (2023). Performance optimization strategies for big data applications in distributed framework. In *Intelligent Technologies: Concepts, Applications, and Future Directions*, Volume *2* (pp. 221–252). Singapore: Springer Nature Singapore.

Islam, M. R., Kabir, M. A., Ahmed, A., Kamal, A. R. M., Wang, H., & Ulhaq, A. (2018). Depression detection from social network data using machine learning techniques. *Health Information Science and Systems*, *6*(1), 8. doi:10.1007/s13755-018-0046-0

Jothi, N., Husain, W., & Rashid, N. A. (2021). Predicting generalized anxiety disorder among women using Shapley value. *Journal of Infection and Public Health*, *14*(1), 103–108. doi:10.1016/j.jiph.2020.02.042

Kaur, H., Ahsaan, S. U., Alankar, B., & Chang, V. (2021). A proposed sentiment analysis deep learning algorithm for analyzing COVID-19 tweets. *Information Systems Frontiers: A Journal of Research and Innovation*, *23*(6), 1417–1429. doi:10.1007/s10796-021-10135-7

Kim, J., Lee, J., Park, E., & Han, J. (2020). A deep learning model for detecting mental illness from user content on social media. *Scientific Reports*, *10*(1), 11846. doi:10.1038/s41598-020-68764-y

Mahdikhani, M. (2022). Predicting the popularity of tweets by analyzing public opinion and emotions in different stages of Covid-19 pandemic. *International Journal of Information Management Data Insights*, *2*(1), 100053. doi:10.1016/j.jjimei.2021.100053

Padurariu, C., & Breaban, M. E. (2019). Dealing with data imbalance in text classification. *Procedia Computer Science*, *159*, 736–745. doi:10.1016/j.procs.2019.09.229

Pradhan, B., Hussain, M. W., Srivastava, G., Debbarma, M. K., Barik, R. K., & Lin, J. C. W. (2022). *A Neuro-Evolutionary Approach for Software Defined Wireless Network Traffic Classification*. IET Communications.

Reddy, K. H. K., Roy, D. S., Mishra, T. K., & Hussain, M. W. (Eds.). (2023). *Handbook of Research on Network-Enabled IoT Applications for Smart City Services*. IGI Global.

Sewnet Amare, N., Nibret Gessesse, D., Solomon Kinfu, Y., Melesew Mekuriyaw, A., Amera Tizazu, M., Mossie Menalu, M., … Gonie Mekonnen, A. (2022). Prevalence of antenatal depression and associated factors among pregnant women during COVID-19 pandemic in North Shewa zone, Amhara region, Ethiopia. *International Journal of Africa Nursing Sciences*, *17*(100459), 100459. doi:10.1016/j.ijans.2022.100459

Srinivasan, R., & Subalalitha, C. N. (2023). Sentimental analysis from imbalanced code-mixed data using machine learning approaches. *Distributed and Parallel Databases*, *41*(1–2), 37–52. doi:10.1007/s10619-021-07331-4

Tao, X., Chi, O., Delaney, P. J., Li, L., & Huang, J. (2021). Detecting depression using an ensemble classifier based on Quality of Life scales. *Brain Informatics*, *8*(1), 2. doi:10.1186/s40708-021-00125-5

Turlapati, V. P. K., & Prusty, M. R. (2020). Outlier-SMOTE: A refined oversampling technique for improved detection of COVID-19. *Intelligence-Based Medicine*, *3*(100023), 100023. doi:10.1016/j.ibmed.2020.100023

Vandana, M. N., & Chaudhary, D. (2023). A hybrid model for depression detection using deep learning. *Measurement. Sensors*, *25*(100587), 100587. doi:10.1016/j.measen.2022.100587

William, D., & Suhartono, D. (2021). Text-based depression detection on social media posts: A systematic literature review. *Procedia Computer Science*, *179*, 582–589. doi:10.1016/j.procs.2021.01.043

Yang, K., Zhang, T., & Ananiadou, S. (2022). A mental state Knowledge–aware and Contrastive Network for early stress and depression detection on social media. *Information Processing & Management*, *59*(4), 102961. doi:10.1016/j.ipm.2022.102961

13

Depression Symptoms Prediction on Online Social Networks Using Machine Learning Algorithms

Oluwafolake Ojo
Federal University of Agriculture, Abeokuta, Nigeria

Inioluwa Adewuyi and Oluwadolapo Oni
Federal University of Agriculture, Abeokuta, Nigeria

Olufunke Oyinloye
University of Ilesa, Ilesa, Nigeria

Idris Gbolade
Federal University of Agriculture, Abeokuta, Nigeria

Abayomi Ojo
Obafemi Awolowo University Teaching Hospital, Ile-Ife, Nigeria

13.1 Introduction: Background and Driving Forces

Capitalizing the fact that the COVID-19 pandemic-related lockdown has led to significant social upheavals and a complete change in lifestyles, social behaviour, and transactions at the global level (Gao, Scullin, 2020; Wen et al., 2021); it severely impacted the general psychological health of most citizens across different countries. The swift dissemination of the virus, coupled with the escalating tally of afflicted individuals and fatalities, instigates profound apprehension and anguish worldwide (Elbay et al., 2020). Consequently, numerous governments had to develop diverse strategies to mitigate the outbreak, including imposing travel restrictions on non-residents, safeguarding public spaces, and even suspending transport systems (Zhu, Tan, 2021; Zhu et al., 2020). Nigeria saw its initial outbreak of COVID-19 in early 2020 (Ohia et al., 2020). Nigeria, along with numerous other nations, implemented a "lock-down" approach to enforce social distancing and significantly curtail the spread of diseases. Indeed, schools were among the myriad of institutions that were compelled to shut down for a prolonged period of time. The shutdown led to the termination of several specialists. COVID-19 has a dual impact on public well-being, affecting both the physical and

DOI: 10.1201/9781032631738-13

psychological aspects (Huang & Zhao, 2020). The emotional well-being of Nigerians has been adversely affected due to the exceptional circumstances of being confined to their homes (Olaseni et al., 2020). The epidemic was frequently associated with adverse economic consequences and an increased prevalence of mental health issues. The COVID-19 epidemic has had a profound impact on mental health, resulting in the emergence of several diseases such as depression, post-traumatic stress symptoms, aggression, dread, boredom, stigma, and insomnia (Gritsenko et al.; 2021). The pandemic has led to a surge in mental health problems (Bérard et al., 2021), including substance misuse and suicidal ideation and behaviour (Sun et al., 2021), particularly among young individuals. Specifically, the COVID-19 epidemic and quarantine were expected to lead to a significant increase in anxiety and depressive symptoms (Fullana et al., 2020). The global prevalence of clinical depression is substantial. According to the World Health Organization, close to half a billion people worldwide have clinical depression (Holt et al., 2014). Depression in middle age heightens the probability of experiencing dementia and cognitive deterioration during old age (Chow et al., 2022). Additionally, the postpartum period is a critical time for the development of psychological illnesses in women. Anxiety and severe depression are prevalent throughout pregnancy and the postpartum period (Harrison et al., 2022), affecting over 20% of women. Furthermore, it has been seen that COVID-19-recovered individuals who also suffer from depression experience more pronounced emotional and physical impairments, necessitating psychological intervention, in comparison to those without depression (Xu et al, 2022). Depression is associated with a history of substance misuse, a decline in social and vocational functioning, and an increase in suicidal behaviour, all of which pose significant risks. Early recognition and prompt response are urgently required to mitigate or prevent the subsequent distress that frequently ensues (Hetrick et al., 2008). During the examination of the enduring effects of the COVID-19 pandemic on mental well-being, scientists discovered that after approximately one year, even the group of individuals without any pre-existing health conditions exhibited heightened levels of sadness and indications of worry. The increasing occurrence of mental health issues in communities that have not previously experienced mental disorders, exhibit severe symptoms or demonstrate obvious effects of the COVID-19 pandemic alarms experts in the field. Efficient online solutions are required to effectively tackle these challenges (Kok et al., 2022). Technological breakthroughs have led to improvements in healthcare systems. E-health refers to the use of information and communication technologies for the administration and supply of healthcare (Yusif et al., 2020). Artificial intelligence (AI) has several uses across various industries and domains. The arrival of AI has transformed medical diagnostics with the ability to access huge databases and the speed of execution of diagnostic procedures (Jiang et al., 2017). As a matter of fact, smart cities innovation (Bibri & Krogstie, 2020) in combination with AI technologies, mainly the complex machine learning (ML) ones, are essential for the development of health services (Reddy et al., 2023), (Pradhan et al., 2022), (Ghazal et al, 2021). Depictive tasks encompass the application of deep learning and computer vision in radiology and dermatology as well as NLP for doing psychological evaluation (Gille et al., 2020). Different AI-driven models are employed by many mobile applications with smart features such as personalized recommendations, chatbots, telecom corporations, and healthcare systems among others (Sarker et al., 2021). With technological advancements, current participants of surveys can now describe their mental health problems precisely and truthfully using their mobile devices (Osotsi et al., 2020). Social media has evolved into a useful data source for health research given the presence of over three billion users worldwide (Oyebode et al., 2022). Contrary to the conventional diagnosis approach, this research proposed a novel scheme that incorporates AI methods, new mobile application features, and social networking to address the challenges related to early warning signs of depression. The integration of these new technologies serves as a self-diagnostic tool capable of assisting online users in their general well-being.

13.2 Existing Research

In this section, previous research investigating the application of smart technology and different AI or ML methods for health monitoring, clinical diagnosis, and predicting or classifying patient mental state are presented. Alvandi et al. examined the impact of digital communication on the emotional state of patients. The investigation results revealed that patients' emotional awareness is directly associated with computer-mediated psychotherapy outcomes. The study showed that there is a high tendency for participants to effectively communicate and concentrate through computer-mediated communication. However, the constraint identified in this approach is that the accuracy of emotional recognition greatly depends on the patient's mood state (positive or negative) before treatment (Alvandi et al., 2019). Elhai et al. (2020) investigated the interrelationship between gender, mental health variables, maturity, and the severity of problematic smartphone use (PSU) among users. The investigation which involved approximately 1000 Chinese students demonstrated that there is a strong correlation between mental health variables and the PSU. A random forest algorithm was proposed by Shen et al. (2020) to predict instances of attempted suicides among Chinese medical students. The results indicated that the ML approach can accurately identify suicidal behaviour or patterns among online users.

An emotional state prediction model using electroencephalography and a multi-modal physiological signals dataset was developed by Zhang et al. (2020); the scheme adopted various AI techniques such as feature extraction, segmentation, and ML classification techniques. Furthermore, an intelligent system for monitoring cyberbullying was designed by the researchers in Balakrishnan et al. (2020). The smart system was trained to analyze the personality traits of social media users while using Twitter as a case study. The empirical results revealed that the use of personality traits and sentiments improved the ability to identify instances of cyberbullying. However, it was observed that emotions did not yield the same outcome.

Additionally, the effectiveness of supervised ML for forecasting early signs of mental health problems among Asian PlayerUnknown's Battlegrounds (PUBG) gamers was examined by some researchers. Through comprehensive experimental analysis, it was established that there is a direct correlation between Internet gaming disorder and attention deficit hyperactivity disorder in the game data of PUBG gamers (Aggarwal et al., 2020). A predictive scheme was developed by the researchers Nemesure et al. (2021) and Hussain and Roy (2023) in ML techniques. The model was trained to perform analysis on electronic health records datasets, thereby, predicting the possibility of psychiatric traits in patients. Similarly, a deep learning model was proposed in another study to determine depression diagnosis among patients using datasets from

Norway. After a thorough investigation, the evaluation results revealed that the depressive symptom feature-based methods outperformed the generic word frequency-based methods (Uddin et al., 2022). Additionally, a review study was conducted by Rivera et al. (2022) which involved the careful selection of over 40 research publications that focused on the assessment and treatment of psychiatric disorders using electroencephalography and deep learning techniques. Another set of researchers investigated the similarity and difference of spatial cubes in brain MRI images that serve as parameters in an ML method for identifying depression signs (Mousavian et al., 2021). Furthermore, an empirical study was conducted to evaluate the effectiveness of depression identification. The study utilized publicly accessible Facebook data and implemented an ML methodology. The findings demonstrated a significant enhancement in accuracy and a decreased occurrence of misclassification (Islam et al., 2018). Also, the researchers in the study by Ashraf et al. (2020) examined the application of ML techniques to create a depression detection model based on photos and video data.

Orabi et al. (2018) proposed a predictive model based on a deep neural network; the model was trained using sparse and unstructured text datasets and it is capable of forecasting the possibility of depression among Twitter users. In another study, researchers examined the feasibility of detecting depression between end-users across social media platforms with the aid of ML methods. The empirical results validate that the approach can accurately identify depression-related posts on social media, even when tested on unrelated datasets and when the training datasets do not contain terms such as "depression" and "diagnosis" (Chiong et al., 2021). Furthermore, a related study examined the application of natural language processing techniques on Twitter data to perform sentiment analysis, with a particular focus on sadness. The tweets were classified as either neutral or negative, employing a meticulously chosen language to detect signs of depression (Deshpande and Rao, 2017). A strategy that utilizes data analytics and ML algorithms to identify depression in individuals was introduced by Al Asad et al. (2019); the model obtained its dataset from user-generated content on two significant social media platforms, specifically Twitter and Facebook. Joshi and Kanoongo conducted an extensive analysis using existing literature on AI and several ML approaches to detect depression (2022). As detailed in a published work by Yalamanchili et al. (2020), the authors performed an empirical investigation using audio information to train a classification model. The goal was to identify people as either depressed or not depressed. In Rejaibi et al. (2022), the authors used a recurrent neural network that made use of Mel-frequency cepstral coefficients to identify depressive symptoms and quantify their severity. By examining EEG data, Sarkar et al. (2022) performed a comparative study on the use of deep learning algorithms for the monitoring of mental depression. Several models were identified as helpful for monitoring mental depression using EEG brain waves.

These models include recurrent neural networks (RNNs), RNN with long short-term memory (LSTM), logistic regression (LR), support vector machines (SVMs), and RNN (which was applied to 40% of the data in the testing set). Psychiatric units, medical diagnostic centres, and hospitals might greatly benefit from automated depression detection systems based on deep learning that use the aforementioned data types. In the study by Li et al. (2022), a model was trained using a method based on ML to find biomarkers of major depressive disorder in brain images that respond to changes in cerebral blood flow.

The study conducted by Martínez-Castaño et al. (2022) utilized a BERT-based classifier to identify initial indications of self-harm and evaluate the intensity of depression symptoms. The experiment findings revealed that BERT-based classifiers, when adequately trained, may proficiently detect persons on social media who might be susceptible to self-harm. A study was done, as mentioned in He et al. (2022), to investigate deep learning methods for automatically detecting depression. The study specifically aimed to extract representations of depression from audio and visual data. In addition, Rodrigues Makiuchi et al. (2019) introduced a multimodal technique for diagnosing depression by combining speech and linguistic representation. A separate study focused on the difficulties of identifying gambling addiction and self-harm, as well as evaluating the intensity of depression using social media posts. This was accomplished by employing pre-trained BERT transformers and automatically extracting data from mental health subreddits. The study yielded good results in all three tasks (Bucur et al., 2021). A prior study developed a technique for deep visual-textual multimodal learning to reveal the psychological status of users on social media platforms (Lin et al., 2020; Jabeen et al., 2023).

The main drawbacks observed from the above literature are lack of a large dataset of mental health data; this negatively affects the ML results and limits research in this domain when compared with other fields. Another limitation identified is that most scenarios in the experiments conducted on using ML to monitor or detect depression on social media platforms are limited to certain groups of users and races. Therefore, it is difficult to generalize the outcomes; this shows the need for further investigation to encompass individuals from a wide range of backgrounds.

13.3 Proposed Depression Detection Model

In this section, the description of the proposed model, dataset, and ML techniques used in this research are presented. The procedure entails the extraction and initial processing of social media postings obtained from Reddit. The posts that have been subjected to filtering are inputted into a BERT model that has undergone training to identify indicators of depression. A user interface has been created to facilitate the acquisition of the psychological state of individuals using online platforms by psychological health specialists, organizations, or caretakers. The system interacts with the system's components and storage system via an application programming interface. The schematic of the model and the constituent parts is shown in Figure 13.1.

13.3.1 Acquiring and Pre-processing Data

The dataset for this research was acquired from Reddit, a platform for aggregating trending topics, debating, and ranking online material, based in the United States. Users who have registered on the website contribute various types of information, such as hyperlinks, words, and visual representations. This content is then assessed by other users using a voting mechanism. Reddit organizes user-generated material into topical boards known as "subreddits". These subreddits include a wide array of topics, such as news, gaming, discoveries in science, visual arts, movies, songs, books, athletic ability, and cuisine. Posts from subreddits are typically extracted by employing web scraping methods, utilizing PRAW, a Python-based wrapper specifically

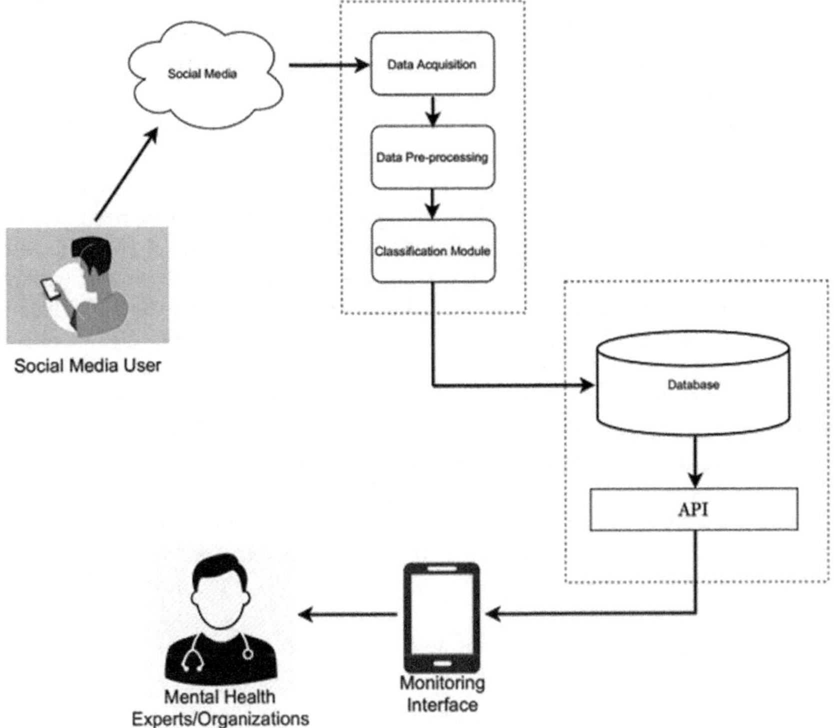

FIGURE 13.1 System architecture and design.

developed for interacting with the Reddit API. The Twitter API was used to collect raw data, which was then utilized to ensure the generalizability and dependability of the data. The raw data was subjected to pre-processing in order to remove unnecessary language. Pre-processing procedures include emotional character removal, connection elimination, tokenization, stop-word deletion, and word normalization. Before being used to generate the list, it was transformed into a string object. Afterward, the string object is used to extract the emoticons. Subsequently, the string is sanitized and segmented into components using a tokenizer that employs regular expressions. Tokenization is the procedure of recognizing and classifying individual words in a text by separating them into distinct components. Subsequently, a list is generated, and all tokens are converted to lowercase. After eliminating the stop words, the list object was lemmatized.

13.3.2 Classification Module

Text categorization entails arranging unstructured text-based content into predetermined categories. By using pre-defined labels or groupings that are suitable for the given context, digital text classification algorithms evaluate, supervise, and classify text-based data. An ML classification system constructed on diverse data sources performs classification tasks in the proposed model. Data that users have supplied has been labelled, trained, and tested. Prior knowledge is sorted as part of the learning process. The BERT model is capable of performing classification tasks. When pre-trained on unannotated data, the BERT model uses deep bidirectional representations, a novel approach to language representation. An innovative model can be created by implementing this method, which eliminates the need for task-specific architectural modifications. Using the BERT architecture, the investigation was conducted. Receiving tokenized postings is the objective of the embedding layer. To capture the sequential sequence of words in a phrase, BERT employs positional embedding.

Through the utilization of segment embedding, the BERT model can efficiently manage sentence pairs for activities pertaining to employment. As the model learns to acquire unique embeddings, it will eventually be able to differentiate between the first and subsequent texts. Tokens, in the context of embedding, denote the WordPiece token vocabulary. The use of a thorough embedding method presents a significant chance to enhance the effectiveness of algorithms that identify sadness by providing important insights. By utilizing a softmax activation function, BERT-encoded representations are employed to forecast post-categories following a linear transformation. One may see the steps to train a model in Algorithm 1.

Among the pre-processing steps are the elimination of emotional characters, connections, stop words, tokenization, and word normalization. The list was created by converting it to a string object first. Extracting the emojis is the next step, using the string object.

The next step is to parse the string into its component elements using a regular expression-based tokenizer. In tokenization, each word in a text is broken down into its distinct components to be recognized and labelled. The next step is to concatenate all the tokens into a lowercase list. The lemmatization of the list object followed the removal of stop words.

ALGORITHM 1: BERT Model Training

Input: Text_Data: $T_1, T_2, \ldots, T_N$

1: START
2: for EPOCH(E)= ai……N {
3: If Text_Data (T) = Training_Data (D_t = 1…..k){
4: B←– BERT (V)//acquire feature vector from BERT model
5: L ←– linear(B) //acquire class prediction by applying a linear layer to B(V)
6: Calculate output B_s (Softmax Output)
7: Find the Optimal S_b value for S_i }
8: If $S_i \approx S_b$ then
9: S_i Obtains quantity B_q from S_b}
10: While (new_dataRequest <= 1){
11: S_i receives B_q from $T_{database}$ }
12: STOP

13.3.3 Depression Tracking Application Interface

The repository is populated with the data acquired from the classification procedure. The database's stored entries can be obtained by utilizing an application package interface (API) that is offered by the monitoring interface. Clinicians, mental health groups, parents, and other interested parties can utilize the monitoring interface to access, track, and observe the depressed states of users on online platforms. The research data utilized for the categorization of text content, which includes both testing and training data, were acquired from a research by Pirina and Coltekin (2018). The Reddit Dataset comprises posts containing potential markers of depression from the "Depression Forum" subreddit, along with posts lacking content related to depressive symptoms from other major subreddits. The dataset comprises around 3000 postings, with over 1300 indicating depression and approximately 1500 suggesting non-depression. Table 13.1 displays the distribution of the dataset in terms of percentages, while Figure 13.2 illustrates the proportion of the dataset that falls into each group. Figure 13.3 presents a comparison between a post exhibiting signs of depression and another post that does not exhibit such signs. Additionally, Figure 13.4 displays the highest-frequency phrases associated with depressive disorders and their occurrences in the Tweets database. Table 13.2 displays the frequency of phrases connected to depression on the social media platform Twitter.

TABLE 13.1
Dataset Statistics

	Training	Validation	Test
Percentage of samples indicating depression	61.62%	62.1%	61.8%
Percentage of samples indicating non-depression	38.38%	37.9%	38.2%

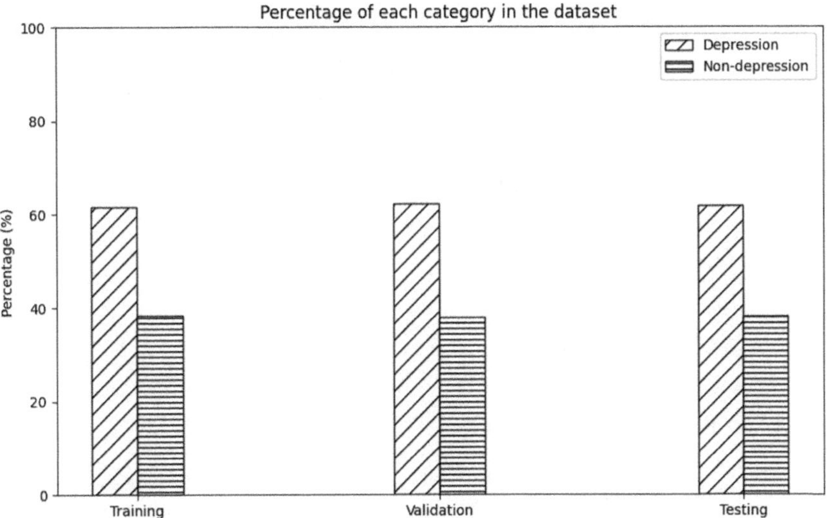

FIGURE 13.2 Proportional distribution of all categories in the dataset.

Post Indicating Depression

Ever just sit there and wonder what's the point? Is it all really worth it? The hard work. At the job, on you're self. And whatever else. I mean if this is all im gonna be as a person even after all this hard work... what's the point. At the end of the day the only thing i really end up looking forward to is sleeping. It's honestly the only time I feel okay. It's all gone when i sleep, I'm at peace. My mind isnt running through everything that makes me feel like trash. Is it worth it to continue working as hard as do at Work? All I ever do is get shafted or picked on. What about going to therapy, is it worth it to keep going? I mean yeah, i have someone to vent to and they listin to me. They don't tell me things like, "you have no reason to feel this way" or things like that. I mean i really don't see a way out of this place. What am I gonna find to "make it go away" Some days are bearable, but some days I just wish i could stay in my dreams all day. Sleeping, no hurting. Just.... peace... If got a few new things to bring up to my therapist in two weeks i guess... Thanks for reading.

Post Indicating Non-depression

Kids- I don't want them...is it likely I will change my mind in the future Hey all! I have felt very strongly that I don't want children for many years now. I don't think there is anything wrong with me not wanting kids. And I don't think there is anything wrong with people that do want kids. I've been wondering how likely it is that I might want kids in the future. Has anyone not wanted kids when they were in their early twenties and then had a change of mind/heart? Just curious! Btw I'm 25 years old.

FIGURE 13.3 Posts showing depressive and non-depressive states.

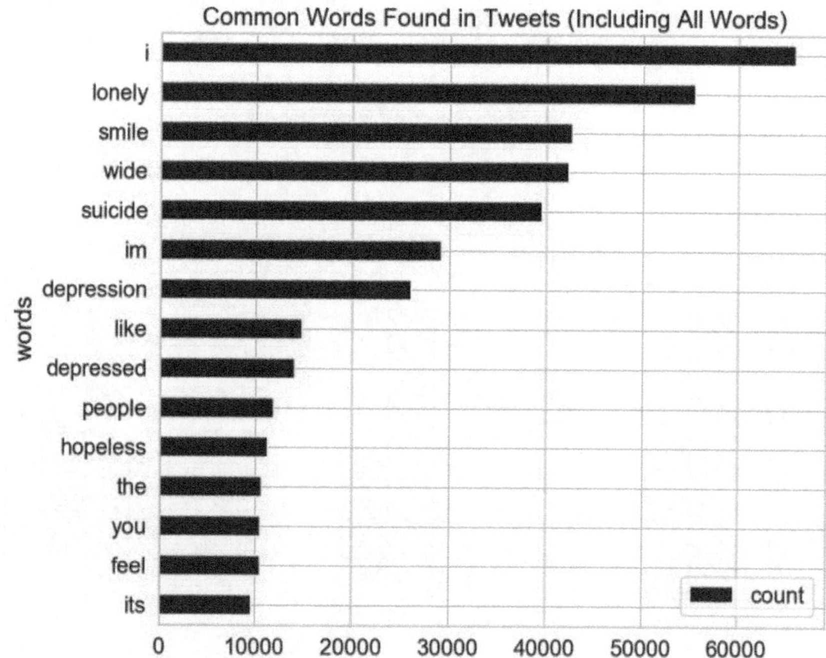

FIGURE 13.4 Depression-related terminology.

TABLE 13.2
Word Count of Depression-Related Words

Words	Count
I	68000
Lonely	57000
Smile	42000
Wide	42000
Suicide	39000
Im	29000
Depression	28000
Like	15000
Depressed	15000
People	12000
Hopeless	12000
The	11000
You	11000
Feel	11000
Its	9000

13.3.4 Evaluation Metrics

i) Precision (P): It shows the fraction of detected depression posts that match the labelled depression posts database. It can be mathematically denoted as

$$P = \frac{TP}{TP + FP} \tag{13.1}$$

TP implies true positive, FP indicates false positive, TN implies true negative, and FN indicates false negative (Ahmed et al., 2023).

ii) Recall (R): It shows the percentage of labelled depression posts that have been detected correctly. It can be mathematically denoted as

$$R = \frac{TP}{TP + FN} \tag{13.2}$$

iii) F1-score: The harmonic average of precision and recall is called the F1-score. The F1-score is a measure of test accuracy; it demonstrates its highest value at 1 and lowest value at 0. F1-score can be mathematically denoted as

$$F1\_score = 2.\frac{precision.recall}{precision + recall} \tag{13.3}$$

Accuracy: It is the percentage of correctly classified depression posts over the total number of depression posts. It can be mathematically denoted as:

$$Accuracy = \frac{TP + TN}{TP + TN + FN + FP} \tag{13.4}$$

13.4 Discussion and Results

The results of the studies that were conducted are summarized in this section. The losses that occurred across the five intervals of the training and verification of the BERT model are shown in Figure 13.5. The validation loss was most advantageous during the third epoch, as illustrated in Figure 13.5. The fact that it produced the most favourable result serves as evidence for this claim. According to the empirical findings depicted in Figure 13.6, the LSTM scheme obtained 50% accuracy rate, 100% precision, a recall of about 21%, and an F1 score of 31%. Furthermore, the examination carried out using the CNN model resulted in a 60% accuracy rate, a 100% precision rate, around a 26% recall rate, and a 41% F1 score. Based on the information provided in Table 13.3, the BERT algorithm demonstrates higher results compared to the two ML algorithms previously discussed. It achieves an accuracy of 92.4%, precision of 92.8%, recall of about 92.1%, and an F1 score of 92.4%. Therefore, it is anticipated that the BERT model will demonstrate outstanding performance in recognizing phrases related to depression. However, it was observed that the BERT model had a comparatively lower precision outcome compared to the other two algorithms, which achieved a precision of 100%. However, the BERT model exhibited superior consistency and achieved the best score in the other three performance metrics, making it the most suitable choice. Furthermore, the TP and FN rows of the confusion matrix, as presented in Table 13.4, offer further evidence substantiating the superiority of the BERT model as the optimal approach for this task. Thus, it can be deduced that the

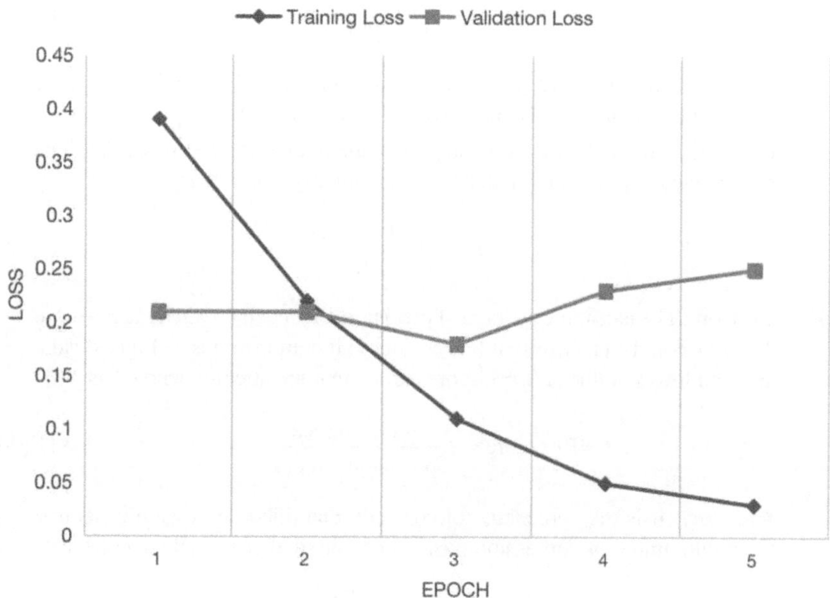

FIGURE 13.5 Loss results for BERT model.

BERT model demonstrated the highest degree of performance in all the evaluated areas. Figures 13.7 and 13.8 illustrate a prototype of a monitoring system that utilizes a graphical user interface. The primary objective of this study was to discern and distinguish instances of depression. The implementation of this method is anticipated to greatly assist in the detection of content connected to depression across various social media platforms.

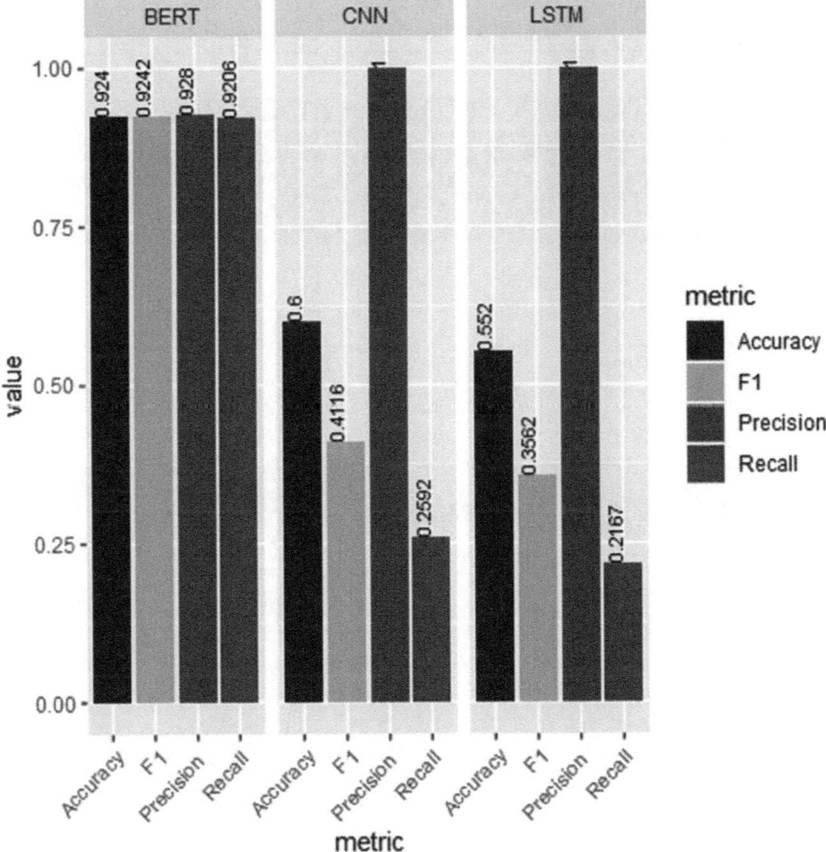

FIGURE 13.6 Evaluation results for the machine learning models.

TABLE 13.3

Performance evaluation for depression detection.

	Accuracy	Precision	Recall	F1
Baselines				
LSTM	0.5520	1.0000	0.2167	0.3562
CNN	0.6000	1.0000	0.2592	0.4116
BERT	0.9240	0.9280	0.9206	0.9242

TABLE 13.4

Confusion Matrix for LSTM, CNN, and BERT

N = 250	Predicted: DEPRESSED		Predicted: NOT DEPRESSED	
Actual: DEPRESSED	LSTM: **31** CNN: **35** BERT: **116**	TP	LSTM: **112** CNN: **100** BERT: **10**	FN
Actual: NOT DEPRESSED	LSTM: **0** CNN: **0** BERT: **9**	FP	LSTM: **107** CNN: **115** BERT: **115**	TN

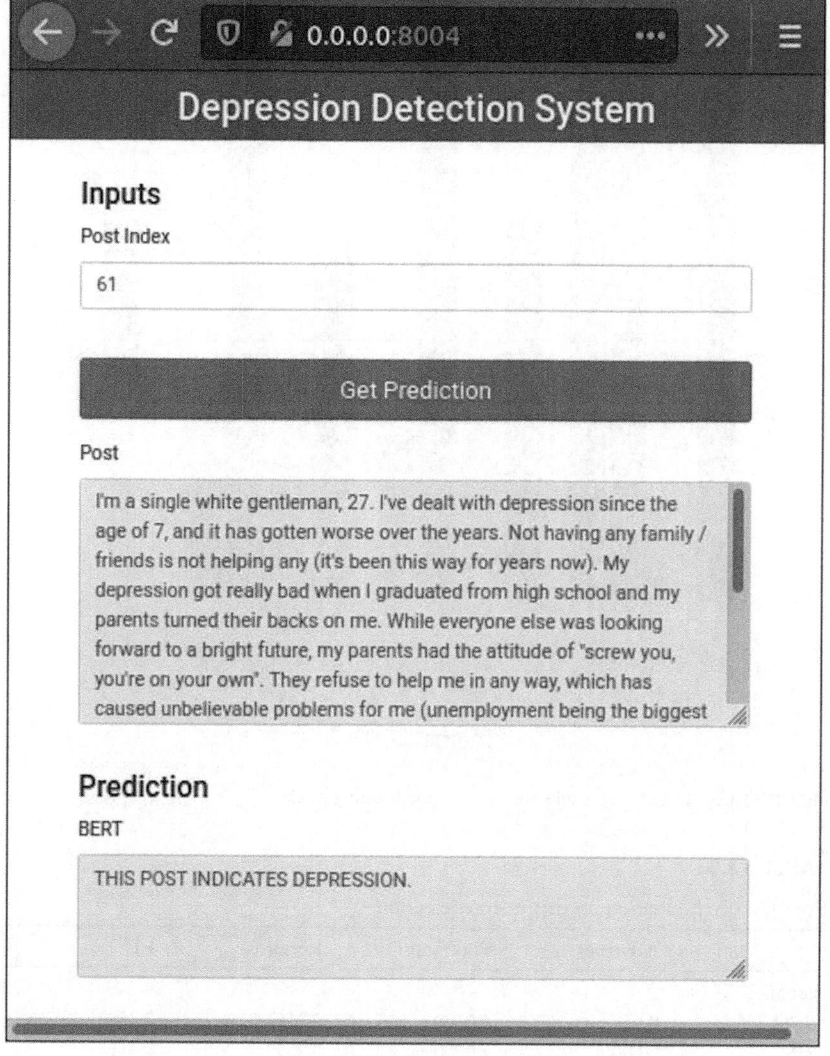

FIGURE 13.7 Tracking application interface with depression posts.

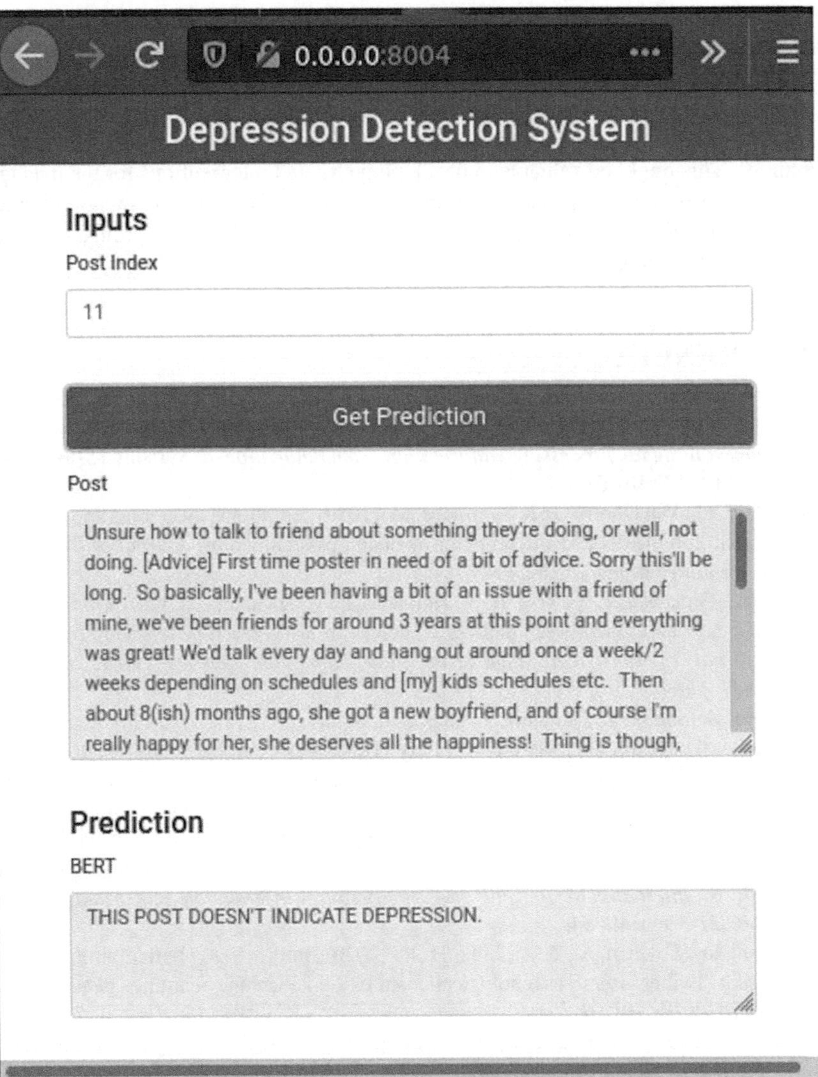

FIGURE 13.8 Tracking application interface with non-depression post.

13.5 Conclusion

In this study, the feasibility of creating an artificial intelligence system to oversee social media engagement and classify postings was examined to detect individuals suffering from depression on these platforms. The model used in this research was based on a dataset that included empirical observations from individuals who were both diagnosed with depression and those who were not. The BERT model outperformed other ML models with an average accuracy rate of 90%. An advantage of

BERT is its bidirectional nature, allowing the model to include information from both preceding and succeeding directions. Experts in public health and mental health will highly value the results of this attempt. Moreover, this work would significantly enhance the field of E-health in smart cities. An in-depth examination of social media data may provide valuable insights into the mental well-being of both people and communities. This might be valuable in developing targeted interventions for the management or prevention of depression. Future studies might focus on investigating the use of photo or video datasets and other social media sites. There is optimism that the BERT paradigm might be extended to include a broad spectrum of mental disorders.

REFERENCES

Al Asad, N., Pranto, M. A. M., Afreen, S., & Islam, M. M. (2019, November). Depression detection by analyzing social media posts of user. In *2019 IEEE international conference on signal processing, information, communication & systems (SPICSCON)* (pp. 13–17). IEEE.

Alvandi, E. O., Van Doorn, G., & Symmons, M. (2019). Emotional awareness and decision-making in the context of computer-mediated psychotherapy. *Journal of Healthcare Informatics Research*, *3*, 345–370.

Ashraf, A., Gunawan, T. S., Riza, B. S., Haryanto, E. V., & Janin, Z. (2020). On the review of image and video-based depression detection using machine learning. *Indonesian Journal of Electrical Engineering and Computer Science (IJEECS)*, *19*(3), 1677–1684.

Aggarwal, S., Saluja, S., Gambhir, V., Gupta, S., & Satia, S. P. S. (2020). Predicting likelihood of psychological disorders in PlayerUnknown's Battlegrounds (PUBG) players from Asian countries using supervised machine learning. *Addictive Behaviors*, *101*, 106132.

Ahmed, R., Bibi, M., & Syed, S. (2023). Improving heart disease prediction accuracy using a hybrid machine learning approach: A comparative study of SVM and KNN algorithms. *International Journal of Computations, Information and Manufacturing (IJCIM)*, *3*(1), 49–54.

Balakrishnan, V., Khan, S., & Arabnia, H. R. (2020). Improving cyberbullying detection using Twitter users' psychological features and machine learning. *Computers & Security*, *90*, 101710.

Bibri, S. E., & Krogstie, J. (2020). The emerging data–driven Smart City and its innovative applied solutions for sustainability: The cases of London and Barcelona. *Energy Informatics*, *3*, 1–42.

Bérard, E., Kai, S. H. Y., Coley, N., Bongard, V., & Ferrières, J. (2021). Lockdown-related factors associated with the worsening of cardiovascular risk and anxiety or depression during the COVID-19 pandemic. *Preventive Medicine Reports*, *21*, 101300.

Bucur, A. M., Cosma, A., & Dinu, L. P. (2021). Early risk detection of pathological gambling, self-harm and depression using bert. arXiv preprint arXiv:2106.16175.

Chiong, R., Budhi, G. S., Dhakal, S., & Chiong, F. (2021). A textual-based featuring approach for depression detection using machine learning classifiers and social media texts. *Computers in Biology and Medicine*, *135*, 104499.

Chow, Y. Y., Verdonschot, M., McEvoy, C. T., & Peeters, G. (2022). Associations between depression and cognition, mild cognitive impairment and dementia in persons with diabetes mellitus: A systematic review and meta-analysis. *Diabetes Research and Clinical Practice*, *185*, 109227.

Deshpande, M., & Rao, V. (2017, December). Depression detection using emotion artificial intelligence. In *2017 International Conference on Intelligent Sustainable Systems (ICISS)* (pp. 858–862). IEEE, Palladam, India.

Elhai, J. D., Yang, H., Rozgonjuk, D., & Montag, C. (2020). Using machine learning to model problematic smartphone use severity: The significant role of fear of missing out. *Addictive Behaviors*, *103*, 106261.

Elbay, R. Y., Kurtulmuş, A., Arpacıoğlu, S., & Karadere, E. (2020). Depression, anxiety, stress levels of physicians and associated factors in Covid-19 pandemics. *Psychiatry Research*, *290*, 113130.

Fullana, M. A., Hidalgo-Mazzei, D., Vieta, E., & Radua, J. (2020). Coping behaviors associated with decreased anxiety and depressive symptoms during the COVID-19 pandemic and lockdown. *Journal of Affective Disorders*, *275*, 80–81.

Gao, C., & Scullin, M. K. (2020). Sleep health early in the coronavirus disease 2019 (COVID-19) outbreak in the United States: Integrating longitudinal, cross-sectional, and retrospective recall data. *Sleep Medicine*, *73*, 1–10.

Gille, F., Jobin, A., & Ienca, M. (2020). What we talk about when we talk about trust: Theory of trust for AI in healthcare. *Intelligence-Based Medicine*, *1*, 100001.

Gritsenko, V., Skugarevsky, O., Konstantinov, V., Khamenka, N., Marinova, T., Reznik, A., & Isralowitz, R. (2021). COVID 19 fear, stress, anxiety, and substance use among Russian and Belarusian university students. *International Journal of Mental Health and Addiction*, *19*, 2362–2368.

Ghazal, T. M., Hasan, M. K., Alshurideh, M. T., Alzoubi, H. M., Ahmad, M., Akbar, S. S., … Akour, I. A. (2021). IoT for smart cities: Machine learning approaches in smart healthcare—A review. *Future Internet*, *13*(8), 218.

Reddy, K. H. K., Roy, D. S., Mishra, T. K., & Hussain, M. W. (Eds.). (2023). *Handbook of Research on Network-Enabled IoT Applications for Smart City Services*. IGI Global.

Hetrick, S. E., Parker, A. G., Hickie, I. B., Purcell, R., Yung, A. R., & McGorry, P. D. (2008). Early identification and intervention in depressive disorders: Towards a clinical staging model. *Psychotherapy and Psychosomatics*, *77*(5), 263–270.

Holt, R. I., De Groot, M., & Golden, S. H. (2014). Diabetes and depression. *Current Diabetes Reports*, *14*, 1–9.

Huang, Y., & Zhao, N. (2020). Generalized anxiety disorder, depressive symptoms and sleep quality during COVID-19 outbreak in China: A web-based cross-sectional survey. *Psychiatry Research*, *288*, 112954.

Harrison, V., Moulds, M. L., & Jones, K. (2022). Perceived social support and prenatal wellbeing; The mediating effects of loneliness and repetitive negative thinking on anxiety and depression during the COVID-19 pandemic. *Women and Birth*, *35*(3), 232–241.

He, L., Niu, M., Tiwari, P., Marttinen, P., Su, R., Jiang, J., … Dang, W. (2022). Deep learning for depression recognition with audiovisual cues: A review. *Information Fusion*, *80*, 56–86.

Islam, M. R., Kabir, M. A., Ahmed, A., Kamal, A. R. M., Wang, H., & Ulhaq, A. (2018). Depression detection from social network data using machine learning techniques. *Health Information Science and Systems*, *6*, 1–12.

Jiang, F., Jiang, Y., Zhi, H., Dong, Y., Li, H., Ma, S., … Wang, Y. (2017). Artificial intelligence in healthcare: past, present and future. *Stroke and Vascular Neurology*, *2*(4), 230–243.

Joshi, M. L., & Kanoongo, N. (2022). Depression detection using emotional artificial intelligence and machine learning: A closer review. *Materials Today: Proceedings*, *58*, 217–226.

Jabeen, S., Li, X., Amin, M. S., Bourahla, O., Li, S., & Jabbar, A. (2023). A review on methods and applications in multimodal deep learning. *ACM Transactions on Multimedia Computing, Communications and Applications, 19*(2s), 1–41.

Kok, A. A., Pan, K. Y., Rius-Ottenheim, N., Jörg, F., Eikelenboom, M., Horsfall, M., … Penninx, B. W. (2022). Mental health and perceived impact during the first Covid-19 pandemic year: A longitudinal study in Dutch case-control cohorts of persons with and without depressive, anxiety, and obsessive-compulsive disorders. *Journal of Affective Disorders, 305*, 85–93.

Lin, C., Hu, P., Su, H., Li, S., Mei, J., Zhou, J., & Leung, H. (2020, June). Sensemood: depression detection on social media. In *Proceedings of the 2020 International Conference on Multimedia Retrieval* (pp. 407–411).

Li, Z., McIntyre, R. S., Husain, S. F., Ho, R., Tran, B. X., Nguyen, H. T., … Chen, N. (2022). Identifying neuroimaging biomarkers of major depressive disorder from cortical hemodynamic responses using machine learning approaches. *EBioMedicine, 79*.

Mousavian, M., Chen, J., Traylor, Z., & Greening, S. (2021). Depression detection from sMRI and rs-fMRI images using machine learning. *Journal of Intelligent Information Systems, 57*, 395–418.

Martínez-Castaño, R., Htait, A., Azzopardi, L., & Moshfeghi, Y. (2022). Early risk detection of self-harm using BERT-based transformers. In *Early Detection of Mental Health Disorders by Social Media Monitoring: The First Five Years of the eRisk Project* (pp. 183–206). Cham: Springer International Publishing.

Nemesure, M. D., Heinz, M. V., Huang, R., & Jacobson, N. C. (2021). Predictive modeling of depression and anxiety using electronic health records and a novel machine learning approach with artificial intelligence. *Scientific Reports, 11*(1), 1980.

Orabi, A. H., Buddhitha, P., Orabi, M. H., & Inkpen, D. (2018, June). Deep learning for depression detection of twitter users. In *Proceedings of the Fifth Workshop on Computational Linguistics and Clinical Psychology: From Keyboard to Clinic* (pp. 88–97).

Olaseni, A. O., Akinsola, O. S., Agberotimi, S. F., & Oguntayo, R. (2020). Psychological distress experiences of Nigerians during Covid-19 pandemic; the gender difference. *Social Sciences & Humanities Open, 2*(1), 100052.

Ohia, C., Bakarey, A. S., & Ahmad, T. (2020). COVID-19 and Nigeria: putting the realities in context. *International Journal of Infectious Diseases, 95*, 279–281.

Osotsi, A., Oravecz, Z., Li, Q., Smyth, J., & Brick, T. R. (2020). Individualized modeling to distinguish between high and low arousal states using physiological data. *Journal of Healthcare Informatics Research, 4*, 91–109.

Oyebode, O., Ndulue, C., Mulchandani, D., Suruliraj, B., Adib, A., Orji, F. A., … Orji, R. (2022). COVID-19 pandemic: identifying key issues using social media and natural language processing. *Journal of Healthcare Informatics Research, 6*(2), 174–207.

Pradhan, B., Hussain, M. W., Srivastava, G., Debbarma, M. K., Barik, R. K., & Lin, J. C. W. (2022). *A Neuro-Evolutionary Approach for Software Defined Wireless Network Traffic Classification*. IET Communications.

Pirina, I., & Çöltekin, Ç. (2018, October). Identifying depression on reddit: The effect of training data. In *Proceedings of the 2018 EMNLP Workshop SMM4H: The 3rd Social Media Mining for Health Applications Workshop & Shared Task* (pp. 9–12).

Rodrigues Makiuchi, M., Warnita, T., Uto, K., & Shinoda, K. (2019, October). Multimodal fusion of bert-cnn and gated cnn representations for depression detection. In *Proceedings of the 9th International on Audio/Visual Emotion Challenge and Workshop* (pp. 55–63).

Rejaibi, E., Komaty, A., Meriaudeau, F., Agrebi, S., & Othmani, A. (2022). MFCC-based recurrent neural network for automatic clinical depression recognition and assessment from speech. *Biomedical Signal Processing and Control, 71*, 103107.

Rivera, M. J., Teruel, M. A., Mate, A., & Trujillo, J. (2022). Diagnosis and prognosis of mental disorders by means of EEG and deep learning: a systematic mapping study. *Artificial Intelligence Review, 55*, 1209–1251.

Shen, Y., Zhang, W., Chan, B. S. M., Zhang, Y., Meng, F., Kennon, E. A., … Zhang, X. (2020). Detecting risk of suicide attempts among Chinese medical college students using a machine learning algorithm. *Journal of Affective Disorders, 273*, 18–23.

Sun, S., Goldberg, S. B., Lin, D., Qiao, S., & Operario, D. (2021). Psychiatric symptoms, risk, and protective factors among university students in quarantine during the COVID-19 pandemic in China. *Globalization and Health, 17*(1), 1–14.

Sarker, I. H., Hoque, M. M., Uddin, M. K., & Alsanoosy, T. (2021). Mobile data science and intelligent apps: Concepts, ai-based modeling and research directions. *Mobile Networks and Applications, 26*, 285–303.

Sarkar, A., Singh, A., & Chakraborty, R. (2022). A deep learning-based comparative study to track mental depression from EEG data. *Neuroscience Informatics, 2*(4), 100039.

Uddin, M. Z., Dysthe, K. K., Følstad, A., & Brandtzaeg, P. B. (2022). Deep learning for prediction of depressive symptoms in a large textual dataset. *Neural Computing and Applications, 34*(1), 721–744.

Wen, J., Kozak, M., Yang, S., & Liu, F. (2021). COVID-19: potential effects on Chinese citizens' lifestyle and travel. *Tourism Review, 76*(1), 74–87.

Xu, F., Wang, X., Yang, Y., Zhang, K., Shi, Y., Xia, L., … Liu, H. (2022). Depression and insomnia in COVID-19 survivors: A cross-sectional survey from Chinese rehabilitation centers in Anhui province. *Sleep Medicine, 91*, 161–165.

Yusif, S., Abdul, H.-B., & Jeffrey, S. (2020). An exploratory study of the readiness of public healthcare facilities in developing countries to adopt health information technology (HIT)/e-Health: the case of Ghana. *Journal of Healthcare Informatics Research 4*, 189–214.

Yalamanchili, B., Kota, N. S., Abbaraju, M. S., Nadella, V. S. S., & Alluri, S. V. (2020, February). Real-time acoustic based depression detection using machine learning techniques. In *2020 International Conference on Emerging Trends in Information Technology and Engineering* (ic-ETITE) (pp. 1–6). IEEE.

Zhang, J., Yin, Z., Chen, P., & Nichele, S. (2020). Emotion recognition using multi-modal data and machine learning techniques: A tutorial and review. *Information Fusion, 59*, 103–126.

Zhu, Y., Wang, C., Dong, L., & Xiao, M. (2020). Home quarantine or centralized quarantine, which is more conducive to fighting COVID-19 pandemic? *Brain, Behavior, and Immunity, 87*, 142.

Hussain, M. W., & Roy, D. S. (2023). Performance Optimization Strategies for Big Data Applications in Distributed Framework. In *Intelligent Technologies: Concepts, Applications, and Future Directions*, Volume 2 (pp. 221–252). Singapore: Springer Nature Singapore.

Zhu, P., & Tan, X. (2021). Is compulsory home quarantine less effective than centralized quarantine in controlling the COVID-19 outbreak? Evidence from Hong Kong. *Sustainable Cities and Society, 74*, 103222.

14

A Sorting Strip Based Body Worn Antenna for Assisting Breast Cancer Detection for a Smart Healthcare Environment

G. Indumathi, G. Sujitha, and K. Vishveswari
Mepco Schlenk Engineering College, Sivakasi, India

14.1 Introduction: Background and Driving Forces

In most of the developed countries, among the worldwide females, breast cancer has been observed in a red alert manner because of its malignancy for the past three decades. Even with the latest treatment modalities, the survival rates of such patients are still lower in developing countries compared to developed nations. This is mainly due to the delayed recognition of the disease and the need of cost-effective treatments. If the malignant tissues presence is detected at the prior stage, then the saving of such patients will be easier. But such things are not so easy if a woman has dense breasts or if the malignancy is present near the underarm.

The cost-expensive imaging methods such as CT or MRI scan may lead to the destruction of the tissue in which they penetrate and make the patient suffer physically, so it introduces some uncomfortable things. Recently, society has been more focused toward healthcare because of the huge growth of population (Reddy et al., 2023). Recently wearable medical appliances are attracting and becoming the most wanted research. The difficulty in such appliances is how to do data transmission along with power capability.

A wearable electronic gadget is a special type of appliance that is attached to the body for its functioning. Kavitha and Swaminathan (2019) proposed one such electronic radiating element which can be attached to the textile fabric for health monitoring and communication. The evolving technology like the Internet of Things (IoT) is utilizing wearable gadget attached to radiating elements. Since the size of such wearable devices is small, the radiating element attached to it should of smaller in size, which makes the researchers work hard to design and implement it. Hence, a compact wearable antenna is designed and proposed in the chapter. The designed antenna has to resonate on the WiMAX band. WiMAX band has many applications such as broadband connections, hotspots, medical applications, and cellular backhaul. Several frequency bands are approved (ITU-R regulations 2022) for biomedical applications,

 DOI: 10.1201/9781032631738-14

including the Medical Device Radio Communication (Med Radio) band (401–406 MHz) and the Industrial, Scientific, and Medical (ISM) bands (433.1–434.8 MHz, 868–868.6 MHz, 902.8–928 MHz, and 2.4–2.5 GHz, 5.7–5.875 GHz) (Bakogianni and Koulouridis, 2016, Ding et al., 2020, FCC.gov, 2012).

An X-ray technology, namely, mammography screening was used in the past to find out the cancer-affected tissues. But it leads to a time-consuming process. Alternatively, an imaging method namely microwave imaging is used by Zerrad et al. (2023), where they discussed the development of a high-frequency imaging system for the finding of malignant tissues in the breast, where they analyzed in terms of both time and frequency domains with high-quality factors. Similarly, Amsaveni et al. (2023) proposed a screening method using patch antenna with an artificial breast phantom model. In their works, they analyzed the tumor locations by comparing them with specific absorption rate (SAR) values. A textile sensor system is proposed under the vision of Smart Bra for easy and simple monitoring of breast in a sustained manner in Elsheakh et al. (2023). Amdaouch et al. (2022) employed less number of antennas to identify the breast cancer. They proposed a technique that incorporates traditional delay and sum algorithm along with SAR values to optimize the cancer tissue locations. A simple microstrip-based patch is employed by Ali and Ahmed (2022) to identify the stage I cancer tissues.

Chirwa et al. (2003) developed an antenna for human intestine monitoring with the help of an implanted source which works at the band of 150 MHz to 1.2 GHz. Many such antennas are proposed to work with multiple operating frequencies but are larger in size (Ali and Ahmed, 2022). The smaller size antennas are found to operate at higher frequencies which induces some loss when it is implanted deeper into the body (Chirwa et al., 2003); additionally, many studies lead to some medical complications due to their operation at the skin level (Kim and Rahmat-Samii, 2004; Luu et al., 2017). Ali et al. (2017) presented a tiny circular antenna to address these concerns. Those antennas were intended to work at two separate resonance frequencies for data and power respectively 403 and 915 MHz. Furthermore, the implanted antenna is placed deep into muscle tissue, making it resistant to changes in implantation depth and hence to environmental changes. The veracity of the foregoing was demonstrated by a complete wave 3D simulation of the worldwide wireless network. Furthermore, the authors presented an elongated version of the above work in Liu et al. (2012) with comparison of simulated work with experimentally tested antenna by immersing it in porcine tissues. The validity of the comparison between numerical reflection coefficient prediction and measurement findings is established. A tiny monopole antenna with a basic shape and lightweight textile materials like Teflon, denim, and FR4 substrate has been presented (Kiourti and Nikita, 2012), which can be employed for body-centric applications and works at 2.4GHz (ISM band). The team of Kavya and Vinu had proposed a triple-band wearable button antenna for body-centric applications (Karacolak et al., 2009) which operates at 2.4, 5.6, and 9.2 GHz.

The work described by Liu et al. (2012) and Karacolak et al. (2009) has been expanded in this study. A wearable miniature circular antenna (Kavya and Vinu, 2018) is designed specifically for breast tumor detection which can be analyzed experimentally using a four-layer breast phantom model. In this chapter, two breast phantom models, one with malignant tissues and another without malignant tissues are considered. A comparison between these two phantom models is carried out based on the numerical prediction of the reflection coefficient.

14.2 Antenna Preface

Any structure or device that collects or radiates electromagnetic waves is known as an antenna. In 1887, Heinrich Hertz created a wireless communication method by creating an electrical stimulus in a dipole antenna. The forms of antennas vary in terms of size and shape. Conventionally TV or telephone system uses an antenna made up of a conducting material like a rod or dish where it can capture RF waves and translate them into an electrical signal.

There are various classifications for antennas. The frequency band of operation is one method, while physical structure and electrical/electromagnetic design are others. Adaptive or smart 8 antennas are the name given to these antennas and the technology that supports them. Some widely used antennas are Microstrip, Reflector, Travelling wave A, half wave dipole (Hertz), aperture, vertical (Marconi) antenna, etc.

14.2.1 Antenna Constraints

Some of the most common constraints that are adopted to verify the successful design and operation of the proposed radiating element are its operating frequency, radiating effects measurements, divergence behaviors, efficacy, etc. As said earlier, antennas are translators which can translate the electromagnetic radiation in an elegant manner. The proper arrangement of the conducting material and the dielectric will reflect an antenna radiating behavior. The operating frequency range is generally defined as bandwidth. Antennas are known for their broadband activity.

The generation of an electromagnetic wave, or antenna radiation, occurs in an uninsulated conducting material when a high-frequency component pass through it. The far field of an antenna is the point where the emission pattern from the antenna whose electric and magnetic fields are completely unrelated.

A 3-dimensional space (x, y, z) represents the azimuth and elevation plane. Such orientation is used for knowing the radiated power. The actual antenna patterns are measured with respect to the isotropic radiator which can do the power emission in all directions. If the power variation is observed in the elevation plane with a fixed azimuthal value, then it is an omnidirectional emission. A dipole radiator is a good example of such radiation. A directional antenna transmits energy primarily in one or more directions.

The oscillating behavior of an antenna in terms of electric and magnetic field is defined as antenna polarization. It may be a linear category if the electric or magnetic field oscillates in a single axis or clockwise/anticlockwise oscillations with an orbit about the origin point. When the electric field spins around the origin perfectly then it is called circular polarization.

The basic measurement of antenna working is antenna efficiency, which tells us how much power is absorbed with respect to the emitted power by an antenna.

The radiating angle of the major power from the radiator is called as the beamwidth. It forms the major portion of the field pattern. The reflecting signal from a radiator with respect to the signal power excluding the radiation loss is measured as reflection coefficient.

The standing wave ratio is another factor for deciding the performance of a radiator which represents the ratio of the highest and lowest voltages created at an antenna's port during a standing wave. An impedance mismatch induces some effect on standing wave ratio due to some misleads in the design part. Antenna gain is a measurement of an antenna's efficiency.

14.3 Wearable Antenna

The antennas that can be worn are called as wearable antennas and are increasing rapidly in consumer electronics, smartwatches with inbuilt Bluetooth antennas, smart glasses, GoPro action, and Nike+Sensor with communication with a smartphone via Bluetooth inserted in a user's shoe are all examples of wearable antenna.

14.3.1 Challenges in Wearable Antennas

- Closeness: Since the electromagnetic (EM) waves are lossy when it is in contact with human physique and influence some heating effects. When a smart wearable device is put close to the body, it loses a significant amount of efficiency.
- Limited quantity: Wearable technologies like Google Glass require a lot of space. As a result, the wearable antenna should be as compact as possible. Industrial and product designers leave minimal room for antennas, posing a severe antenna design challenge

14.3.2 Effects of Antenna on Human Body

The sound, light, and microwave signals can vibrate the energies but not possible to convert them. The effects of rising temperatures on human tissues are numerous, the most common of them is the electrical phenomena. SAR denotes how much energy the human tissue absorbs over the specified volume or mass of the body. SAR values more than the specified can create some ruinous concerns for the human tissues.

14.3.3 Wearable Antenna Effects on Human Body

Generally, the communicating path between the wearable antenna and the receiving device is lossy. Variations in input impedance, frequency shifts, and lower antenna effectiveness may be caused due to the lossy high dielectric behavior of the human body. Various strategies can be adopted to address such consequences based on the application requirements. One of the most important considerations is antenna placement and direction. When the antenna is properly placed in the correct position, and based on the distance between the antenna and the human body, such impacts can be minimized.

14.4 Proposed Antenna Design

The proposed antenna is composed of ground, a patch, at a substrate, a superstrate, a ground wire, and a coaxial feeding. A sorting strip is employed to make contact between a circular patch and the ground. The sorting strip is used to reduce the antenna structure. A sandwich of patch and ground with a substrate in between and a superstrate over the patch is considered. Both the substrate and superstrate are made up of Teflon. The circular slots in the patch are necessary for the patch to operate at the relevant frequencies. The coaxial feeding point is terminated with a 50-Ohm impedance. Table 14.1 gives the dimensional values of the parametric structure adopted in this work.

A female breast phantom model made up of four layers (skin, fat, glandular tissues, and muscle) is considered. The exterior section of the breast tissues is created with dimensions of roughly 10 cm in length and 4 cm in width, with depth determined by the thickness of each layer. The proposed miniaturized antennas are made to have contact with the skin layer of the four-layered phantom model for stimulation.

The electrical specifications of the various tissues of the phantom model are obtained through the literature survey (Kiourti and Nikita, 2012; Karacolak et al., 2009; Shamed & Sharawi, 2017; Ding et al., 2019).

14.5 Results and Discussions

High Frequency Structure Simulator (HFSS) is the software used for simulation. The return loss or reflection coefficient is a metric used for identifying the amount of EM wave reflections due to the mismatch in the transmission medium impedance and is also used to identify the antenna's operating frequency. Figure 14.1 (a and b) depicts the return loss behavior of the proposed radiating structure when placing it in contact with a phantom model without and with malignant tissues. As here, S11 of an antenna is −13 dB at 5.6 GHz with tumor and −17 dB at 5.6 GHz without tumor, which covers the entire corresponding authorized band. There should be no reflected power and 100% power to be sent to the antenna in the ideal situation. Here, the reflected powers for the antenna with the presence of malignant tissues and without malignant tissues is below −10 dB. It is discovered that when malignant tissues are present, the antenna's reflection coefficient increases. This is because of the higher conductivity of the tumor cells.

It's not necessary for an antenna to have a higher gain always. If the direction of an antenna is known then it is better to have a higher gain. Otherwise, if the direction is not known, then there is no need for a higher gain it is better to possess lower gain. The gain of an antenna without and with a tumor is shown in Figure 14.2(a and b). At 5.6

TABLE 14.1

Adopted Dimensional Values

Parameters	Values (mm)	Parameters	Value deg)
r1	10	θ1	70
r2	8	θ2	18
W1	0.3	θ3	163
W2	0.5	θ4	109
T1	1.28	r3	1.2
T2	1.28	W3	0.2

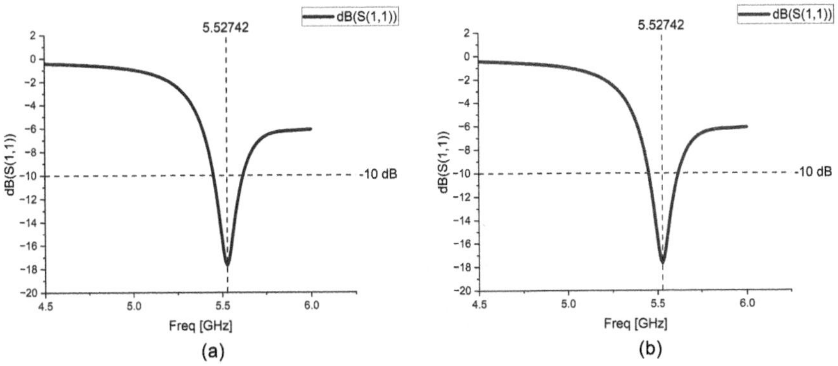

FIGURE 14.1 (a) Return loss without tumor and (b) return loss with tumor.

GHz, the suggested antenna achieves a gain of 4.9 dB with tumor and 3.1 dB without tumor.

The Voltage Standing Wave Ratio (VSWR) of the proposed radiating element is achieved to be 1.56 at 5.6 GHz with the presence of tumor and 1.32 at 5.6 GHz without the presence of tumor cells. Those observed values are very close to the ideal values and are therefore acceptable.

SAR is a critical measure that defines a wearable antenna's level of safety. Figure 14.3(a and b) shows the SAR values of an antenna that falls within the permissible range, i.e., 0.9876 and 1.1874 W/kg, respectively, without and with a tumor. The simulated antenna analysis outcome without considering tumor and with tumor is tabulated in Tables 14.2 and 14.3.

.The E-field distribution is observed without tumor as 53088.98, and it is noticed to be decreased to 52091.86 V/m when kept in contact with tumor. The strength of a magnetic field (H) is measured in amperes per meter (A/m). The time rate of energy transfer is referred to as power. This also applies to waves. The power emitted by a radiation source (antenna) and transmitted through space by an electromagnetic wave is known as radiated power. From the H field of an antenna, it is observed without and with tumor as 82.82 and 41.06 A/m, respectively. The measures of the simulation and fabricated antenna are compared in Table 14.4.

14.6 Conclusion and Future Scope

For the development of smart healthcare applications, a miniaturized circular antenna that operates at Wimax band and can be used as an assisting device for breast tumor detection is proposed in this report. The frequency range for Wimax band is 5.6–5.72 GHz with a center frequency of 5.66 GHz. Since the proposed antenna resonates at 5.66 GHz, it is suitable for body-centric communication and wireless communication. This antenna is made up of teflon as a material for both the substrate and superstrate, as it is more flexible in the case of wearable antenna for healthcare applications. The proposed antenna provides suitable return loss, gain, VSWR, and SAR values. This

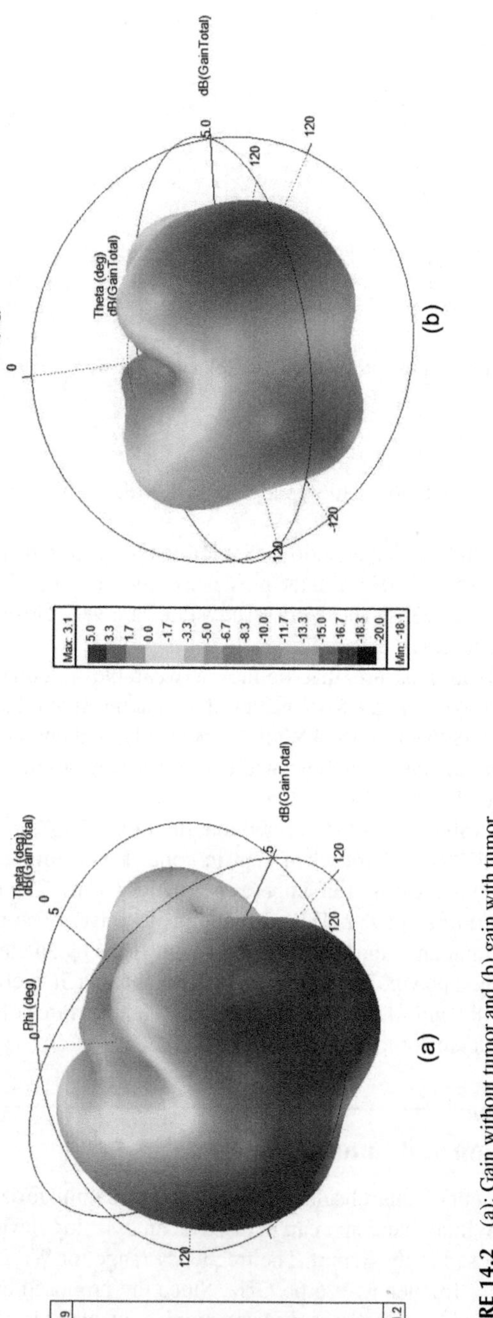

FIGURE 14.2 (a): Gain without tumor and (b) gain with tumor.

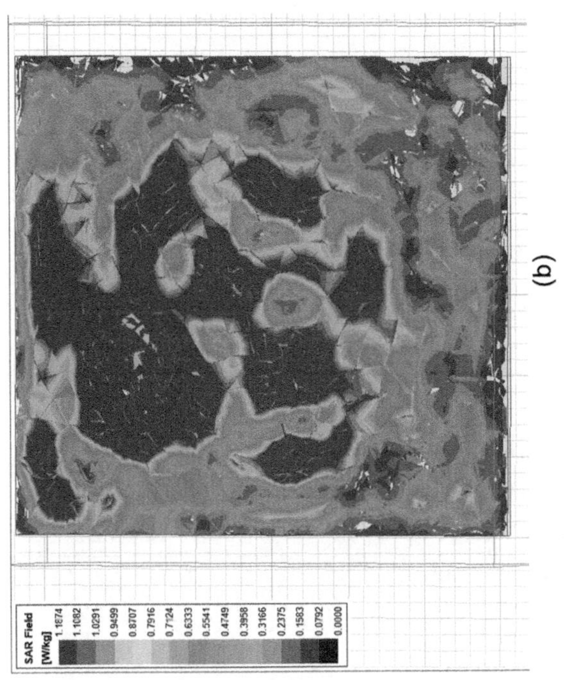

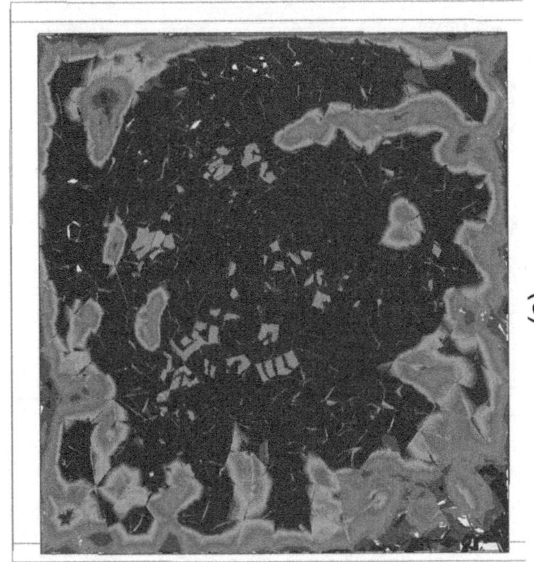

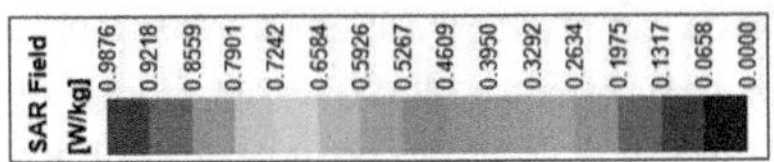

FIGURE 14.3 (a) SAR without tumor and (b) SAR with tumor.

TABLE 14.2

Simulation Outcome of the Antenna without Tumor Condition

Quantity	Value
Peak directivity (dB)	5.70428
Peak gain (dB)	3.09858
Peak realized gain (dB)	−4.83891
Radiated power (mW)	1.79002
Accepted power (mW)	3.26158
Incident power (mW)	20.2851
Radiation efficiency	0.54882
Front-to-back ratio	7.09758
System power (mW)	20.2851
Peak system gain (dB)	−4.83891

TABLE 14.3

Simulation Outcome of the Antenna with Tumor Condition

Quantity	Value
Peak directivity (dB)	6.23323
Peak gain (dB)	4.93547
Peak realized gain (dB)	−3.53227
Radiated power (mW)	2.14124
Accepted power (mW)	2.88697
Incident power (mW)	20.2869
Radiation efficiency	0.741692
Front-to-back ratio	12.6818
System power (mW)	20.2869
Peak system gain (dB)	−3.53227

TABLE 14.4

Analysis of the Simulated Antenna and Tested Antenna without Tumor Condition

	Value	
Quantity	Simulation	Testing
Reflection coefficient (dBi)	−17.4	−14.3 dBi
VSWR	1.32	1.4963

antenna possesses the satisfied SAR. The proposed reading element is analyzed in the presence of tumor cells and without the presence of tumor cells and the difference in the antenna parameters are analyzed. The antenna possesses different results with and without the presence of tumor. Since the characteristics of the tumor cells vary from the normal cells, as the tumor cells have high conductivity, so there will be changes in antenna parameters. From this variation, we can the proposed radiating element as an assisting device to predict the malignancy.

In the future, various stages of the tumor can be detected due to the change in the electrical properties of the tissue cells. From the literature survey, we understood that slotted monopole antennas and Vivaldi antennas in an array form are suited to be placed in a hemispherical configuration. Further work can be extended in the above-mentioned antenna structures. Further, for a smart life, bras with flexibility can be designed with different sizes by incorporating an optimal array of structures for better patient monitoring and performance.

REFERENCES

Ali, N. and Ahmed, J., "Microstrip Patch Antenna Design For Breast Cancer Detection," 2022 *International Conference on Engineering & MIS (ICEMIS)*, Istanbul, Turkey, 2022, pp. 1–4. https://doi.org/10.1109/ICEMIS56295.2022.9914365

Ali M. M., Bashar M. E. I., & Hosain M. K., Circular Planner Inverted-F Antenna for Implantable Biomedical Applications, *2nd International Conference on Electrical & Electronic Engineering (ICEEE)*, *1*, pp. 1–4, 2017.

Amdaouch, I., Saban, M., Gueri, J. E., Chaari, M. Z., Alejos, A. V. Alzola, J. R., Munoz, A. R., and Aghzout, O., "A novel approach of a low-cost UWB microwave imaging system with high resolution based on SAR and a new fast reconstruction algorithm for early-stage breast cancer detection." *J. Imaging*, *8*(.10), 264, 2022. https://doi.org/10.3390/jimaging8100264

Amsaveni, A., Kaiser, A., Harish, L., & Rashmi, S., "Double Layered Hexagonal Slot Antenna for Breast Cancer Detection using Microwave Imaging," *2023 2nd International Conference on Advancements in Electrical, Electronics, Communication, Computing and Automation (ICAECA), Coimbatore*, India, pp. 1–5, 2023. https://doi.org/10.1109/ICAECA56562.2023.10200648

Bakogianni, S., and Koulouridis, S., "An implantable planar dipole antenna for wireless med radio-band biotelemetry devices," *IEEE Antennas Wireless Propag. Lett.*, *15*, 234–237, 2016.

Chirwa L. C., Hammond P. A. Roy S., and Cumming D. R. S. "Electromagnetic radiation from ingested sources in the human intestine between 150 MHz and 1.2 GHz." *IEEE Transactions on Biomedical Engineering*, *50*(4), 484–492, 2003.

Ding, S., Koulouridis, S., and Pichon, L., "A Dual-Band Miniaturized Circular Antenna for Deep in Body Biomedical Wireless Applications," *13th European Conference on Antennas and Propagation (EuCAP)*, Krakow, Poland, pp. 1–4, 2019.

Ding, S., Koulouridis, S., and Pichon, L. (2020). Design and characterization of a dual-band miniaturized circular antenna for deep in body biomedical wireless applications. *International Journal of Microwave and Wireless Technologies*, *12*(6), 461–468.

Elsheakh, D. A., Mohamed, R. A., Fahmy, O. M., Ezzat, K., and Eldamak, A. R. "Complete breast cancer detection and monitoring system by using microwave textile based antenna sensors." *Biosensors*, *13*(1), 87, 2023. https://doi.org/10.3390/bios13010087.

FCC. *Federal Communications Commission* 2012. Washington, D.C., USA. Online: https://www.fcc.gov

"International Telecommunications Union-Radio communications (ITU-R), radio regulations, section 5.138 and 5.150," ITU. Geneva, Switzerland, 2022.

Karacolak, T., Cooper, R., and Topsakal, E., Electrical properties of rat skin and design of implantable antennas for medical wireless telemetry. *IEEE Transactions on Antennas and Propagation*, *57*(9), 2806–2812, 2009.

Kavitha, A. and Swaminathan, J. N., "Design of flexible textile antenna using FR4, jeans cotton and Teflon substrates," *Microsystem Technologies, 0123456789*, 1311–1320, 2019.

Kavya, R. and Vinu, R., "Wearable Triple Band Button Antenna" *International Conference on Emerging Trends and Innovation in Engineering and Technological Research (ICETIETR)*, pp. 1–5, 2018.

Kim J. and Rahmat-Samii Y., Implanted antennas inside a human body: Simulations, designs, and characterizations. *IEEE Transactions on Microwave Theory and Techniques, 52*(8 II), 1934–1943, 2004.

Kiourti A., and Nikita K. S., Miniature scalp-implantable antennas for telemetry in the MICS and ISM bands: Design, safety considerations and link budget analysis. *IEEE Transactions on Antennas and Propagation, 60*(8), 3568–3575, 2012.

Liu C., Guo Y. X., and Xiao S, Compact dual-band antenna for implantable devices. *IEEE Antennas and Wireless Propagation Letters, 11*, 1508–1511, 2012.

Luu, Q. T., Koulouridis, S., Diet, A., Le Bihan, Y., and Pichon, L., Investigation of inductive and radiating energy harvesting for an implanted biotelemetry antenna, *11th European Conference on Antennas and Propagation*, EUCAP 2017, pp. 160–163, 2017.

Reddy, K. H. K., Roy, D. S., Mishra, T. K., & Hussain, M. W. (Eds.). (2023). *Handbook of Research on Network-Enabled IoT Applications for Smart City Services*. USA, IGI Global.

Shamed, A. E. and Sharawi, M. S. Miniaturized dual wideband circular patch antenna for biomedical telemetry. *11th European Conference on Antennas and Propagation (EUCAP)*, pp. 1027–1030, 2017.

Zerrad, F.-E., Taouzari, M., Makroum, E. M., Aoufi, J. E., Qanadli, S. D., Karaaslan, M., Al-Gburi, A. J. A., and Zakaria, Z. Microwave imaging approach for breast cancer detection using a tapered slot antenna loaded with parasitic components. *Materials, 16*(4), 1426, 2023. https://doi.org/10.3390/ma16041496

15

Artificial Intelligence Prediction of the Risk of Ovarian Cancer at an Early Stage in Smart Cities

J. M. Sheela Lavanya and P. Subbulakshmi
Vellore Institute of Technology, Chennai, India

15.1 Introduction

In recent years, the integration of artificial intelligence (AI) in healthcare has witnessed unprecedented advancements, offering innovative solutions to long-standing challenges. In this context, our research delves into the domain of predictive medicine, specifically focusing on the early detection of ovarian cancer using AI-driven models. It is often difficult to effectively treat ovarian cancer in its advanced stages, and patient survival rates are low. Addressing this critical issue, our study aims to harness the power of AI to develop a robust predictive model capable of identifying potential cases at an early stage.

As we embark on this journey toward improved healthcare outcomes, it is imperative to consider the broader societal context in which these advancements unfold. The paradigm of smart cities emerges as a pertinent framework where technological innovations synergize with urban development goals (Reddy et al., 2023). Citizens' quality of life can be enhanced by leveraging data analytics, AI, and the Internet of Things (IoT). This research positions itself at the intersection of AI-driven healthcare and the broader smart city initiative, recognizing the potential for our predictive model to seamlessly integrate into intelligent urban ecosystems.

Beyond the confines of traditional healthcare paradigms, our exploration into the implications of AI in predicting ovarian cancer risk aligns with the visionary ethos of smart cities. By merging these two spheres, we aim to contribute not only to advancements in healthcare but also to the realization of proactive and responsive urban environments. This introduction sets the stage for a comprehensive examination of how our AI model may play a pivotal role in shaping the future of healthcare within the dynamic context of smart cities.

Female reproductive systems consist of the ovary, which produces the ovum. Whenever the ovary is affected in any way, it causes direct damage to the reproductive

DOI: 10.1201/9781032631738-15

system. There are several types of disorders that are caused by uncontrolled cell growth, but cancer is the most common. Any part of the human body can be affected by this growth. There is a growing number of cells in the ovary that are contributing to the development of ovarian cancer (Momenimovahed et al., 2019). In the world, cancers such as ovarian cancer are among the most common, are deadly diseases, and are very common among women. Cells that grow and multiply uncontrollably inside the ovaries or fallopian tubes are considered to be ovarian cancers. As one of the most common types of cancer, ovarian cancer ranks fifth in terms of prevalence among women worldwide. *Proceedings of National Academy of Sciences* recently published a study which indicates that ovarian cancer may be caused by six types of cells. Most of the ovarian malignancies originate in the fallopian tubes. Transporting eggs from the ovary to the uterus is done by fallopian tubes when they are developing. Ovarian cancer can be classified into three types: (1) epithelial ovarian cancer (cancer that develops outside of the ovaries); (2) endometrial ovarian cancer (originating inside the ovaries); (3) stromal cancer (arises from the cells of the ovary producing hormones); (4) germ cell cancer (it develops from the egg cells). Most cases of ovarian cancer occur in women who are postmenopausal. In recent years, however, young women have also been diagnosed with ovarian cancer as a result of an unhealthy lifestyle. It is not possible to determine any particular symptoms in association with ovarian cancer. A recent report prepared for the American Cancer Society estimates that there will be approximately 19,710 cases of ovarian cancer diagnosed in the United States by the year 2022. A total of 13,270 women died as a result of ovarian cancer. An important aspect of early detection of ovarian cancer is screening. There are eight out of ten patients with ovarian cancer that have been diagnosed too late and thus die from the disease.

Various risk factors are associated with ovarian cancer development. According to the blood test and the protein analysis results, according to the results obtained from these tests, there are many parameters that can be used in order to predict cancer. CA-19 and CA-125 are the most common proteins used for identifying cancerous cells. Through algorithms of machine learning (ML), it can be used for predicting the stages of ovarian cancer in its early stages by analyzing the diverse parameters found in the blood report, including the albumin–globulin (GA) ratio as well as the alkaline globulin (AG). Invasive methods are used to diagnose ovarian cancer, which is an expensive and unpleasant procedure. Thus, it is necessary to develop a method that is noninvasive and less expensive for detecting ovarian cancer.

A ML algorithm consists of algorithms that extract useful information from data in an automated manner (Badillo et al., 2020; Pradhan et al., 2022; Hussain and Roy, 2023). There are a number of algorithms that can be learned from data in order to perform tasks such as prediction and classification in an efficient manner. Computers are capable of learning from data, identifying patterns, and reaching conclusions without the assistance of humans. Algorithms of ML are primarily focused on the estimation of relationships between independent variables and dependent variables in a dataset, which is called a model. Model estimation serves both predictive and inferential purposes. Essentially, prediction involves predicting something that has not yet occurred, while inference is the process of identifying a hidden pattern within a dataset. ML algorithms (Jenhani et al., 2008) can be separated into the following four categories based on the way they are classified:

(i). *Supervised learning*: As the name implies, supervised learning algorithms deal with labeled data. There is a primary purpose to this learning method which is to make predictions. The supervised learning method covers both regression and classification issues. In addition to these methods, there are a few others like random forests, simple linear regressions, decision trees (DTs), ridge regressions, and support vector machines (SVMs) that make up these systems.

(ii). *Unsupervised learning*: The unsupervised learning method is concerned with unlabeled data. A large collection of unknowable data can be analyzed using this method in order to uncover relevant insights and hidden patterns. This learning can be applied when input data is available without corresponding output data. The analysis is further broken down into two categories: cluster analysis and association analysis. A number of methodologies have been employed in this study, including Principal Component Analysis (PCA), Independent Component Analysis (ICA), K-means clustering, neural networks, anomaly detection, and K-nearest neighbors (KNNs).

(iii). *Reinforcement*: An important part of reinforcement learning is determining the actions required to improve performance. In this type of learning, no specific results are expected.

(iv). *Semi-supervised learning*: Both supervised and unsupervised learning take place at this intermediate stage. Both labeled and unlabeled data can be used to facilitate its learning process.

This research has several key highlights, including the following:

i) To review and acknowledge the earlier works on the prediction of ovarian cancer by various authors.
ii) The proposed model for predicting the ovarian cancer risk is introduced.
iii) Evaluation of the proposed model in comparison against existing algorithms for ML.

This chapter has been meticulously organized according to the following structure: Section 15.2 presents a thorough analysis of the various methodologies utilized by researchers in the study of ovarian cancer, each characterized by different levels of accuracy. Section 15.3 outlines the primary objective of this research endeavor and provides intricate information regarding the dataset employed. Detailed explanations of the methodologies and models are provided in Section 15.4. Detailed explanations of the reasoning behind the model are provided in Section 15.5. Furthermore, Section 15.6 of this encompasses a comprehensive examination of diverse parameters for evaluating the models, ultimately leading to the conclusion of the research project, accompanied by the outcomes of the model and potential avenues for future research.

15.2 Related Work

In Lu et al. (2020), the utilization of the minimum redundancy-maximum relevance (MRMR) technique was carried out by the authors to distinguish the most pertinent characteristics from the data. Following this, a model was established using a DT, utilizing these selected pertinent characteristics, with the objective of classifying benign ovarian tumors and ovarian cancer. After evaluating the DT model, the author measured the accuracy, in comparison to the risk of ovarian malignancy algorithm (ROMA), resulting in a success rate of 87%.

In an attempt to ascertain the indicators accountable for identifying high-grade serous ovarian cancer, computational forecasting (Akter and Akhter, 2022) was formulated. The authors harnessed the publicly accessible HGSOC proteomic dataset to construct decision support systems (DSS). They opted for a two-step elimination technique, centering the Pearson coefficient and the relief method. Subsequently, a dichotomous classification assignment (tumor or non-tumor) was executed. This proposed method has proven instrumental in the discovery of new medical symptoms and biomarkers.

The researcher conducted a study in which the dataset used involved the analysis of the dataset of PLCO with the utilization of screening by transvaginal ultrasonography (TVUS) to detect ovarian cancer at an early stage. This particular dataset was obtained from the United States National Cancer Institute (NCI). The research specifically focused on three distinct features of each sample. The Prostate, Lung, Colorectal, and Ovarian cancer screening trial (PLCO) dataset, which had limited accessibility, presented a significant number of missing values. These missing values were addressed through the implementation of KNN imputers, while the imbalanced data within the dataset was managed using SMOTE. In order to conduct their analysis, the authors employed three algorithms, namely, random forest, XGBoost, and KNN.

According to the study performed by the authors in Thabtah et al. (2019), a dataset of ovarian cancer samples was employed. This dataset composed of 202 samples obtained from the Tokyo Women's University Medical Centre East. Through incorporating medical examination data of the patients, the researchers utilized five distinct ML techniques to forecast instances of cancer. Of the various characteristics considered, the CA125 characteristic was found to be particularly significant. Notably, XGBoost demonstrated the highest accuracy, reaching 80%.

During the study by Akazawa and Hashimoto (2020), the authors investigated postoperative complications and hospital readmissions within 30 days of surgery. In order to carry out this examination, information from Northwestern Medicine Enterprise Data Warehouse (NMEDW) was retrieved, specifically the preoperative CT scan. An analytical approach was used to analyze the unstructured data by converting it into variables using natural language processing (NLP). To predict the occurrence of significant postoperative issues, various classification algorithms including random forest, XGBoost, and SVMs can be utilized. Based on the results of the study, out of 291 people who underwent surgery, 25 required rehospitalization and 45 encountered complications.

The researchers in Barber et al. (2021) employed seven supervised learning algorithms to furnish predictive insights for individuals afflicted with epithelial ovarian cancer. In addition, the researchers also factored in the magnitude of the remaining tumor. Ultimately, it was inferred that the gradient boosting technique demonstrated the highest level of efficacy in prognosticating epithelial ovarian cancer.

In Kawakami et al. (2019), the authors made the decision to choose the gene associated with ovarian cancer as a means of providing compelling evidence that these genes act as indicators of patient survival. To ascertain the clinical facts and genes that have a significant impact on estimating patient survival after ovarian cancer surgery, both univariate and multivariate regression analyses were carried out in conjunction with combined regression analysis. Meanwhile, in Hossain et al. (2019), the authors developed a system for detecting ovarian cancer by using the ML mechanism by combining five classifiers. Based on the Gini Index, DTs with maximum information gain were employed as classifiers along with memory-based learning techniques. It is worth noting that feature selection was not undertaken by the authors due to the fact that the utilized dataset solely consisted of pertinent attributes. Moreover, a pre-processing method for the data was executed in order to eradicate any absent values and anomalies from the dataset.

The study executed (Wang et al., 2019) deep learning algorithms in order to extract the most pertinent information for clinical interpretation from preoperative CT scans in order to enhance the prompt detection for high-grade serous ovarian cancer (HGSOC). The aim of their investigation was to construct and evaluate a model for prognostic purposes, integrating an appropriate method for selecting relevant features. By employing clinical data and diverse classification models, it becomes feasible to accurately and economically predict ovarian cancer occurrence. In addition to CA-125, numbers of neutrophils in the bloodstream (NEU), albinism (ALB), and blood protein report's specific aspects are addressed in these learning techniques. In order to assess the effectiveness of various methodologies, precision, accuracy, recall, and the F1-score are utilized. The purpose of these methodologies is to assist in detecting ovarian cancer at an early stage.

In Bebortta et al. (2023a), a health service provider (HSP) system that collects patient data in real-time is critical for identifying diseases early and treating them promptly. However, healthcare systems are complex, making it difficult to flow user data seamlessly. As a method to handle sparse SVMs and improve the interpretability of classification results, the cluster primal–dual splitting (cPDS) algorithm has been developed. A fully-centralized and a fully-decentralized conurbation can be accommodated by our proposed approach due to its intrinsic adaptability. According to predictive accuracy evaluations, this model consistently shows superior prediction capabilities. In the field of transmission costs, our method is the golden standard of computing efficiency and is also a reliable approach for predicting hospitalizations caused by heart disease. With the combination of EHR data and IoT data, the proposed methodology can improve cardiac illness prediction and detection. However, the cPDS has scaling issues and the EHRs and IoT-generated health data are not complete and varied enough.

The article by Tripathy et al. (2023) has outlined the significant role of fog computing in revolutionizing healthcare, particularly in the context of IoT-based applications for remote patient monitoring and smart healthcare systems. The integration of fog and cloud computing in healthcare has been explored, highlighting the potential for improved data management, analytics, and real-time decision-making. The proposed model, HealthFog, represents a notable advancement, leveraging deep learning and edge computing to offer real-time data processing and diagnosis of cardiac conditions. Through the utilization of deep Q network ensemble methods, this model demonstrates promising accuracy rates, lower energy consumption, and advanced throughput when compared to traditional cloud-based healthcare systems.

The article by Bebortta et al. (2023b), "DeepMist: Toward Deep Learning Assisted Mist Computing Framework for Managing Healthcare Big Data" introduces the concept of DeepMist, a mist computing framework designed for the management of healthcare big data. The framework leverages deep learning technologies to optimize data processing and analysis in healthcare settings. The potential applications of DeepMist in improving data management, analysis, and decision-making within the healthcare domain are likely to be discussed, along with the benefits and challenges associated with integrating deep learning into mist computing for healthcare big data management.

In Tripathy et al. (2022), smart healthcare assistants are a highly sensitive and complex project. The current research work proposes a fog-computing-enabled smart healthcare system that uses AI to perform an automated diagnosis of heart disease using IoT-enabled resources and incorporates the latest technology, namely, a deep-learning ensemble method. Based on different QoS characteristics and fog-cloud cost models, this research proposed to enhance HealthFog by allowing cost-optimal execution and using more intelligent ensemble models with advanced security capabilities.

While these studies contribute valuable insights, our focus extends to the early identification of ovarian cancer risks, providing a more comprehensive understanding of potential risk factors at the nascent stages. However, the amalgamation of AI in healthcare and smart city initiatives remains an underexplored territory in the literature. Our study takes a pioneering approach by not only advancing the frontier of AI-driven disease prediction but also proposing a synergistic integration of these predictive models into the fabric of smart city initiatives. This multidisciplinary approach positions our research at the forefront of innovation, laying the groundwork for a future where the symbiosis of AI and smart city principles reshapes the landscape of healthcare delivery and urban well-being.

15.3 Methodology

As an integral component of the research approach, this study incorporates

- Gathering of data
- Prepossessing of the data
- Splitting of data
- Feature selection process
- Algorithms for ML
- The proposed model
- Methodology for evaluating performance

15.3.1 Gathering of Data

In the present investigation, a collection of ovarian cancer data was obtained from the renowned platform known as Kaggle. This specific dataset comprises a collective sum of 349 samples, with each individual sample harboring 49 unique attributes. Out of these 349 samples, it was discovered that 57% had received a diagnosis of ovarian cancer, while the remaining individuals were deemed cancer-free. The collection of data was obtained from individuals ranging in age from 23 to 68. Among the 349 patients, a total of 234 were identified as being in the postmenopausal stage. The dataset encompassed a variety of blood routine examinations, protein analyses, and a collection of general chemistry tests. These attributes encompassed a range of factors, including Alpha Feto Protein (AFP), AG ratio, age (years), albumin (ALB) being a gene that codes for a protein alkaline phosphate (ALP), alkaline transaminase (ALT), which is an enzyme that can be found in the liver, aspartate aminotransferase (AST), an enzyme primarily found in the liver but also present in all other organs, Basophils (BASO), a specific type of white blood cell, blood urea nitrogen (BUN), level of calcium in blood (Ca), and more.

15.3.2 Prepossessing of the Data

A preliminary step entails transforming data into a format that can be interpreted by a machine, for instance, Comma-Separated Values (CSV).

- Data cleaning: This method entails the elimination of records and columns that are sparsely distributed and the replacement of missing data points. Through the utilization of data cleansing methodologies, inaccurate information, such as absent, contradictory, and unfinished values, has been eradicated from the dataset.
- Standardization: The utilization of the min–max standardization procedure has been determined in order to guarantee that the attributes of the ovarian cancer dataset do not engage in detrimental interactions with other attributes in relation to distance. In this process, features are standardized or scaled by applying the following formula in order to adjust their values range from 0 and 1.

$$F\left(X = \frac{X - \min(X)}{\max(X) - \min(X)}\right) \tag{15.1}$$

Assuming that the minimal and maximal values of feature X are denoted as min(X) and max(X), respectively, it is referred to as standardization or feature scaling. This process involves transforming the numeric values of the dataset to a range between 0 and 1.

Upon completion of the preprocessing phase, the final dataset becomes devoid of noise, exhibits consistency, and is standardized. The preprocessed dataset is composed of 349 instances with 48 attributes each, in addition to a single target variable.

15.3.3 Splitting of Data

The dataset has been divided into two distinct portions: one is allocated for the purpose of training the model, commonly referred to as the training set, while the other is utilized to evaluate the accuracy of the employed model, known as the testing set. The training dataset comprises 80% of the total data, whereas the testing dataset accounts for the remaining 20%.

Feature selection serves as a vital process within the realm of ML, as it aims to enhance the efficiency of the model by carefully choosing the most pertinent features from the available data (Boehm et al., 2022). The random forest feature selection method entails a bootstrap aggregation process, wherein the most effective features are determined by following a series of iterative steps. The initial step of this method involves the selection of threshold values, which subsequently dictate the inclusion or exclusion of specific features.

The subsequent steps of the random forest feature selection method are as follows:

(i). Establish a fixed standard threshold value.

(ii). One can determine the Gini impurity by employing the given formula, in which C denotes the aggregate number of categories and pi signifies the likelihood of a data point being affiliated with category i.

$$\mathrm{Gini}(p) = \sum_{i=1}^{C} 1 - (p_i)^2 \tag{15.2}$$

(iii). Organize the Gini impurity scores in a sequential manner, starting from the lowest value and progressing toward the highest.

(iv). Select the characteristics that demonstrate a Gini impurity score surpassing the predetermined threshold value.

(v). Discard the characteristics that are situated beneath the predetermined threshold value. By adhering to this course of action, it is plausible to procure a dataset that is endowed with a diminished quantity of variables, all the while conserving the variability.

15.3.4 Model

For the purpose of comparing the results with the proposed model, three classification techniques are utilized, namely, logistic regression (LR), DTs, and SVMs.

15.3.4.1 Logistic Regression

For the purpose of solving classification problems within the field of ML (Charbuty and Abdulazeez, 2021), we employed a supervised learning technique. This particular approach to learning expands upon the principles of linear regression, wherein the dependent variable exhibits a categorical and non-continuous nature. Within the framework of LR, two distinct categories can be identified: binary LR, which applies to situations involving two levels, and multinomial regression, which is more applicable to scenarios involving two or more stages. A LR model's primary goal is to predict the category to which a novel observation will be assigned, instead of merely allocating the finding to an established group. Rather than directly estimating a class, the LR approach calculates probabilities that the given features belong to it. Binary classification problems are particularly well suited to LR. In the context of LR, the training data are categorized using logit or sigmoid functions, as shown in equation (15.3).

$$\sigma(x) = \frac{1}{\left(1 + e^{-(a+bx)}\right)} \tag{15.3}$$

If in this case, the variables designated for binary autonomous factor are expressed in 0 and 1. In the LR equation, with 1 indicating a probability of achieving a positive result and 0 denoting the absence of such, the creation of the LR equation can be expressed in the following manner:

$$P\left(Y = 1 / X = x;\beta\right) = P\left(x;\beta\right) = \frac{1}{\left(1 + e^{-\left(\beta^T x\right)}\right)} \tag{15.4}$$

The equation provided above illustrates the probability that data point x_i belongs to category 1. The parameters β are represented as

$$\beta = \left(\beta_0\ \beta_1\beta_2\ldots\beta_p\right)$$

Following this, the likelihood that the data points are part of category value 0 can be articulated as:

$$P\left(Y = 0 / X = x;\beta\right) = 1 - P\left(x;\beta\right) = \frac{e^{-\left(\beta^T x\right)}}{\left(1 + e^{-\left(\beta^T x\right)}\right)} \tag{15.5}$$

Equations (15.3) and (15.4) can be combined to form equation (15.6):

$$P\left(Y = y / X = x;\beta\right) = \left(P\left(x;\beta\right)\right)^y \left(1 - P\left(x;\beta\right)\right)^{(1-y)} \tag{15.6}$$

Equation (15.6) functions as the model for classification, with a dependency on the parameter β. The determination of β can be achieved by employing the method of maximum likelihood.

15.3.4.2 Support Vector Machine

For the purpose of addressing problems associated with classification and regression (Zhang and Han, 2020), SVM, which employs supervised learning techniques, is utilized. The utilization of SVMs entails the pursuit of two complementary objectives.

(i). The first objective is to maximize the accuracy by ensuring that the correct labels are assigned to the new data.
(ii). The second objective is to optimize the reproducibility of the classifier, ensuring its generalizability to new data.

The primary objective of this methodology is to ascertain a decision function, commonly known as the hyperplane, which segregates the data values into distinct categories. Multiple alternative hyperplanes can be utilized to discriminate between the different classes of data points. Nevertheless, the primary objective is to ascertain the hyperplane that demonstrates the utmost margin, thus guaranteeing that the most closely related data points belonging to a specific category are positioned at the maximum distance from the hyperplane. Hyperplane functions as delineation boundaries which facilitate the classification of the data points into multiple categories. The dimensionality of the dataset is defined by the number of attributes it possesses.

Given a training dataset $D = (x_i, d_i)_{i=0}^{N}, x_i \epsilon R^n, d_i \epsilon -1,1$ the objective is to ascertain the corresponding response $d\epsilon -1,1$ for a pattern $x\epsilon R^n$, where $x = x_i$ for every i.

Let $\alpha = \alpha_0 \alpha_1 \alpha_3 \ldots \alpha_p$

The expression representing the equation of the hyperplane that separates can be stated as follows:

$$\alpha_1 x_1 + \alpha_2 x_2 + .. + \alpha_p x_p - b = 0 \tag{15.7}$$

Consequently, a hyperplane equation is expressed as follows:

$$P_0 : \alpha^T x + b = 0 \tag{15.8}$$

Moreover, it is necessary to generate two parallel hyperplanes in relation to the hyperplane that has been constructed.

$$P_1 : \alpha^T x + b = 1 \tag{15.9}$$

$$P_2 : \alpha^T x + b = -1 \tag{15.10}$$

This transformation has currently undergone a progression into an optimization problem, as the requirement for identifying the optimal hyperplane has arisen. Furthermore, SVMs can be categorized into two distinct types:

- Linear SVM
- Nonlinear SVM

Linear SVM is suitable for cases where the data objects can be linearly separated in this problem of two-class classification. On the contrary, in cases where the data is not capable of being separated by a straight line, it is possible to utilize a collection of mathematical functions referred to as kernels in order to convert the training set which is nonlinear into a linear format. This ultimately allows for the categorization of the data values into distinct categories.

15.3.4.3 Random Forest

An adaptable form of supervised learning, known as the random forest algorithm, is utilized for the purposes of both classification and regression (Liaw and Wiener, 2002). In the random forest classifier, multiple DTs are constructed using distinct subsets, with the objective of enhancing accuracy by means of averaging. This methodology harmonizes the creation of DTs with the utilization of ensemble learning techniques. The execution of this method involves several steps:

- Root node: The root node is established by inputting the complete training set.
- Splitting: The identification of the most suitable division can be ascertained by employing the Gini equation (15.2) and the entropy approach, which

evaluates the degree of randomness and ambiguity present in the information. The computation of this partition can be accomplished via the subsequent formulation (15.11).

$$E(p) = \sum_{i=1}^{C} -p_i \left(\log_2 p_i\right) \tag{15.11}$$

The symbol pi is utilized to denote the likelihood of a specific data point being classified as belonging to class i.

- Decision node: Establish decision points that function as links to the terminal points.
- Leaf node: The culmination of the classification procedure, which finalizes the entire operation through the act of forecasting.

15.4 Proposed Model

The cohesive system suggested in this investigation amalgamates both the process of identifying salient attributes and methods of categorization for predicting the occurrence in the early stages of ovarian cancer. The operational methodology of the suggested framework is elucidated in six sequential stages, as delineated.

(i). Gathering of data: The dataset on ovarian cancer was acquired from the platform Kaggle.
(ii). Prepossessing of the data: This particular stage incorporates the procedure of data cleansing and the application of the min–max standardization approach to achieve standardization.
(iii). Feature selection process: The feature selection method of random forest is employed for the purpose of selecting the most important features.
(iv). Splitting of data: After the process of selecting the features, datasets are split into two components: the training component and the testing component.
(v). Algorithms for ML: The employment of the random forest classification technique is pursued with the objective of making predictions.
(vi). Methodology for evaluating performance: The evaluation of the model is conducted utilizing diverse arithmetical metrics.

The operational mechanism of the model that has been suggested is observed in Figure 15.1

15.5 Evaluation Parameters

To visually represent and provide a concise summary of the classification algorithm's performance, we employ the utilization of a confusion matrix (Lavanya and Subbulakshmi, 2023). This matrix serves as a means to analyze the effectiveness of the

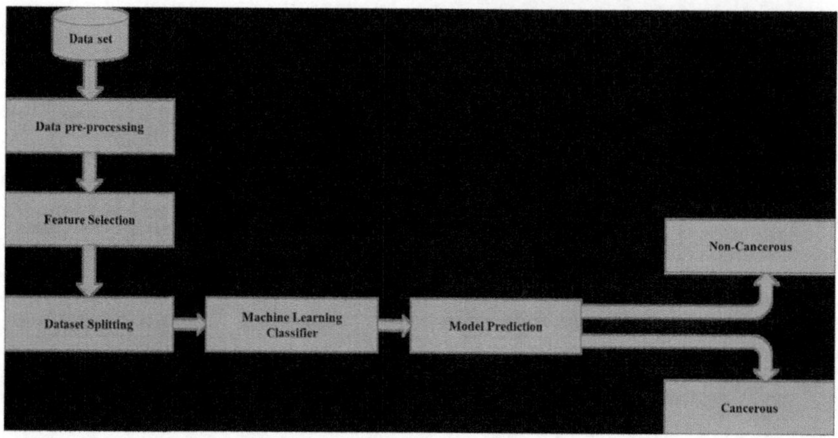

FIGURE 15.1 Proposed system model.

deployed ML techniques. The evaluation of the model's efficiency is based on four parameters:

- True positive (Tp): This parameter aims to forecast the occurrence of an event with increased precision.
- False positive (Fp): Its purpose lies in detecting the presence of inaccurate event data values.
- True negative (Tn): This metric is utilized to predict the absence of event data values.
- False negative (Fn): This is employed when erroneously predicting the absence of event values.

In order to establish the confusion matrix, it is necessary to determine the performance metrics. These metrics encompass the F1-score, accuracy, recall, and precision.

(i). Precision: This metric represents the level of excellence of the model and measures the ratio of accurate positive predictions in relation to all positive predictions (Parameswari et al., 2021).

$$\text{Precision} = \frac{T_p}{T_p + F_p}$$

(ii). Recall: Recall computes the ratio of true positive forecasts among all existing positive occurrences (Josephine et al., 2022). It evaluates the model's capacity to accurately detect all the occurrences of ovarian cancer in the dataset.

$$\text{Recall} = \frac{T_p}{T_p + F_n}$$

(iii). F1-score: As an integral component of this performance, consideration is given to both the occurrence of Fn and Fp outcomes (Godbin and Jasmine, 2022). This allows it to maintain its efficacy across both balanced datasets and unbalanced datasets.

$$\text{F1-score} = \frac{2(\text{Precision} * \text{Recall})}{\text{Precision} + \text{Recall}}$$

(iv). Accuracy: In order to ascertain it, it becomes imperative to partition the aggregate quantity of accurately recognized instances by the complete amount of specimens.

15.6 Result and Discussion

The experiment made use of the ovarian cancer open dataset provided by Kaggle. A variety of medical factors present in the dataset were employed with the aim of ascertaining the existence of ovarian cancer. The variables were utilized with the aim of classifying into type 1, indicating the presence of malignancy, while type 0 represented individuals who did not possess any form of cancer. Within the dataset, there were six instances that exhibited the absence of values, and these values were estimated by the process of computing the average of the already present characteristics. Moreover, in order to maintain a dataset that is consistent, any data that contained noise was eliminated. Leading to the generation of a comprehensive dataset that is devoid of any instances of noisy or missing values techniques like standard scaling were implemented on the dataset. The model that was suggested for predicting ovarian cancer was executed and contrasted against alternative classifiers, including LR, DTs, and SVM. The most optimal indicators for prediction, as identified through the implementation of the random forest feature selection approach, are visually presented in Figure 15.2.

The assessment of performance has been carried out employing F1 measures, precision, recall, and accuracy as quantitative indicators. The indicators of performance that have ensued are provided in (Table 15.1) henceforth. As a result of this model, as shown in Figure 15.3, 91% accuracy, 91% precision, 90% recall, and 93% F1 measure were achieved. The proposed approach, illustrated in Figure 15.3, demonstrates a superior level of accuracy in comparison to the other two traditional methodologies. A comparison between the results of both existing ML algorithms and the proposed model is presented in Figure 15.3 by computing the four evaluation metrics.

TABLE 15.1

Comparative Analysis of Various Model's Accuracy

Model	Precision	Recall	F1-score	Accuracy
Logistic regression	0.86	0.83	0.82	0.81
Support vector machine	0.92	0.9	0.86	0.84
Decision tree	0.92	0.9	0.86	0.83
Proposed model	0.91	0.9	0.93	0.91

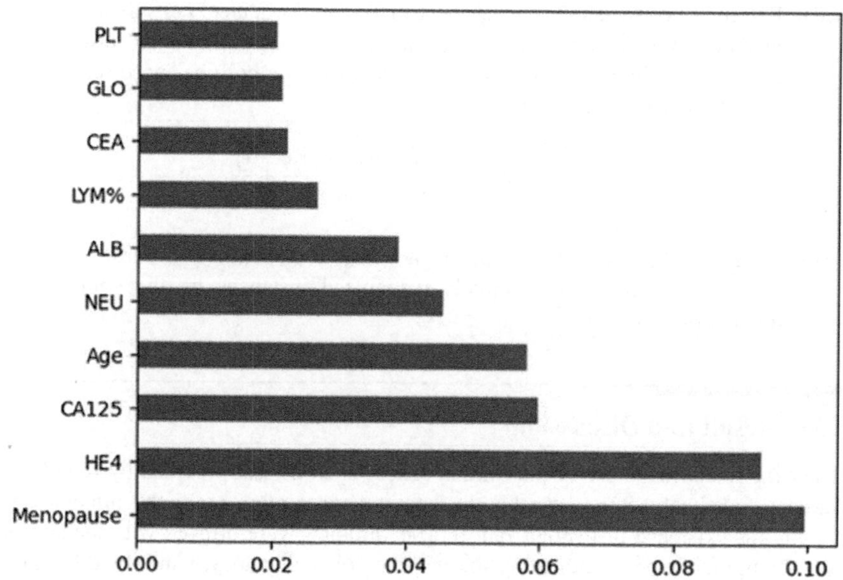

FIGURE 15.2 Ten out of 49 features showed the greatest predictive value through random forest feature selection.

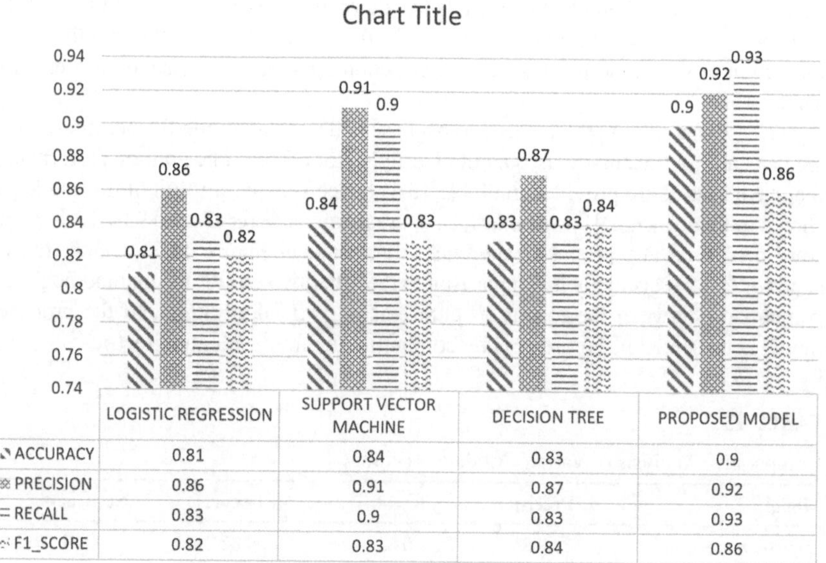

	LOGISTIC REGRESSION	SUPPORT VECTOR MACHINE	DECISION TREE	PROPOSED MODEL
ACCURACY	0.81	0.84	0.83	0.9
PRECISION	0.86	0.91	0.87	0.92
RECALL	0.83	0.9	0.83	0.93
F1_SCORE	0.82	0.83	0.84	0.86

FIGURE 15.3 Performance comparisons.

15.7 Conclusion

Women with ovarian cancer are at a higher risk of death as a result of a delayed diagnosis of this disease. A new research work has been published in which it proposes the use of ML methodologies to contribute to medical science in the attempt to overcome this deadly condition. In spite of the fact that these methods are not intended to replace doctors, in remote areas without adequate access to modern medical facilities, technological developments can nonetheless be of value. Furthermore, doctors may be able to make more informed decisions with the help of a medical decision-making app. There are also a few limitations to the proposed techniques, as they can only be used to detect whether or not someone has cancer, as they can only be used to detect the presence of cancer. Hence, it won't be able to identify the severity of the disease. It is conceivable that in subsequent times, the application of this approach could be expanded, thereby enabling the prospect of generating even more precise prognostications and determining appropriate methodologies for feature selection that could be applied to the accurate diagnosis of ovarian cancer in a more facile and less convoluted manner. Moreover, if this proposed methodology is extended to other categories of chronic diseases, it could also be utilized to identify other enduring ailments. Our research marks a significant stride in leveraging AI for the detection and prediction of early-stage ovarian cancer, offering a beacon of hope for improved healthcare outcomes. The success of our predictive model underscores the transformative potential of AI in reshaping disease diagnosis and prognosis. As we navigate the complex landscape of healthcare innovation, it becomes evident that our model not only contributes to early-stage ovarian cancer detection but also aligns seamlessly with the broader vision of smart cities.

REFERENCES

Akazawa, M., & Hashimoto, K. (2020). Artificial intelligence in ovarian cancer diagnosis. *Anticancer Research, 40*(8), 4795–4800.

Akter, L., & Akhter, N. (2022). Ovarian cancer prediction from ovarian cysts based on TVUS using machine learning algorithms. In *Proceedings of the International Conference on Big Data, IoT, and Machine Learning: BIM 2021* (pp. 51–61). Springer Singapore.

Badillo, S., Banfai, B., Birzele, F., Davydov, I. I., Hutchinson, L., Kam-Thong, T., … & Zhang, J. D. (2020). An introduction to machine learning. *Clinical Pharmacology & Therapeutics, 107*(4), 871–885.

Barber, E. L., Garg, R., Persenaire, C., & Simon, M. (2021). Natural language processing with machine learning to predict outcomes after ovarian cancer surgery. *Gynecologic Oncology, 160*(1), 182–186.

Bebortta, S., Tripathy, S. S., Basheer, S., & Chowdhary, C. L. (2023a). FedEHR: A Federated Learning Approach towards the Prediction of Heart Diseases in IoT-Based Electronic Health Records. *Diagnostics, 13*(20), 3166.

Bebortta, S., Tripathy, S. S., Basheer, S., & Chowdhary, C. L. (2023b). *DeepMist: Towards Deep Learning Assisted Mist Computing Framework for Managing Healthcare Big Data. IEEE Access.*

Boehm, K. M., Aherne, E. A., Ellenson, L., Nikolovski, I., Alghamdi, M., Vázquez-García, I., … Shah, S. P. (2022). Multimodal data integration using machine learning improves risk stratification of high-grade serous ovarian cancer. *Nature Cancer*, *3*(6), 723–733.

Charbuty, B., & Abdulazeez, A. (2021). Classification based on decision tree algorithm for machine learning. *Journal of Applied Science and Technology Trends*, *2*(01), 20–28.

Godbin, A. B., & Jasmine, S. G. (2022). Screening of COVID-19 based on GLCM features from CT images using machine learning classifiers. *SN Computer Science*, *4*(2), 133.

Hossain, M. A., Islam, S. M. S., Quinn, J. M., Huq, F., & Moni, M. A. (2019). Machine learning and bioinformatics models to identify gene expression patterns of ovarian cancer associated with disease progression and mortality. *Journal of Biomedical Informatics*, *100*, 103313.

Hussain, M. W., & Roy, D. S. (2023). Performance Optimization Strategies for Big Data Applications in Distributed Framework. In *Intelligent Technologies: Concepts, Applications, and Future Directions*, Volume *2* (pp. 221–252). Singapore: Springer Nature Singapore.

Jenhani, I., Amor, N. B., & Elouedi, Z. (2008). Decision trees as possibilistic classifiers. *International Journal of Approximate Reasoning*, *48*(3), 784–807.

Josephine, D. J., Wise, D. J. W., Verunathi, A. R., SheelaLavanya, J. M., SterlinRani, D., & Saravanan, K. G. (2022, January). A Novel Approach of Applying Rank Ordering Clustering Algorithm in Agricultural Data. In *2022 4th International Conference on Smart Systems and Inventive Technology (ICSSIT)* (pp. 456–459). IEEE.

Kawakami, E., Tabata, J., Yanaihara, N., Ishikawa, T., Koseki, K., Iida, Y., … Okamoto, A. (2019). Application of artificial intelligence for preoperative diagnostic and prognostic prediction in epithelial ovarian cancer based on blood biomarkers. *Clinical Cancer Research*, *25*(10), 3006–3015.

Lavanya, J. S., & Subbulakshmi, P. (2023, January). Machine Learning Techniques for the Prediction of Non-Communicable Diseases. In *2023 International Conference on Artificial Intelligence and Knowledge Discovery in Concurrent Engineering (ICECONF)* (pp. 1–8). IEEE.

Liaw, A., & Wiener, M. (2002). Classification and regression by random Forest. *R News*, *2*(3), 18–22.

Lu, M., Fan, Z., Xu, B., Chen, L., Zheng, X., Li, J., … & Jiang, J. (2020). Using machine learning to predict ovarian cancer. *International Journal of Medical Informatics*, *141*, 104195.

Momenimovahed, Z., Tiznobaik, A., Taheri, S., & Salehiniya, H. (2019). Ovarian cancer in the world: Epidemiology and risk factors. *International Journal of Women's Health*, 287–299.

Parameswari, M., Balaji, S., Josephine, D. J., Rani, M. D. S., Lavanya, M. J. S., & Wise, D. J. W. (2021). Robust heart disease diagnosis and analysis system using data mining. *Annals of the Romanian Society for Cell Biology*, 9461–9466.

Pradhan, B., Hussain, M. W., Srivastava, G., Debbarma, M. K., Barik, R. K., & Lin, J. C. W. (2022). *A Neuro-Evolutionary Approach for Software Defined Wireless Network Traffic Classification*. IET Communications.

Reddy, K. H. K., Roy, D. S., Mishra, T. K., & Hussain, M. W. (Eds.). (2023). *Handbook of Research on Network-Enabled IoT Applications for Smart City Services*. IGI Global.

Thabtah, F., Abdelhamid, N., & Peebles, D. (2019). A machine learning autism classification based on logistic regression analysis. *Health Information Science and Systems*, *7*, 1–11.

Tripathy, S. S., Imoize, A. L., Rath, M., Tripathy, N., Bebortta, S., Lee, C. C., … & Pani, S. K. (2022). A novel edge-computing-based framework for an intelligent smart healthcare system in smart cities. *Sustainability*, *15*(1), 735.

Tripathy, S. S., Rath, M., Tripathy, N., Roy, D. S., Francis, J. S. A., & Bebortta, S. (2023). An Intelligent Health Care System in Fog Platform with Optimized Performance. *Sustainability*, *15*(3), 1862.

Wang, S., Liu, Z., Rong, Y., Zhou, B., Bai, Y., Wei, W., … Tian, J. (2019). Deep learning provides a new computed tomography-based prognostic biomarker for recurrence prediction in high-grade serous ovarian cancer. *Radiotherapy and Oncology*, *132*, 171–177.

Zhang, Z., & Han, Y. (2020). Detection of ovarian tumors in obstetric ultrasound imaging using logistic regression classifier with an advanced machine learning approach. *IEEE Access*, *8*, 44999–45008.

16

Chatbot Enable Brain Cancer Prediction Using Convolutional Neural Network for Smart Healthcare

Sima Das
Bengal College of Engineering and Technology, West Bengal, India

Vikash Kumar
National Institute of Technology Rourkela, Odisha, India

Giovanni Cicceri
University of Palermo, Italy

16.1 Introduction

The disease, which is widely affecting and has a massive impact on humankind without any sustenance, and which has become a primary concern all over the globe, is known as cancer. Cancer is almost a life-threatening disease; patients are losing their lives due to it. The number of affected people who have come up is astonishing on its own. The number of people who are diagnosed with cancer each year is ten million all over the globe; not only this, but the number of patients dying from cancer is more than half of the number ten million. Cancer has become the second life-threatening disease, and it affects the patient more deeply. Deep down, we all think about how to deal with this disease in a more advanced and intelligent way. A convolution neural network (CNN) has proved essential in cancer-related prediction (Alawad et al., 2021; Bilgıç, 2021; Cao et al., 2019; G. Chen et al., 2019; Huo, 2021; Ketout et al., 2011; Kido et al., 2018; Kollias & Zafeiriou, 2021; Lee et al., 2019; J. Li, 2018; L. Lu et al., 2019; Y. Lu, 2021; Saric et al., 2019; Sedigh et al., 2019; Senarathna, 2021; Tanna & Sharma, 2021; Yanagisawa et al., n.d.). It is implemented to emphasize the healthcare sector regarding cancer and optimize treatment. With the help of the CNN model, researchers can analyze and classify the outcome of the study of genes for cancer. This is how we can efficiently and significantly make this sector more advanced and reliable in smart cities (Reddy et al., 2023). The present research involves developing an

DOI: 10.1201/9781032631738-16

automation system to detect and categorize brain tumors and help accomplish better treatment in less time for smart health care (Das et al., 2022; Das, Adhikary, et al., 2023a, Das, Malick, et al., 2023b; Ghosh et al., 2022; Sima et al., 2023).

Deep learning (DL) is the sub-extension of artificial intelligence (AI) and comes under the clan of neural networks, which signifies the strand of learning from the big data. DL has the same process as machine learning (ML); DL includes the data set as a given input, and then, with the help of DL algorithms, it predicts the output of the given data set input. DL has been referred to as the more inclusive model with a huge amount of data and information, and then DL gives us precise and significant predictions. The device or application of DL used currently is far better than the previous method and application. DL has been implemented in healthcare very broadly these days. It also helps in the medicinal design and the prediction of cancers according to their types; not only this, but it also helps to identify the future course of patients and helps them manage and maintain their health in smart cities. From the prediction, it provides the best suggestions and methods for the durability of the patient. DL gives the best and most exact prediction result for the cancer patient, and this helps the patients get positive energy and benefits. The other benefit of DL is that it can acquire different forms or formats of data input.

Nowadays, chatbots have been used very broadly and widely. This is a complex computational program made by humans. It can copy the human conference and discussions. Currently, this has been widely used in the customer center to assist the customer and guide them to browse the menu and select; generally, in the customer support system, users are asked to choose any option or to press any key of the keypad then after the next operation and process is going to execute, this is how the chatbot guides a user without any failure. It is even used in industry to guide the user. People are also using this in their day-to-day lives while working through laptops and computers; examples of chatbots that are being used in laptops and computers are Siri (Apple), Cortana (windows), and many more. This guides the user of laptops and computers and, amazingly, the car driver. Car drivers use this technology for many things; if they want to pick up the call, they use voice commands; rather than using their hands, they don't move their hand from steering to pick up the call.

Digitalization is increasing day-by-day, and the world is becoming more and more advanced. Chatbot technology is now embedded and used in IoT as well. Chatbots are used in the Internet of Things (IoT) paradigm because they have the acumen to exchange data and information from various other devices and systems.

Application programming interface (API) is the center of web services in our day-to-day lives. API refers to the protocols or rules and criteria followed in web service applications. The APIs that are used to develop the functionality or system in IoT are referred to as IoT API; hence, they are used in web service applications programming interfaces. It is very useful for designing hi-tech and advanced applications that can be easily embedded with web services. They also help data to flow effortlessly in the HTTP paradigm. API also allows the IoT device to perform more securely, and with the help of API, the maximum possibility of cyber-attack is avoided; the most famous attack is a Distributed Denial of Service (DDOS) attack, and the chances of a DDOS attack become minimal; it also helps to improvise the flexibility.

Advantages of API in IoT

- For any application, a developer has to embed some rules or protocols in the system, and it is essential to make the process efficient and manageable. The developer must have the authority to manage the token as well. So, to manage all these things parallelly, we need speed. And this provides better efficiency as well.
- The API is beneficial in the early detection of loss and failure. It helps to manage the system.
- It also helps improve the scalability and make things better and easier for developers.
- It is also language-independent, so developers feel more comfortable and can code any of the languages they feel like.

Cancer is a life-threatening disease worldwide. To tackle this problem, many advanced technologies, systems, and devices are emerging quickly. The reason behind this is very simple: to help mankind and make life better and easier. The evolution in the digital world regarding new technologies and ideas is executing very fast as they are in parallel and ready for fabrication. This is all due to the modern ideas of the technologies and their dedicated involvement in strengthening the healthcare system's roots. Healthcare is a very important sector, and in this field, the involvement and contribution of technology must be superior. A result must be adequate enough from the technology, and the accurate and exact predicted result can determine this; ultimately, the result will signify whether the technology is acceptable or good enough to use. NLP stands for natural language processing and is a sub-part of AI, though AI is a broad spectrum. NLP makes oncologic detection and investigation more efficient these days. The subtle and nuanced data was the strand then; these are the unshaped, static, and no interpretation data, which are very raw. Previously, processing these data into meaningful and executable delineated data or information was not accessible. NLP helps in the transformation of subtle or nuanced data and information into executable delineated data and information. With the help of NLP and powerful algorithms, the practice of oncology becomes easier, and it also emphasizes the healthcare sector, especially oncology. Cancer is the most menacing and life-threatening disease. It is developed by the body's unconditional and abnormal cell division at a specific place. This can arise due to the consumption of alcohol and tobacco, less physical activity, irregular diet, and less protein and nutrient supplements like fruits and vegetables. According to WHO, the most common and famous cancers these days are breast cancer, lung cancer, rectum, prostate, skin, and colon cancer. The factors that cause cancers are ultraviolet rays, radiation, tobacco, and some bacteria and viruses.

The chapter is organized as follows: Section 16.2 will be a discussion on the literature survey, followed by proposed work and results comparison considering testing and validation of CNN and ANN techniques in Sections 16.3 and 16.4, respectively, and last but not least, we will summarize the conclusion.

16.2 Literature Survey

Protein–protein connections carry out leading roles from the beginning to the developing of most cancer-associated paths. The protein–protein interplay may perform distinctive roles in numerous cancers kinds. Hence, prioritizing every type of cancer could assist in locating most cancer-related ways, inventing a good knowledge of most cancers, and easing treatment detection. Few researchers have anticipated computational procedures for removing the PPI essentialness of dissimilar cancers. Most cancers are built and are totally taking place in the PPI community. An important downside of this research is that it doesn't always use a rich source together with genomics variation information. An amino acid series translates beneficial evidence approximately protein construction and performance. They denote every amino acid series constructed on its editions in seven one-of-a-kind methods: binary vectors, pathogenicity ratings, binding affinity modifications on mutations, gene expression built on a network of the communications, biophysicochemical belongings, g-hole dipeptide, and one-warm vectors. Constructed on those illustrations, they plan and consider seven specific deep-learning replicas. They also examine the precision of methods in predicting 20 distinct cancer sorts since the TCGA cohort (Abdollahi et al., 2021).

Most cancers are harmful by worst predictions. The bad prediction and struggle to beneficial sensory systems had been related to TP53 mutation. Compulsive checkups like biopsies cannot be commonly accomplished in medical training; hence, non-invasive and reproducible procedures remain favored. However, automated forecast strategies primarily built on imagination have limitations, including harmful 3D data usage, minor illustration length, and ineptness in multimodal combinations. In this look, they anticipated a model-pushed multimodal deep studying scheme to overwhelm those challenges. The spiral revolution might be used to practice 3D information efficaciously with fewer computational assets and easily augment the statistics length with high pleasantness. Moreover, version-driven gadgets have been designed to introduce previous expertise in the deep getting-to-know multimodal fusion framework. A bilinear assembling module was presented to advance the performance of first-class-grained prediction. The experimental results show that the anticipated prototype gives the favored concert in forecasting TP53 mutation in pancreatic cancer, suggesting a new method for non-invasive gene estimation (X. Chen et al., 2021).

The classifiers are based totally on genetic signatures wherein numerous microarray studies are examined to forecast medical consequences for most cancer sufferers. However, the signatures from specific research had promoted with low-intensity ratio all through the class of man or woman datasets, which has been taken into consideration as a tremendous point of studies. Hence, to triumph over the trouble mentioned above, this chapter offers a DL Framework that associates an algorithm of linear discriminant analysis (LDA) and autoencoder (AE) neural network to categorize exclusive capabilities inside the gene expression profile. Hence, a complicated ensemble category has been proposed based totally on the DL set of rules to evaluate the final medical results of breast cancer. Lastly, the test effects display that the DL model exhibits better (98%) accuracy as compared to other methods (Zhang et al., 2020).

Brain imaging technologies perform a critical role in health analysis by presenting new perspectives of the brain structure, providing more information on the brain's state and functions. Image processing is used in clinical technology to help in the initial recognition and treatment of existing important infections. The author focused on cancer detection primarily based on brain magnetic resonance imaging (MRI), the usage of an aggregate of the convolutional neural community (CNN), and a sparse stacked AE. The model provides a full-size impact in enhancing the precision and efficacy of the model. The consequences prove that the developed model is very robust in categorizing and grouping tumor in MRI pictures (Thachayani & Kurian, 2021).

Gastric cancer is one of the most uncommon cancers, accounting for the second highest number of deaths worldwide. The proposed method uses unique layers architectures for improved function. The proposed framework is based on the publicly accepted BOT gastric slice dataset. The consequences show that the deep mastering framework achieves higher than modern-day networks like DenseNet and ResNet with an accuracy of a hundred % for slice-based type (Y. Li et al., 2018).

Previous studies have shown a substantial variation in the MRI imaging pattern of body tissue with and without diseases. A few research studies have demonstrated that enhancing the ML model leads to earlier identification and treatment of disease as compared to traditional techniques. In this chapter, the ML models, i.e., ANN and CNN, which are used to distinguish the imaging pattern of tumorous and non-tumorous tissue of the brain, are developed and compared. The data sets obtained from the free available domain (Nickparvar Masoud, 2021) are initially used to train the DL model. The trained DL model is used further to differentiate the imaging pattern of tumorous and non-tumorous tissue of the brain. The developed model predicts brain cancer using a convolutional neural network at an early stage and direct messages utilizing a chatbot IoT interface so that proper therapy may be provided at the right moment and the lives of the individuals can be saved. The motivation behind the work involves developing an automation system to detect and categorize brain tumors and help accomplish better treatment in less time. The suggested DL algorithm yielded encouraging results, correctly distinguishing the presence and specific location of brain tumors in patients.

16.3 Proposed Work

Imaging is generally used in the dedicated monitored treatment of cancer. MRI is the technique where we use the imaging process that contains strong magnetic and radio waves to develop the best way of MRI for body scanning purposes. MRI is safer to use and also not harmful to pregnant women. It is also used for diagnosing tumors, as well as for the spinal cord and brain. ML techniques are developing rapidly as they have powerful and effective algorithms (Pradhan et al., 2022; Hussain and Roy, 2023). One of the algorithms is the decision support system. It is the most useful and effective algorithm that is widely used to recognize the pattern and outcome of the given input, and this prediction is not easy for humans to analyze and predict. DL generally works with a huge cluster of data and information, but it is quite impossible for human beings to work along with the same huge cluster of data in a specific manner. Hence, DL is more efficient for such a large cluster of data. This tends to more uses of ML and AI in the medical sector and pharmacy business. DL is very efficient, and its data are also beneficial for predicting and diagnosing the patient in the proper manner. The patient can make the appropriate decision from the outcome to aid themselves in an efficient way. The proposed chatbot system is shown in Figure 16.1 to predict brain cancer using a convolutional neural network.

16.3.1 Dataset Collection

MRI uses a prevailing magnetic field, radio waves, and a processor to provide special snaps of the interior of patient's brain. In order to obtain a comprehensive interpretation of data and supervision-associated practices, only a lively researcher utilizing MRI has been used. Data were collected from the participants who had given their consent and were in the age group above 18 years. Data from contributors whose norms were not met or who completed much less than a single segment of the survey were excluded from succeeding analyses.

16.3.2 Feature Extraction

This dataset includes MRI pix of human brain tumors. There are folders; one represents the normal brain photograph and the other represents the tumor pictures. Totally, there are 1064 snapshots in each of those folders. A total of 604 tumorous and 460 non-tumorous snapshots are reserved. The images are of different shapes, which are resized to 256 × 256 pixels for training, 175 photos for validation, and 300 for testing.

16.3.3 Classification

Convolutional neural networks (CNNs) are emerging techniques in the medical sector for diagnosing cancer. In many sectors, we use CNN, such as bioinformatics, for scrutinizing materials, image recognition and analysis in medical, recognition of speech, and recognition of audio. Various sets of models have been developed to analyze and predict cancer. The numerous models target the specific sector of the gene expression data. CNN helps us to understand the relation and co-relation between genes. The deeper CNN models are used to accomplish the classification and accuracy in computer vision. The present study uses the CNN and ANN models to predict brain cancer disease. In the present proposed work, CNN exhibits better results compared to ANN.

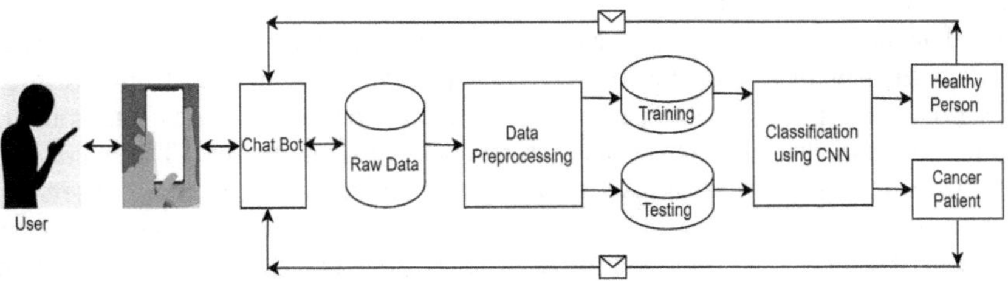

FIGURE 16.1 Flowchart of the proposed chatbot system.

16.3.4 Metrics Evaluation

Researchers have used a variety of criteria (Singh et al., 2024) for the evaluation of the model's efficacy, such as precision (PN), recall (RL), sensitivity (ST), specificity (SY), accuracy (AY), and F1 score. The matrices are evaluated by considering a total of 1064 snapshots, computing positively true (PT), negatively true (NT), positively false (PF), and negatively false (NF) data. PT denotes the existence of a tumor and is recognized positively, whereas PF denotes a non-tumorous case but is acknowledged wrongly as a tumor. NT and NF represent non-tumorous cases and tumors that are unrecognized/missed throughout the process, respectively. Meanwhile, FPR and FDR denote false positives and discovery rates. Equations (16.1)–(16.7) are used to evaluate the overall performance of the developed model.

$$\mathrm{PN} = \frac{\mathrm{PT}}{\mathrm{PT} + \mathrm{PF}} \tag{16.1}$$

$$\mathrm{RL\ and\ ST} = \frac{\mathrm{PT}}{\mathrm{PT} + \mathrm{NF}} \tag{16.2}$$

$$\mathrm{SY} = \frac{\mathrm{NT}}{\mathrm{NT} + \mathrm{PF}} \tag{16.3}$$

$$\mathrm{AY} = \frac{\mathrm{PT} + \mathrm{NT}}{\mathrm{PT} + \mathrm{NT} + \mathrm{PF} + \mathrm{NF}} \tag{16.4}$$

$$\mathrm{F1\ Score} = \frac{2(\mathrm{PT})}{2(\mathrm{PT}) + \mathrm{PF} + \mathrm{NF}} \tag{16.5}$$

$$\mathrm{FPR} = \frac{\mathrm{PF}}{\mathrm{PF} + \mathrm{NT}} \tag{16.6}$$

$$\mathrm{FDR} = \frac{\mathrm{PF}}{\mathrm{PF} + \mathrm{PT}} \tag{16.7}$$

16.3.5 Send Message Using Bot

The software manages the bot in the telegram; people do not manage this bot. This is based on the characteristics and features of AI. They are multitaskers and can do tasks like giving commands to the IoT, teaching, playing, searching, and broadcasting. Users can also get news, notifications, messages, weather reports, and alerts from the bot. Users can also play games and get paid services from the bot. The interaction from this bot is straightforward: users have to send instructions to the bot, or users can add them to a clan or group. Telegram is a very popular paradigm and platform in Instant Messaging (IM), and users also do not have to worry about storage because the messages are stored in the cloud. Users can operate Telegram from any operating system like Windows, Android, IOS, and other platforms, including the web version.

Users can build the chatbot on Telegram, and it is a straightforward process also; it takes very little time, only a few steps, and will be completed within a very minimum amount of time.

Factors that tend to work chatbot in IoT

- Actually, it does not require memorizing the different ingredients, languages, and keys to operate smart IoT systems and devices. People efficiently manage IoT devices using day-to-day languages and do not need to memorize the instructions and several commands. Normally, one can communicate easily and efficiently with the devices and system to fabricate and execute the task.
- The chatbot has the ability to learn on its own or self-learning. The chatbot is designed in such a way that it can comprehend the commands and injunction in normal and straightforward languages, not only languages but also gestures. So, the interaction between humans and chatbots becomes wider; the plurality also increases in communication. Increasing plurality means we do not have to inject full command or instruction; it can easily understand you better and more efficiently.
- Chatbot also purifies the serving request over the IoT paradigm, making for a better communication channel. While under some process, if the user acquires or obtains some sort of information, instruction, or request, then the user can easily interrogate or ask its queries and doubts regarding requests in ordinary language, and the chatbot will guide the user very efficiently.

16.4 Result

The results computed from the different developed models are compared and shown in Figures 16.2 and 16.3. The accuracy for testing the convolutional neural network obtained is 98.23%, where the artificial neural network is 82.63%, and the precision is 95% for CNN, where the ANN is 80%. Similarly, recall and specificity for the CNN model are 94% and 96.6%, respectively, while for the ANN model are 75% and 79%, respectively. The FPR and FDR remain at 0% and 0.035% for CNN and ANN models, respectively. So, after forecasting, it can be observed that the CNN DL technique is more accurate in predicting brain cancer.

16.5 Conclusion and Future Direction

This paper includes the study for the help of cancer-related technology fields and digital industrial sectors. This technology will help everyone those are in a dilemma, and it is very efficient and easy to use. The world of technology is growing too fast and new technologies are evolving. They are not only evolving but also fabricating themselves in a very successful manner. This technology is helping the world to become a better place; from the past, many problems and problem statements have been solved with the help of technology for smart health in smart cities. One of the life-threatening

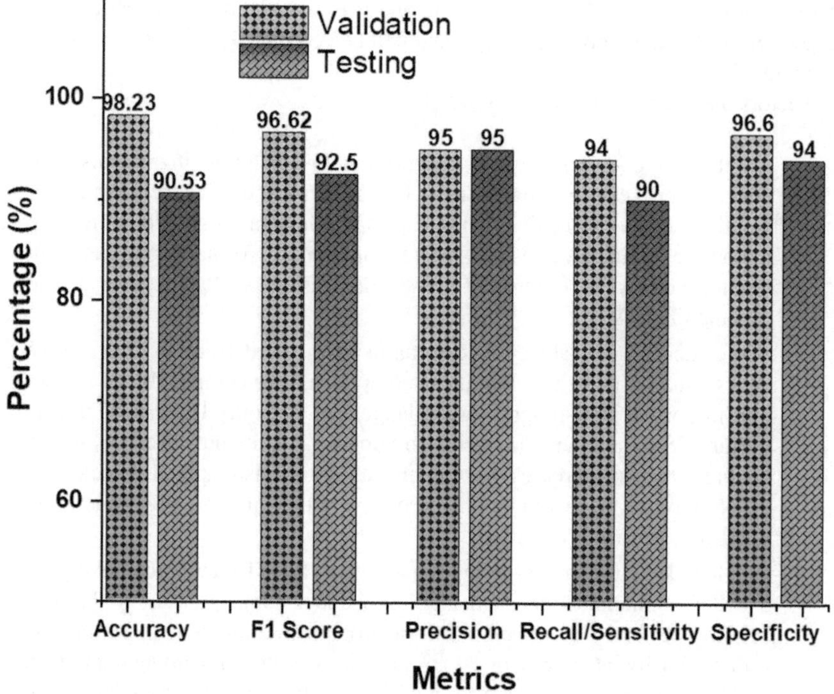

FIGURE 16.2 Prediction using CNN.

diseases is cancer, and it is challenging in today's life. The present work proposed a model that predicts brain cancer using a convolutional neural network at an early stage and direct messages utilizing a chatbot IoT interface so that proper therapy may be provided at the right moment and the lives of the individuals can be saved. The suggested DL algorithm yielded encouraging results, correctly distinguishing the presence and specific location of brain tumors in patients. In this chapter, major topics like DL, MRI, API, and IoT have been covered for early detection and diagnosis of brain cancer. Additionally, the idea and technology of chatbots in association with IoT paradigm have been discussed briefly. Essential topics covered in the proposed methodology are feature extraction, classification, and metrices evaluation. In the future, different methodologies can be proposed to develop a new and advanced device that can detect different types, classification, and stages of cancer. Not only this but the different medication for the different types of cancer patients can also be suggested by utilizing chatbots in association with IoT paradigm. There is enormous scope in the future to merge new and advanced technology into the healthcare sector, especially in the cancer-related field.

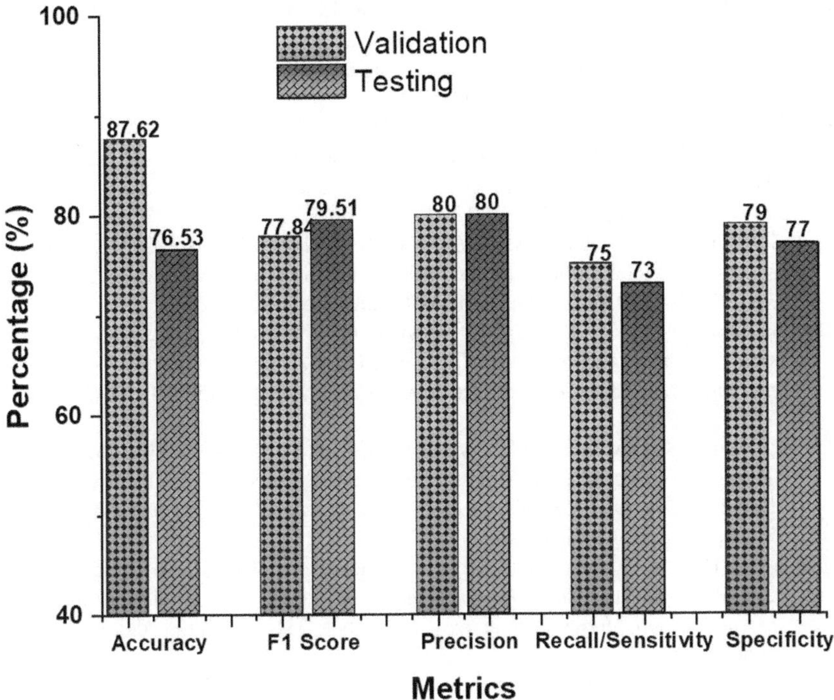

FIGURE 16.3 Prediction using ANN.

REFERENCES

Abdollahi, S., Lin, P.-C., & Chiang, J.-H. (2021). WinBinVec: Cancer-Associated Protein-Protein Interaction Extraction and Identification of 20 Various Cancer Types and Metastasis Using Different Deep Learning Models. *IEEE Journal of Biomedical and Health Informatics*, *25*(10), 4052–4063. https://doi.org/10.1109/JBHI.2021.3093441

Alawad, M., Yoon, H., Gao, S., Mumphrey, B., Wu, X., Durbin, E. B., Jeong, J. C., Hands, I., Rust, D., Coyle, L., Penberthy, L., & Tourassi, G. (2021). Privacy-Preserving Deep Learning NLP Models for Cancer Registries. *IEEE Transactions on Emerging Topics in Computing*, *9*(3), 1219–1230. https://doi.org/10.1109/TETC.2020.2983404

Bilgıç, B. (2021). Derin Öğrenme Yöntemi Kullanılarak Göğüs Kanseri ve Deri Kanseri Teşhislerinin Karşılaştırılması Comparison of Breast Cancer and Skin Cancer Diagnoses Using Deep Learning Method. *2021 29th Signal Processing and Communications Applications Conference (SIU)*, 1–4. https://doi.org/10.1109/SIU53274.2021.9477992

Cao, G., Ieee, M., & Song, W. (2019). Gastric Cancer Diagnosis with Mask R-CNN. *2019 11th International Conference on Intelligent Human-Machine Systems and Cybernetics (IHMSC)*, *1*, 60–63. https://doi.org/10.1109/IHMSC.2019.00022

Chen, G., Chen, Y., Yuan, Z., Lu, X., Zhu, X., & Li, W. (2019). Breast Cancer Image Classification based on CNN and Bit-Plane slicing. *2019 International Conference on Medical Imaging Physics and Engineering (ICMIPE)*, 1–4. https://doi.org/10.1109/ICMIPE47306.2019.9098216

Chen, X., Lin, X., Shen, Q., & Qian, X. (2021). Combined Spiral Transformation and Model-Driven Multi-Modal Deep Learning Scheme for Automatic Prediction of TP53 Mutation in Pancreatic Cancer. *IEEE Transactions on Medical Imaging*, *40*(2), 735–747. https://doi.org/10.1109/TMI.2020.3035789

Das, S., Adhikary, A., Laghari, A. A., & Mitra, S. (2023a). Eldo-care: EEG with Kinect sensor based telehealthcare for the disabled and the elderly. *Neuroscience Informatics*, *3*(2), 100130. https://doi.org/10.1016/j.neuri.2023.100130

Das, S., Ghosh, A., & Saha, S. (2022). A review on gaming effects on cognitive load for smart healthcare and its security. *Using Multimedia Systems, Tools, and Technologies for Smart Healthcare Services*, December, 1–28. https://doi.org/10.4018/978-1-6684-5741-2.ch001

Das, S., Malick, S., Dey, S. S., Sarkar, A., Hossain, F., & Samad, A. (2023b). Game-Stress-Tracker: EEG-Based Smart Advisor Bot for Stress Detection During Playing BGMI Game. *International Conference on Signals, Machines, and Automation*, 391–399. Singapore: Springer Nature.

Ghosh, A., Das, S., & Saha, S. (2022). Stress detection for cognitive rehabilitation in COVID-19 scenario. *Smart Health Technologies for the COVID-19 Pandemic: Internet of Medical Things Perspectives*, December, 331–357. https://doi.org/10.1049/pbhe042e_ch12

Huo, Y. (2021). Full-Stack Application of Skin Cancer Diagnosis Based on CNN Model. *2021 IEEE International Conference on Computer Science, Electronic Information Engineering and Intelligent Control Technology (CEI)*, 754–758. https://doi.org/10.1109/CEI52496.2021.9574583

Hussain, M. W., & Roy, D. S. (2023). Performance Optimization Strategies for Big Data Applications in Distributed Framework. In *Intelligent Technologies: Concepts, Applications, and Future Directions*, Volume *2* (pp. 221–252). Singapore: Springer Nature Singapore.

Ketout, H., Gu, J., & Horne, G. (2011). MVN_CNN and UBN_CNN for endocardial edge detection. *2011 Seventh International Conference on Natural Computation, July 2011*, 781–785. https://doi.org/10.1109/ICNC.2011.6022163

Kido, S., Hirano, Y., & Hashimoto, N. (2018). Detection and classification of lung abnormalities by use of convolutional neural network (CNN) and regions with CNN features (R-CNN). *2018 International Workshop on Advanced Image Technology (IWAIT)*, 1–4. https://doi.org/10.1109/IWAIT.2018.8369798

Kollias, D., & Zafeiriou, S. (2021). Exploiting Multi-CNN Features in CNN-RNN Based Dimensional Emotion Recognition on the OMG in-the-Wild Dataset. *IEEE Transactions on Affective Computing*, *12*(3), 595–606. https://doi.org/10.1109/TAFFC.2020.3014171

Lee, M., Lee, J., Kim, J., Kim, B., & Kim, J. (2019). The Sparsity and Activation Analysis of Compressed CNN Networks in a HW CNN Accelerator Model. *2019 International SoC Design Conference (ISOCC)*, *255*, 255–256. Korea (South): Jeju.

Li, J. (2018). IF-CNN: Image-Aware Inference Framework for CNN With the Collaboration of Mobile Devices and Cloud. *IEEE Access*, *6*, 68621–68633. https://doi.org/10.1109/ACCESS.2018.2880196

Li, Y., Li, X., Xie, X., & Shen, L. (2018). Deep learning based gastric cancer identification. *2018 IEEE 15th International Symposium on Biomedical Imaging (ISBI 2018), 2018-April(Isbi)*, 182–185. https://doi.org/10.1109/ISBI.2018.8363550

Lu, L., Yi, Y., Wang, K., & Wang, Q. I. (2019). Integrating Local CNN and Global CNN for Script Identification in Natural Scene Images. *IEEE Access*, *7*, 52669–52679. https://doi.org/10.1109/ACCESS.2019.2911964

Lu, Y. (2021). Breast Cancer Classification Based on CNN and ESIM Model. *2021 IEEE International Conference on Computer Science, Electronic Information Engineering and Intelligent Control Technology (CEI)*, 742–746. https://doi.org/10.1109/CEI52496.2021.9574530

Nickparvar Masoud. (2021). *Brain Tumor MRI Dataset*. https://Www.Kaggle.Com/

Pradhan, B., Hussain, M. W., Srivastava, G., Debbarma, M. K., Barik, R. K., & Lin, J. C. W. (2022). *A Neuro-Evolutionary Approach for Software Defined Wireless Network Traffic Classification*. IET Communications.

Reddy, K. H. K., Roy, D. S., Mishra, T. K., & Hussain, M. W. (Eds.). (2023). *Handbook of Research on Network-Enabled IoT Applications for Smart City Services*. IGI Global.

Saric, M., Russo, M., Stella, M., & Sikora, M. (2019). CNN-based Method for Lung Cancer Detection in Whole Slide Histopathology Images. *2019 4th International Conference on Smart and Sustainable Technologies (SpliTech)*, 1–4. https://doi.org/10.23919/SpliTech.2019.8783041

Sedigh, P., Sadeghian, R., & Masouleh, M. T. (2019). Generating Synthetic Medical Images by Using GAN to Improve CNN Performance in Skin Cancer Classification. *2019 7th International Conference on Robotics and Mechatronics (ICRoM), ICRoM*, 497–502. https://doi.org/10.1109/ICRoM48714.2019.9071823

Senarathna, S. A. D. L. V. (2021). Lung Cancer Detection and Prediction of Cancer Stages Using Image Processing. *2021 3rd International Conference on Electrical, Control and Instrumentation Engineering (ICECIE)*, 1–9. https://doi.org/10.1109/ICECIE52348.2021.9664658

Sima, D., Kitmo, & Chandra, G. N. (2023). Emotion Detection Using EEG-Based Brain-Computer Interaction. In *Cognitive Cardiac Rehabilitation Using IoT and AI Tools* (p. 10). IGI Global. https://doi.org/10.4018/978-1-6684-7561-4

Singh, P., Kourav, P. S., Mohapatra, S., Kumar, V., & Panda, S. K. (2024). Human heart health prediction using GAIT parameters and machine learning model. *Biomedical Signal Processing and Control*, *88*(PA), 105696. https://doi.org/10.1016/j.bspc.2023.105696

Tanna, R., & Sharma, T. (2021). Binary Classification of Melanoma Skin Cancer using SVM and CNN. *2021 International Conference on Artificial Intelligence and Machine Vision (AIMV)*, 1–4. https://doi.org/10.1109/AIMV53313.2021.9670894

Thachayani, M., & Kurian, S. (2021). AI Based Classification Framework For Cancer Detection Using Brain MRI Images. *2021 International Conference on System, Computation, Automation and Networking (ICSCAN)*, 1–4. https://doi.org/10.1109/ICSCAN53069.2021.9526456

Yanagisawa, H., Yamashita, T., & Watanabe, H. (n.d.). A Study on Object Detection Method from Manga Images using CNN. *2018 International Workshop on Advanced Image Technology (IWAIT)*, 1–4. https://doi.org/10.1109/IWAIT.2018.8369633

Zhang, X., He, D., Zheng, Y., Huo, H., Li, S., Chai, R., & Liu, T. (2020). Deep Learning Based Analysis of Breast Cancer Using Advanced Ensemble Classifier and Linear Discriminant Analysis. *IEEE Access*, *8*, 120208–120217. https://doi.org/10.1109/ACCESS.2020.3005228

17

Federated Learning for Heart Disease Detection in Smart Healthcare: A Survey

Dulani Meedeniya, Roshinie Jayasundara, Meelan Bandara, and Isuru Ariyarathne
University of Moratuwa, Moratuwa, Sri Lanka

17.1 Introduction

With technical advancement, smart city applications have evolved as an innovative approach to improve the quality of life and promote sustainable development (Reddy et al., 2023). This has paved the way for smart healthcare systems integrated with the Internet of Medical Things (IoMT) (Jalal et al., 2022). By merging healthcare and IoT technologies, the IoMT is a mature medical device ecosystem. Many such networks include a variety of devices ranging from wearable fitness trackers and smartwatches to implantable sensors (Sakib et al., 2021). Moreover, IoMT helps enhance the facilities provided to healthcare workers while improving patient outcomes and fostering innovations in diagnostics, treatment, and medical delivery.

Healthcare systems in smart cities can predict and diagnose a variety of diseases accurately. These include lung diseases (Meedeniya et al., 2022), heart ailments, and brain cancers (Wijethilake et al., 2021). For a more accurate diagnosis, a large amount of medical data is required. This is achieved by collecting data through IoMT and other available infrastructures. Among the different diseases, cardiovascular diseases (CVDs) can be considered more threatening. CVDs include many health conditions such as Arrhythmia, heart attacks, and heart failure (Khan et al., 2023). The World Health Organization has indicated that CVDs are one of the leading causes of global death. CVDs are responsible for about 17.9 million deaths each year, which is nearly one-third of all global mortality (Yaqoob et al., 2022). Considering the major influence that these diseases have on human health and the world economy, early detection and management before they develop into full clinical abnormalities become very important.

To develop prediction models for monitoring CVD conditions, traditional machine learning (ML) approaches have been heavily dependent on a huge volume of user data (Hussain and Roy, 2023). However, this conventional approach presents some major challenges, especially in the case of sensitivity and also availability of biomedical data.

DOI: 10.1201/9781032631738-17

Additionally, it involves central storage of data for model training that poses significant privacy issues with security and regulatory compliance (Guerra- Manzanares et al., 2023). Further, a conventional ML system trained in one region may significantly lose effectiveness in another, raising concerns about its global applicability.

With the many challenges being inherent, federated learning (FL) is a very powerful solution to such problems (Meedeniya et al., 2022). FL enables the use of heterogeneous datasets that are widely geographically dispersed to produce globally optimum models. FL has a privacy-preserving architecture in which the data remains on the devices while only model weights are shared with a centralized server. The application of FL systems can also deal with challenges such as sensitivity and the heterogeneity of medical records that are generated by institutes and IoMT devices. Hence, extensive ongoing research efforts are dedicated to designing FL-based smart healthcare systems for the accurate detection and diagnosis of CVDs.

Three major survey papers which provide a thorough overview of FL and related applications can be identified (Yoo et al., 2021a; Li et al., 2021; Wang et al., 2023). Moreover, a significant number of studies that explore the detection of CVDs using ML techniques are available (Katarya and Srinivas, 2020; Ahsan and Siddique, 2022). However, to our awareness, there is a lack of survey papers explicitly discussing the application of FL in the context of heart disease prediction. Motivated by this observation, this study explores the cutting-edge techniques employed by researchers in the development of federated heart disease detection. Through an in-depth analysis, this paper seeks to comprehensively review the state-of-the-art advancements, challenges, and potential future directions in the domain of FL specifically tailored for heart disease prediction.

This chapter is organized as follows: Section 17.1 presents an overview of heart disease detection using FL. Section 17.2 outlines the research methodology employed. An overview of federated heart disease detection is covered in Section 17.3, while Section 17.4 presents publicly available datasets and their limitations. Section 17.5 concentrates on the FL techniques utilized in existing implementations. Recommendations, open challenges, and future directions are discussed in Section 17.6. The chapter concludes in Section 17.7.

17.2 Research Method

In order to comprehensively explore the domain, it was identified that no survey papers explicitly addressed the use of FL for heart disease detection. However, the broader field of smart healthcare has witnessed a boost of survey papers discussing various aspects of FL. Consequently, we set out to bridge this knowledge gap using the implementation papers on heart disease detection using FL.

17.2.1 Research Question

The first step in our research methodology was formulating a set of research questions that effectively encapsulate the breadth and depth of the literature. We outlined four distinct contexts to guide our exploration, each with relevant research questions.

RQ1: What is the background for FL?
- What problems were addressed using FL?

RQ2: What are the considerations of FL implementation?
- What are the different types of FL architectures?
- How is FL practically implemented?
- How is communication maintained?

RQ3: What are the available datasets?
- What are the datasets used?
- What are the challenges of existing datasets?

RQ4: What are the considerations of the ML framework?
- What ML models are used for structured data?
- What ML models are used for unstructured data?
- How are model performances evaluated?

17.2.2 Search Process

In this literature survey, we thoroughly examined related research work to comprehend the current state-of-the-art techniques. As FL gained prominence after its introduction in 2016, we limited our search from January 1, 2017, to August 30, 2023. To ensure a comprehensive search, we used advanced search options on Google Scholar, employing Boolean "AND" and "OR" expressions. We used "('heart disease' OR 'cardiovascular') AND ('Federated Learning') AND ('detection' OR 'prediction' OR 'recognition' OR 'identification')" as the search query. Therefore, our analysis will provide an overview of the current state of FL usage in heart disease detection. It is crucial to note that our search was narrowly tailored to focus exclusively on implementing FL in the context of heart disease detection. Our search encompassed titles, abstracts, and keywords, adhering to a rigorous screening process.

As depicted in Figure 17.1, the flow diagram provides a comprehensive overview of the article selection process, presenting a holistic view of the statistics related to article inclusion in our survey. After the initial search operation, we subjected the collected articles to a rigorous selection, as elaborated in the subsequent sections.

17.2.3 Inclusion and Exclusion Criteria

Solid inclusion and exclusion criteria play a major role when conducting a successful literature search. They prevent information overload and ensure the selected articles align closely with the research objectives while maintaining the integrity of the selection process.

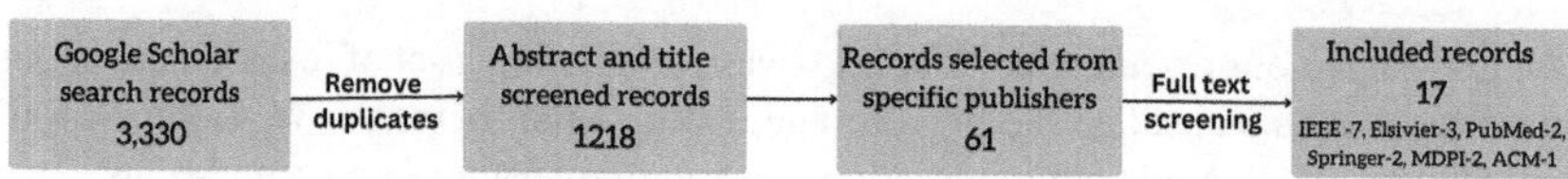

FIGURE 17.1 Article search process.

The inclusion criteria used for this study are as follows:

- Articles that explore heart disease-related datasets.
- Articles that involve the development of ML models within the FL framework.
- Articles wherein FL represents a focal point in the findings, including result analysis and comparison.

The exclusion criteria used for this study are as follows:

- Articles reliant on private datasets for ML models.
- Studies that lack a primary focus on FL and heart disease data.
- Articles introducing hybridization or significant modifications to the FL theme (e.g., federated reinforcement learning).
- Articles lacking a clear presentation of results.

17.2.4 Data Extraction

The selected research articles were required to be carefully analyzed to understand the state-of-the-art practices followed for FL-based heart disease detection. Thus, a careful data extraction phase was carried out under a pre-determined structure that includes the following:

- Document title, publication year, and journal/conference name.
- Details regarding the employed datasets and their respective federated settings.
- Insights into the security or privacy protocols employed within the FL framework.
- A comprehensive overview of the algorithms utilized for training ML models.
- An exact evaluation of the performance of the FL models.

The summarized overview gathered through this phase helped the study to formulate the structure and present the findings more concisely.

17.2.5 Taxonomy

The taxonomy for FL-based heart disease detection is presented in Figure 17.2. It structures the considerations that govern the domain in a hierarchical arrangement. As shown in the figure, FL-based heart disease detection follows one of the three architectures: horizontal federated learning (HFL), vertical federated learning (VFL), and federated transfer learning (FTL). Implementation of these FL architectures involves leveraging techniques like federated averaging and its variants as well as Bayesian inferencing strategies and will be discussed in depth in the later sections. Being a distributed system, any FL infrastructure depends heavily on the network arrangement. Hence, this study explains the usage of centralized, decentralized, and heterogeneous network configurations presented in the related studies.

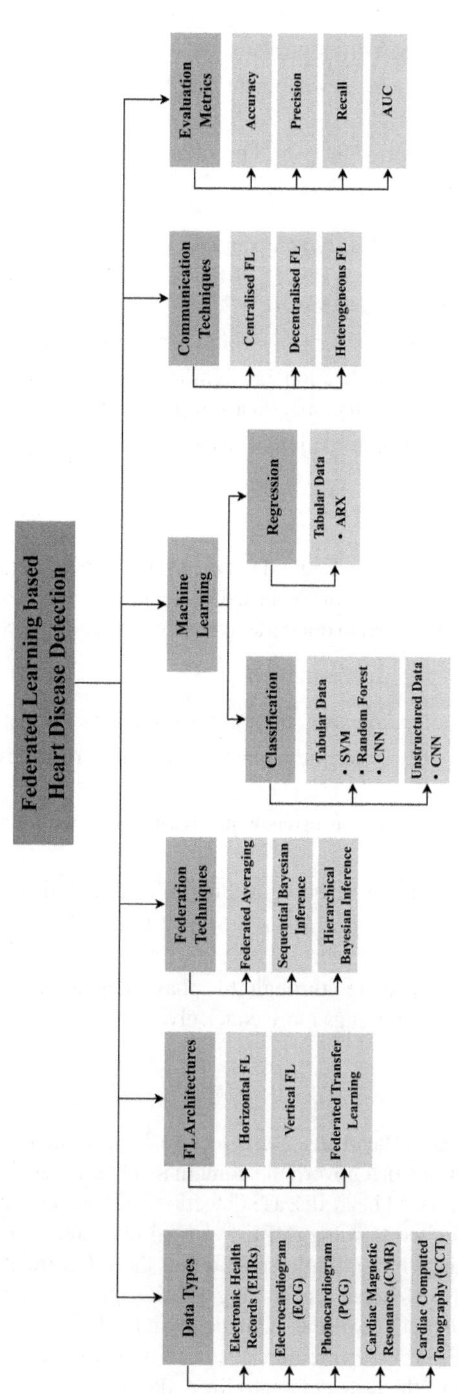

FIGURE 17.2 Taxonomy.

The types of data which are suitable to be ingested through an ML pipeline are available under the scope of CVDs spread in a large range, including structured data in the form of tabular health records, time series data, 2D images, and MRI images. Any ML-based infrastructure depends heavily on the data that it learns and hence this study provides an analytical overview of the existing datasets used by the researchers.

Both classification and regression-based ML techniques have been used to extract the underlying relationships in these datasets. Under the classification domain, researchers have utilized both structured and unstructured data (Pradhan et al., 2022). Commonly employed models include support vector machines (SVMs), random forests, deep neural networks (DNNs), and convolutional neural networks (CNNs). While autoregression with exogenous (ARX) variables have proven effective for regression tasks. Because the medical domain is very sensitive to the predictions yielded by the systems, proper evaluation metrics need to be established for monitoring the prediction strength. Therefore, the taxonomy includes many metrics such as accuracy, F1-score, precision, and recall which were used in the selected studies.

17.3 Federated Learning

In order to develop models with strong generalization capabilities, traditional ML pipelines often rely on centralized datasets. Although the required data can be gathered from multiple sources, privacy concerns and data diversity pose significant challenges. FL can be identified as a robust framework specifically designed to address such challenges (Li et al., 2020). This section discusses different architectures and the methodologies researchers employ for federated heart disease detection.

17.3.1 Overview of Federated Learning

FL is an ML technique that attempts to create models in a distributed network of devices or servers by using localized, private data. It enables multiple devices to learn jointly from their local data without sending them to a central server. In FL, privacy is preserved by transferring only the model parameters/weights to the central location rather than the raw data. This method is highly advantageous in situations when the data is confidential, like the case of healthcare because it allows for the training of smarter and personalized AI models. One of the highly recognized applications of FL is heart disease detection which helps increase the accuracy of the prediction while protecting patient privacy (Khan et al., 2023; Brisimi et al., 2018; Linardos et al., 2022; Jalal et al., 2022; Yaqoob et al., 2022). In prior research, techniques such as asynchronous FL (Khan et al., 2023), decentralized frameworks like cluster primal dual splitting (cPDS) (Brisimi et al., 2018), and hybrid methods (Yaqoob et al., 2022) are applied to improve predictive models, optimizing communication efficiency and maintaining the security of sensitive healthcare data (Jalal et al., 2022).

Figure 17.3 presents the overall architecture of FL. Accordingly, a general FL network consists of two key components: first, a central device, often hosted on a powerful server or cloud, coordinating the FL process, initializing the global model, aggregating updates, and distributing the improved global model. Second, distributed devices, including smartphones, IoT devices, or edge computing systems, represent

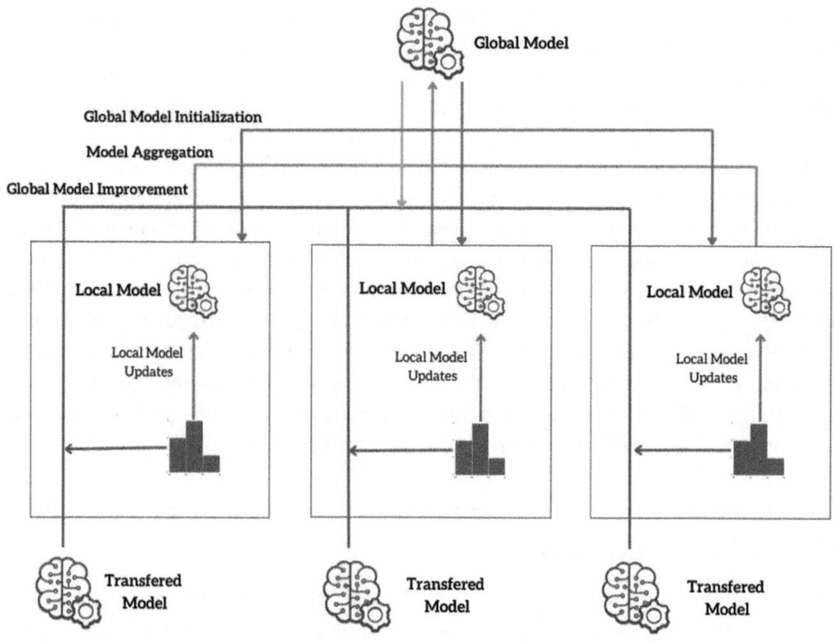

FIGURE 17.3 Fundamental concept of FL.

network nodes, each with a subset of relevant data. These devices train the model locally without sharing sensitive information. Overall, the FL procedure can be summarized into four distinct phases as below (Sohan and Basalamah, 2023).

Global model initialization: Initially, a global ML model is created and distributed to all participating devices. This global model initialization is crucial since it serves as a starting point for the training phase. Typically, the model is designed to be more generic but is not personalized to any specific user or device.

Local model updates: Each device, such as a user's smartphone or a hospital's server, trains the copy of the global model using its local data. This local training process helps to revamp the global model by updating the knowledge of specific patterns and characteristics in that device's data.

Model aggregation: After local training, only the model updates (usually in the form of updated model parameters) are sent back to the central server. These updates capture the insights gained from each device's local data without exposing raw data.

Global model improvement: The central server effectively integrates the knowledge from each device, by combining the model updates received from each participant node. This process iterates over multiple rounds, continually refining the global model based on the collective intelligence of all participating devices.

Personalization emerges over time and through multiple rounds of training, each local model becomes more personalized for each device. It adapts to the specific trends and variations present in the user data while utilizing the collaboratively learned knowledge for better inference potential. In the context of heart disease detection in smart healthcare (Nguyen et al., 2022), this approach allows healthcare providers to offer tailored risk assessments and treatment recommendations based on individual health data. Patients benefit from personalized care, while healthcare institutions can collectively improve their heart disease detection models without sharing sensitive patient information.

17.3.2 Types of Federated Learning

Based on the nature of the feature space and the sample space used in the development of an FL system, three major FL architectures can be recognized as HFL, VFL, and FTL (Jalal et al., 2022), (Meedeniya, 2023).

Horizontal federated learning: Clients have their own data source and in each client, data is presented according to the same feature space (or with a majority overlap). However, the data instances vary from one client to another. HFL starts with multiple models trained on the client side and the model gradients are shared to develop a global model collaboratively. The global model is then sent to the clients to continue fine-tuning. This process iterates until the global model results in good convergence.

Vertical federated learning: Clients have their data source; each client's data is presented with different feature spaces. To provide the ability to jointly analyze the data and build a shared model each client describes the same data instances (or with a majority overlap) according to their feature space. VFL starts with an agreed-upon model architecture at each client location and the client-side-trained model gradients are shared to build the global model which can provide inference on an extended feature space.

Federated transfer learning: For HFL to work, a majority overlap in the feature space among the clients is required, whereas a majority overlap in data instances is required for VFL. FTL requires only a minor overlap among feature spaces and the data instances. FTL starts by training a model at one client, and then the trained model is fine-tuned at another client, using its local data. For this to successfully integrate, it is better if the source domains of the data available at the two clients are similar.

17.3.3 FL Techniques

As explained above, different architectures of FL can be identified in the current research domain and researchers have utilized various techniques to implement such architectures practically. Under the scope of FL-based heart disease detection, three such techniques can be identified from the existing studies (Fang et al., 2021).

Federated averaging: Stochastic gradient descent (SGD) is a frequently employed iterative optimization technique in ML for model parameter tuning. In the FL context, SGD can be adapted by computing gradients for the loss function on a subset of clients rather than using a batch of the entire training dataset. FedAvg [FedAvg] employs a similar approach, enabling clients to execute multiple local iterations before transmitting their updated model weights to a central server. This collaborative process is helpful when constructing a more comprehensive model.

Sequential Bayesian inference: This is an analytical method used for updating the probability distribution of a hidden state variable when new observations are received sequentially. In FL, the posterior probability distribution of one client becomes the prior probability distribution for another client. This allows the clients to share information without having to share their data.

Hierarchical Bayesian inference: This organizes the model into two tiers. The first tier consists of individual nodes or clients equipped with a unique set of model parameters. Above that an elevated layer, with shared hyperparameters, is developed. This hierarchical arrangement allows every participant node to perform local computations independently, resulting in parallel processing. Unlike sequential Bayesian inference, where nodes handle data sequentially, hierarchical Bayesian inference allows for concurrent and decentralized computation, making it a more efficient and collaborative approach in the FL framework.

17.3.4 Communication Strategies

FL has three key communication protocols, namely, centralized, decentralized, and heterogeneous. These protocols are used to efficiently distribute the weights of client ML models to build the global model. Hence, they offer unique flexibility and adaptability to network architectures and client scenarios by enabling efficient and robust ML in distributed environments.

Centralized federated learning: In this architecture, a central server serves as a major part of the pipeline. It carries out functions of the FL algorithm, including selection of participating nodes and the aggregation of model updates. However, this centralization can lead to challenges. As an example, when many nodes are involved, the central server becomes a bottleneck, potentially impeding the efficiency of the learning process. Similarly, it can affect the effectiveness and the reliability of the overall system as well (Witt et al., 2023).

Decentralized federated learning: In this architecture, interacting nodes in the network engage with each other to learn and obtain an independent global model. This alternative approach does away with the need for a centralized design where one server is used to manage the whole process. This de-centralization eliminates the threat of single point failure making the system more stable. However, the type of network topology implemented in the decentralized FL may affect its overall performance (Witt et al., 2023).

Heterogeneous federated learning (HeteroFL): This solution addresses cases that feature different clients, including mobile devices and IoT devices with variable computing and communication capabilities. While traditional FL assumes uniform model architecture across all local models, HeteroFL accommodates the diversity in the network. It enables the development of heterogeneous local models that deal with computation strength variations and data intricacies across the clients, leading to one precise global inference model.

This strategy is very valuable in the use cases that involve constantly changing client heterogeneity (Yu et al., 2020).

17.4 Heart Disease Datasets

In FL-based heart disease detection, the choice of a dataset plays a crucial role. Technological advancements have led to extensive collections of biomedical data, through examinations conducted at healthcare facilities and wearable health monitoring devices. Due to the heterogeneity of such datasets and the privacy considerations, combining data sources to develop generalized prediction systems presents a challenge. This section summarizes publicly available datasets utilized in the related studies while describing the challenges incorporated.

17.4.1 Characteristics of Federated Datasets

Under a FL configuration, training data comes from participant nodes and they provide different behavior compared to a central data source used in traditional ML. This decentralized nature of the data introduces unique characteristics and challenges that need careful interventions. One of the defining attributes of a distributed dataset is the non-independently and identically distributed (non-IID) nature. Non-IID data provides individual data points that are not independent and identically distributed. This means that there is a structure or correlation among the data. This property violates the assumption of independence in statistical analysis. Hence, it becomes essential to account for the non-IID data distribution when training any FL system.

A system participating in FL possesses data from different geographical locations. Authors (Qiu et al., 2022) have utilized a heart sound dataset consisting of records from seven different countries which were collected using different types of medical equipment. As a result, data points followed different formats and required a significant effort to standardize before training a model. Similarly, datasets used in FL often exhibit heterogeneity due to variations in data types, formats, and distributions across different local sources. Apart from the standardization aspects the principle design architecture of a FL system also depends on the overlaps that exist between each client dataset. Hence, understanding these characteristics helps design practical and highly secure FL systems.

17.4.2 Heart Disease Datasets for Federated Learning

Researchers have employed various datasets to train and evaluate their FL-based heart disease detection systems. Varying types of health data including electronic health records (EHRs), electrocardiogram (ECG), phonocardiogram (PCG), electroencephalogram (EEG), echocardiogram (Echo), and cardiac magnetic resonance (CMR) has been used as the foundation for developing such datasets. Table 17.1 summarizes different data sources available in existing literature for CVD diagnosis.

Due to the low availability of datasets designed explicitly for predicting heart diseases, researchers have employed various strategies to combine existing datasets. Such datasets comprise information from diverse locations sourced from devices like

TABLE 17.1

Summary of Different Data Sources

Data Type	Description	Advantage	References
Electronic Health Records (EHRs)	Comprehensive medical history, including treatment history, diagnostic test results, medications, and allergies	Large data volume, quick and easy access	Bharathi et al. (2022), Qiu et al. (2022), Jalal et al. (2022), Brisimi et al. (2018), Khan et al. (2023), Jafari and Adibnia (2023), Salmeron et al. (2023), Obeidi (2023)
Electrocardiogram (ECG)	Electrical activity of the heart through repeated cardiac cycles	Non-invasive, important in early disease detection, widely available, low-cost	Sakib et al. (2021), Yaqoob et al. (2022), Zou et al. (2022), Goto et al. (2022)
Phonocardiogram (PCG)	Visual representation of cardiac sounds	Cost-effective, non-invasive, used for better prediction	Qiu et al. (2022)
Cardiac Magnetic Resonance (CMR)	High-resolution diagnostic images of the heart	Non-invasive, able to discover abnormalities obscured by bone, more detailed images	Linardos et al. (2022)
Echocardiogram (Echo)	Visual images of heart structure and blood vessels obtained through high-frequency sound waves	Non-invasive, real-time visualization of heart anatomy	Goto et al. (2022)
Cardiac-computed tomography scan (CCT scan)	High-quality, three-dimensional (3D) images of the heart	Non-invasive provides important prognostic information	Misonne and Jodogne (2022)

smartwatches, pacemakers, Holter monitors (portable ECGs), and other medical equipment. Table 17.2 illustrates the utilization of datasets in related studies, and it showcases that some studies have relied solely on a single dataset while others have combined multiple datasets to reach the required evaluation metrics.

17.4.3 Challenges in Existing Datasets

In the generic scope of ML, publicly available datasets are not specially generated to cater to the requirements of a FL system. Hence, the researchers are usually required to restructure existing datasets or to combine multiple datasets into the federated configuration. These manual interventions make it very inconvenient to compare results across different research efforts. The non-IID nature of data when collected from varying sources and their different geolocation features, impacts the accuracy and generalization of models. The distribution of data across different nodes can be imbalanced,

TABLE 17.2

Datasets Used in Existing Literature

Data Set with URL	Description	Data Properties	References
Heart disease dataset of UCI https://archive.ics.uci.edu/dataset/45/heart+disease	Include databases from Cleveland, Hungary, Switzerland, and VA Long Beach	303 records with 13 features, tabular data, EHR	Bharathi et al. (2022), Yaqoob et al. (2022), Khan et al. (2023), Jafari and Adibnia (2023), Salmeron et al. (2023), Obeidi (2023)
PhysiioNet/CinC Challenge Heart sound dataset (Physionet/CinC) https://physionet.org/content/challenge-2016/1.0.0/	Include 8 independent datasets, collected from 7 different countries	4,430 heart sound recordings taken from 1,072 patients, PCG	Qiu et al. (2022)
MIT-BIH Supraventricular Arrhythmia database (DS1) https://physionet.org/content/svdb/1.0.0/	Include recordings from Boston's Beth Israel Hospital	78 ECG recordings each 30 minutes long	Sakib et al. (2021)
MIT-BIH Arrhythmia database (DS2) https://www.physionet.org/content/mitdb/1.0.0/	Include recordings from Boston's Beth Israel Hospital Arrhythmia Laboratory	48 ECG recordings each 30 minutes long taken from 47 patients	Sakib et al. (2021)
INCART 12-lead arrhythmia database (DS3) https://physionet.org/content/incartdb/1.0.0/	Include recordings from the St. Petersburg Institute of Cardiological, Russia	75 ECG recordings each 30 minutes long extracted from 32 Holter records	Sakib et al. (2021)
Sudden Cardiac Death Holter database (DS4) https://physionet.org/content/sddb/1.0.0/	Include recordings from Boston Hospitals	23 Holter recordings	Sakib et al. (2021)
Heart Failure Prediction Dataset (HFP) https://www.kaggle.com/datasets/fedesoriano/heart-failure-prediction	Combination of Statlog, Cleveland, Hungary, Switzerland, and VA Long Beach datasets	1190 records with 11 features, tabular data, her	Yaqoob et al. (2023), Jalal et al. (2022)
M&M dataset https://www.ub.edu/mnms/	Data from 6 clinical centers in Spain, Canada, and Germany	375 CMR images	Linardos et al. (2022)
ACDC (Automated Cardiac Diagnosis Challenge) dataset https://paperswithcode.com/dataset/acdc	Clinical records from the University Hospital of Dijon	150 CMR images taken from 100 patients	Linardos et al. (2022)

(*Continued*)

TABLE 17.2 (Continued)

Data Set with URL	Description	Data Properties	References
Congestive Heart Failure RR Interval Database (CHF-RR) https://archive.physionet.org/physiobank/database/chf2db/	Include recordings from the New York Medical Centre	29 ECG recordings from 21 patients	Zou et al. (2022)
Normal Sinus Rhythm RR Interval Database (NSR-RR) https://physionet.org/content/nsr2db/1.0.0/	Include recordings from Washington and New York centers	54 ECG recordings from 54 patients	Zou et al. (2022)
South Africa Heart Disease Dataset (SAHDD) https://www.openml.org/search?type=data&sort=runs&id=1498&status=active	Clinical records of males from the Western Cape	462 records with 10 features, tabular, EHR	Obeidi (2023)
Heart failure clinical records dataset from Pakistan (HF-Pakistan) https://archive.ics.uci.edu/dataset/519/heart+failure+clinical+records	Records from Faisalabad Institute of Cardiology, Pakistan	299 records with 12 features, tabular, her	Obeidi (2023)

leading to challenges in model training as well. Further ensuring privacy and security while data is in transit and at rest also becomes a significant challenge. Overall, there is a clear requirement for a benchmark dataset specifically designed for heart disease detection in a federated configuration.

17.5 Machine Learning for Heart Disease Detection

Heart diseases, being a global health problem, receive significant attention, and hence numerous studies have been performed to develop state-of-the-art heart disease detection systems. Among the rich literature, FL-based heart disease detection systems can also be identified in limited numbers. This section explores the ML techniques followed in those studies and the evaluation metrics utilized. Due to the different types of datasets, the content is classified under ML for structured (tabular) data and ML for unstructured data (ECG, MRI, CT, etc.) A summary of the findings for structured data is presented in Table 17.3, and a summary for unstructured data is presented in Table 17.4.

17.5.1 ML Techniques for Structured Data

A recent study (Yaqoob et al., 2023) has employed a radial basis SVM (RB-SVM) to effectively identify heart diseases by leveraging a consolidated dataset that combines information from the Cleveland, Statlog, Hungary, Long Beach, and Switzerland

TABLE 17.3

Overview of ML Techniques for Structured Data

Study	Type	FL	Model	Dataset	Accuracy
Qiu et al. (2022)	Binary classification	FedAvg	Logistic regression	UCI – Cleveland	82.38%
			SVM		90.3%
Sakib et al. (2021)	Binary classification	FedMA	Bayesian	UCI – Cleveland	92.89%
Linardos et al. (2022)	Binary classification	FedMA	SVM RB	HFP	93.8%
			SVM		91.7%
		FedAvg	SVM		91.3
Goto et al. (2022)	Binary classification	-	Random forest	HFP	87.77%
Misonne and Jodogne (2022)	Multiclass classification	FedAVG + PCFM	CNN	Private	
				3 Class	73.68%
				2 Class	90.70%
Fang et al. (2021)	Regression	Sequential Bayes	ARX	Private	3.16
		Hierarchical Bayes			3.04
Salmeron et al. (2023)	Binary classification	AccFedAvg	DNN	UCI	89.02%
Obeidi (2023)	Multiclass classification	Batch aligned	Global layers	UCI – Cleveland	81.18%
		FedAVG		SAHDD	63.22%
				HF – Pakistan	75.15%

TABLE 17.4

Overview of ML Techniques for Unstructured Data

Study	Type	Model	Dataset	Accuracy
Qiu et al. (2022)	Multiclass sound classification	CNN	Physionet/CinC	72.1%
Sakib et al. (2021)	Multiclass ECG classification	CNN	DS2	89.14% (AFL - 6)
			DS3	89.89% (AFL - 10)
			DS4	76.93% (AFL - 8)
Linardos et al. (2022)	Multiclass MRI classification	3D - CNN	M&M ACDC dataset	AUC 0.77
Goto et al. (2022)	ECG/echocardiogram	CNN	Private dataset of ECG and echocardiogram	AUC 0.93 0.96
Misonne and Jodogne (2022)	Heart segmentation	U - Nets	NSCLC-radiomics	0.879
			Pediatric-CT-SEG	0.940
			Lung CT 2017	0.922

Heart disease datasets. To facilitate the development of a federated global heart disease detection model, the authors have harnessed the power of FedMA resulting in a robust and accurate global model. At the client level, the authors have implemented the Modified Artificial Bee Colony (M-ABC) algorithm. This aids in the recognition of the most impactful features within the dataset, thereby enhancing the model performance by correctly recognizing heart disease cases. The proposed FedMA M-ABC RB-SVM model has achieved an accuracy threshold of 91%, 37.8% faster than the conventional FedAvg SVM method. In a similar effort, another study (Yaqoob et al., 2022) has focused solely on the Cleveland heart disease dataset. In their work, they report a 24.3% decrease in the time required to attain an accuracy threshold of 90% when compared to the FedSGD approach.

In another study (Jalal et al., 2022), authors manually created a dataset by combining data from various sources, including Cleveland (303 samples), Hungarian (294 samples), Switzerland (123 samples), Long Beach (200 samples), and Statlog (270 samples) datasets. Data from the Cleveland and Hungarian datasets were used to simulate two client nodes, while the remaining datasets were used to train the central ML model. During data preprocessing, the authors found outliers when looking at how age and cholesterol, as well as resting blood pressure and cholesterol, relate to the target class. They employed the Z-score to eliminate these outliers, generating a reliable dataset to train a random forest classifier. Based on that basis, authors implemented a horizontal FL system achieving an overall accuracy of 87.77%.

Logistic regression (LR) and SVM are used for the binary classification of the UCI – Cleveland dataset in Bharathi et al. (2022). As the first step, the researchers removed outliers based on the interquartile range. Then they performed a log transformation accompanied with Z-score normalization on the numerical features. After the completion of preprocessing, a federated averaging strategy was utilized to implement a horizontal FL network with one central server and five client nodes. The authors report that they obtained an accuracy of 82.38% for the LR-based model while the SVM-based model obtained an accuracy of 90.3%. The study conducted centralized training for both models and reports that the LR-based model achieves the highest accuracy at 95.8%. Though the accuracy has dropped by a significant margin, the balance between data privacy and generalizability showcases the capacity of FL to yield promising results.

The cPDS algorithm offers a powerful decentralized framework using sparse SVMs (sSVMs) (Brisimi et al., 2018). The study was conducted based on the medical data collected at the Boston Medical Center, from patients with heart-related diagnoses between 2005 and 2010. According to the experiments carried out by the authors, cPDS exhibited improved convergence rates and flexibility in processing data either at the patient level or at the hospital level. By utilizing sSVM, authors were able to develop interpretable classifiers with reduced feature sets, optimizing the designed binary classification. The authors conducted several experiments to identify the best performing configuration for the task and the random graph topology built with 10 hospitals and 13 edges, achieved the highest AUC value of 0.7806 in just 544 seconds of training time.

Yoo et al. (2021b) used a CNN for the classification of a multiclass tabular dataset. First, they preprocessed each row of the dataset into a 2-dimensional array to utilize the potentials of CNNs for high-level feature extraction. To implement the FL architecture, federated averaging was used and a hierarchical clustering procedure was followed to convert the global model into personal federated cluster model (PFCM).

Authors, as opposed to the federated averaging of model weights, calculated the differences between the global and client-learned weights. These disparities were then grouped through the weight updates using hierarchical clustering, resulting in PFCM. The proposed 3-class PFCM was able to complete the inference stage with an accuracy of 73.68%. When the task was reduced to a binary classification, the authors obtained an accuracy of 90.7%, which was better than the metrics reported in other studies with comparable conditions and datasets.

A robust Bayesian inference framework was presented by Fang et al. (2021) for the FL-based heart rate prediction applications. They based their method on an ARX model. The study presented two distinct Bayesian FL techniques: an approach that was built by using the sequential Bayesian process (FD Seq Bayes) and another approach based on an empirical-Bayes type hierarchical method (FD HBayes-EB). The FD Seq Bayes model was intended to provide a statistically rigorous integration of the local models, and the FD HBayes-EB was developed as a scalable method in the framework of hierarchical modeling. In order to identify the efficiency of the Bayesian inferencing strategies, researchers conducted experiments using real outdoor running exercise data from 10 subjects which were collected during actual operation. This information encompassed the duration of exercise, running pace, and heartbeat rate. The outcomes showed that the FD Seq Bayes and FD HBayes-EB algorithms surpassed the simple FedAvg by a large margin in different types of errors. For example, FD Seq Bayes and FD HBayes-EB provide significant decreases of –0.16 and -0.47 in the mean training error.

In the study by Salmeron et al. (2023), five novel federation strategies were proposed based on a standard FedAvg algorithm. To formulate these techniques, authors have employed five metrics. They are client dataset size, inverse accuracy on local data, combined local size and accuracy, normalized inverse of local–global loss difference (contribution), and inverse of contribution. Their experimentation involved a DNN with five dense layers followed by ReLU non-linearity and dropout for regularization, applied to a binary classification task from the UCI dataset. The federation network employed a centralized architecture with five client nodes. During the observations, the researchers consistently noticed that accuracy-based federated aggregation enhanced the global model. Notably, they achieved the highest global accuracy of 89.02% using the size-based federation mechanism.

A novel approach to personalized model training using global layers (GL), which remains robust even when faced with changes in the joint distribution P(X, Y) and mixed input/output spaces X × Y across different clients (Obeidi, 2023). GL can accommodate both client-exclusive features and classes. The training algorithm they propose, known as BatchAlignedFedAvg, builds upon the standard FedAvg method but includes two key modifications. First, instead of specifying a fixed batch size, they opt for a hyperparameter that determines the total number of batches for each local epoch, ensuring a consistent number of local gradient updates across all clients. This prevents issues related to local under or oversampling, which can distort the client distribution, especially when sample sizes are small or imbalanced among clients. Second, the aggregation step is performed each time all clients finish a local pass on their respective batches. This divergence from the traditional FedAvg process helps maintain synchronization and alignment in the model aggregation.

To evaluate the GL architecture, the authors introduce two new benchmark experiments specifically designed for FL. These experiments utilize tabular data naturally partitioned from existing real-world datasets, the UCI Covertype and UCI Heart Disease datasets. Based on the area under the receiver operating characteristic curve (AUROC), GL demonstrates an average improvement of around 4% compared to the next highest scores among the local and FedAvg baselines for the Covertype dataset. For the heart disease dataset, the improvement is approximately 1%. These empirical results, obtained in a full-participant setting, underscore that GL consistently outperforms both federated averaging (FedAvg) and local-only training, with some clients even surpassing their performance compared to a centralized baseline.

17.5.2 ML Techniques for Unstructured Data

The Physionet/CinC Challenge 2016 comprises of 3,240 audio records collected from 764 subjects. These records are categorized into two groups based on expert assessments: "Normal" for records from healthy individuals and "Abnormal" for records from subjects with heart valve defects and coronary heart disease. Qiu et al. (2022) employed continuous wavelet transform (CWT), with a sampling frequency of 2 kHz to convert the audio into image representations. The resulting image dataset was used to train a series of CNN-based models arranged in a horizontal FL framework. The authors report that the experiments conducted using the HFL framework achieved the highest accuracy of 72.1%.

In Sakib et al. (2021), a customized lightweight CNN designed to process single-lead raw ECG heartbeats was employed. The training was done based on the MIT-BIH Supraventricular Arrhythmia database (DS1). To evaluate the efficacy of their techniques, the authors tested the system using the MIT-BIH Arrhythmia database (DS2), INCART 12-lead Arrhythmia database (DS3), and the Sudden Cardiac Death Holter database (DS4). Two types of FL architectures were developed through the study named: synchronous FL (Sync-FL) and asynchronous FL (Async-FL). Notably, Sync-FL outperforms Async-FL when there is a relatively low number of Edge Nodes. But when the number of edge nodes is increased, the classification accuracy becomes superior in the case of Async-FL for all the tested datasets. For DS2, Async-FL with 6 edge nodes achieves the highest accuracy of 89.14%, while for DS3 and DS4, Async-FL with 10 and 8 edge nodes, respectively, achieves accuracy values of 89.89% and 76.93%.

A novel approach to federated heart disease identification using MRI data is presented in (Linardos et al., 2022). The authors initiated the process by applying N4 bias field correction to mitigate the inherent non-uniformities of low frequencies present in MRI images. To ensure consistency in data representation, they resampled the MRI volumes to 1×1×1 mm^3 across all the datasets. They explored three distinct setups for their dataset: (1) a baseline using only the 1-channel MRI image, (2) an MRI image multiplied by a segmentation mask, and (3) the MRI image split into three channels representing the left ventricle blood pool, the right ventricle blood pool, and myocardium. The usage of induced priors derived from the segmentation masks can be identified as a key innovation in their methodology. As the M&M dataset consists of a limited amount of data, authors have employed different data augmentation techniques. These techniques not only increased the effective shape of the training set but also introduced domain shift effects, enhancing model generalization to unseen datasets. The augmentation setups included basic transformations like random rotations and flips, as well as more complex deformations like elastic deformation and the introduction of artefacts and noise. They used AUC with cross-validation and leave-center-out cross-validation techniques to rigorously assess their model's performance.

Goto et al. (2022) primarily aim to develop an ML model capable of detecting hypertrophic cardiomyopathy (HCM) using both ECGs and Echos. They collected a substantial dataset, including 74376 ECGs from 56129 patients and 8392 Echos from 6825 patients. Initially, when the model was tested within their respective institution, it demonstrated excellent performance in identifying HCM, with discrimination scores (C statistics) ranging from 0.88 to 0.93. However, when a model developed in Japan was evaluated in the United States it showed lower discrimination scores (C statistic, 0.79–0.82), revealing the limitations in model generalization.

To overcome these limitations, the authors employed a FL approach. With this method, the discrimination of HCM improved significantly across all centers, achieving high C statistics ranging from 0.90 to 0.96 for both ECG and Echo models. This improved performance extended to different subgroups of patients. Furthermore, when assessing paired data of ECGs and Echos from 11823 patients from an external institution, the automated HCM detection exhibited higher sensitivity at a given positive predictive value compared to human cardiologists. Specifically, the ECG model achieved a sensitivity of 0.98 versus 0.81 at a positive predictive value of 0.01, while the Echo model reached 0.78 versus 0.59 at a positive predictive value of 0.24.

The U-Net architecture, characterized by its distinctive "U" shape, is widely used in medical image segmentation tasks. It initially employs a contraction path to extract high-level features from input images and then follows with an expansion path to generate segmentation masks. This approach efficiently considers the global spatial structure of medical images and is significantly faster than traditional sliding-window methods. In another study (Misonne and Jodogne, 2022), U-Net models are trained on axial slices of segmented CT scan data, aiming to minimize a variant of the 2D Dice loss function. However, applying the classical federated averaging algorithm can pose challenges when the local datasets from different hospitals exhibit significant imbalances. The algorithm tends to prioritize updates from larger datasets, potentially impacting the model's performance on smaller datasets. To mitigate this, the authors introduce the federated equal chances algorithm. Here, each client augments their original dataset with information-preserving transformations, such as rotations and random flips, until they match the size of the largest dataset. Regarding the training time, centralized learning for 535 patients took 9 hours, while local datasets for NSCLC-Radiomics (127 patients), Pediatric-CT-SEG (349 patients), and LCTSC (59 patients) required 0.8, 5.3, and 0.5 hours, respectively. The federated average consumed 18.3 hours, while the federated equal-chances approach accumulated a total of 30.5 hours.

17.5.3 Evaluation Metrics

The assessment of performance in a heart disease detection system is a critical component, serving as a cornerstone for model refinement. Under the considered scope 12 classifications, 1 regression and 1 segmentation-based study were analyzed. For the evaluation of the regression-based ARX model (Fang et al., 2021), the mean squared error was employed to measure the performance.

For classification tasks, a confusion matrix can be used to obtain a summary of prediction results. The metrics true positive (TP), true negative (TN), false positive (FP), and false negative (FN) can be used to extract complex evaluation metrics. All the 12 studies that present classification-based predictions implement multiple metrics which are derivatives as explained earlier. Accuracy (Qiu et al., 2022; Sakib et al., 2021; Yaqoob et al., 2022; Yaqoob et al., 2023; Jalal et al., 2022; Linardos et al., 2022; Khan et al., 2023; Jafari and Adibnia, 2023, Obeidi, 2023) is the most utilized metric and significant usage of recall (Qiu et al., 2022; Sakib et al., 2021; Yaqoob et al., 2023; Jalal et al., 2022; Linardos et al., 2022; Jafari and Adibnia, 2023, Yoo et al., 2021b), precision (Sakib et al., 2021; Yaqoob et al., 2023, Jalal et al., 2022, Khan et al., 2023, Jafari and Adibnia, 2023), specificity(Qiu et al., 2022; Yaqoob et al., 2023; Linardos et al., 2022; Yoo et al., 2021b), AUC (Sakib et al., 2021; Linardos et al., 2022; Goto et al., 2022; Obeidi, 2023), and F1-score (Yaqoob et al., 2023; Jalal et al., 2022; Khan et al., 2023) can also be identified. As special use cases, the 3D dice similarity coefficient has been used in another study (Misonne and Jodogne, 2022), as the study works with 3D CT scan images of the heart for a segmentation task.

The design of FL incorporates a centralized global model and distributed local models deployed on client devices. The global model relies on local models to complete training phases and share model weights. Consequently, a temporal impact becomes a critical factor. Inefficiently designed architectures can lead to prolonged convergence times for the global model. Thus, as a supplementary performance metric, the studies (Yaqoob et al., 2022; Jalal et al., 2022; Brisimi et al., 2018) also record the time expended during the training process.

17.6 Discussion

17.6.1 Study Contribution and Lessons Learned

In this research, we have examined the application of FL in heart disease detection. The study begins by offering a thorough introduction to FL, followed by a discussion of the common architectures and techniques used to effectively manage an FL network. We also explain how communication can be established centrally or in a decentralized manner. The study proceeds to introduce various datasets that have been employed in related research to support FL systems. We provide a comprehensive explanation of different data sources found in these datasets and conclude by highlighting the challenges associated with these datasets. As mentioned earlier, FL for heart disease detection involves both structured and unstructured data. Therefore, we provide a comprehensive overview of ML algorithms utilized for both data types. Before concluding, the study summarizes its contributions, identifies open challenges, and outlines future research directions.

Through the study, we have identified the standard practices followed in the domain and Figure 17.4 presents our recommendations. Our approach begins with a group of nodes with the same domain data and a shared goal of collaboratively constructing a generalized model based on their data. The initial step involves analyzing the feature spaces and sample spaces of these clients. If there is a significant overlap in feature spaces, we opt for HFL. Conversely, if most of the sample spaces overlap, VFL

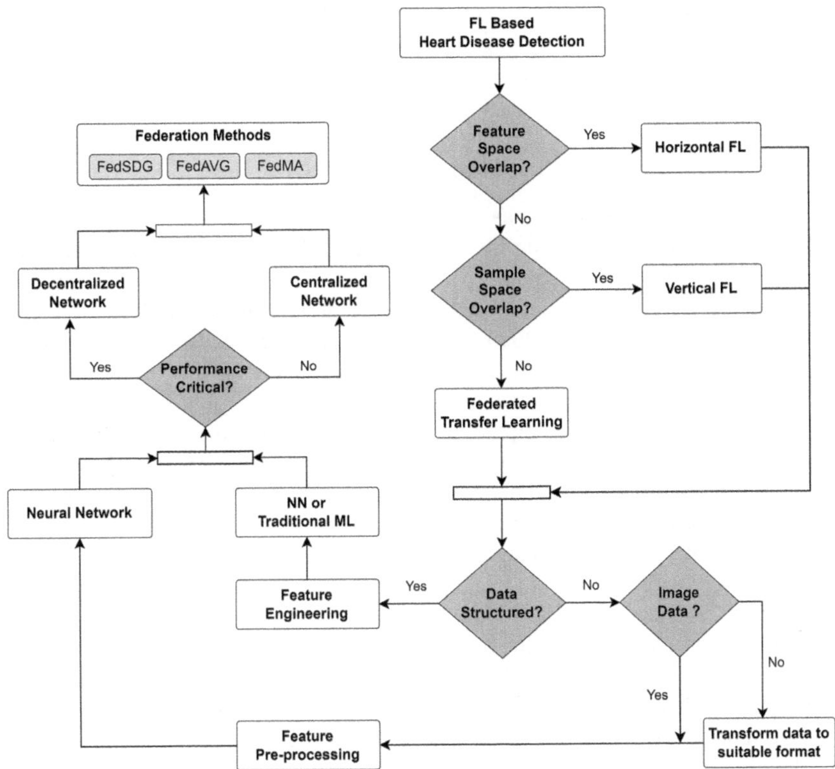

FIGURE 17.4 Recommended techniques to use in heart disease detection using FL.

becomes the preferred choice. In cases where only minor overlaps exist, but the data share similarities, FTL can be employed.

Following the determination of the FL architecture, we turn our attention to data format considerations. For structured data (tabular), we recommend building an advanced feature engineering pipeline, leveraging domain expertise. This is followed by selecting either a traditional ML model or a DNN. A conversion to a suitable format compatible with neural networks is necessary for unstructured data. For instance, image data can be used directly with CNNs, while audio data, such as heart sounds, can be transformed into representative images using techniques like wavelet transforms. After transformation, further feature preprocessing can be applied as needed, and the design of the neural network for data processing should be carefully considered.

Once the model and feature engineering pipeline are agreed upon, the next consideration is whether specific performance requirements exist. If performance is a critical factor, a decentralized FL network design is recommended. Alternatively, selecting a centralized network is preferable when prioritizing manageability as the top concern. As the last step, the selection of a federation technique for aggregating models is required. Several techniques, like FedSDG, FedAVG, FedMA, and even Bayesian

Inferencing, can be used depending on specific requirements. Overall, researchers can follow these steps as a guide for making decisions about the development of federated heart disease detection systems.

17.6.2 Open Challenges and Future Research Directions

Privacy and security concerns

Detecting heart disease using FL is accompanied by a high focus on privacy and security aspects. Some of the approaches used by researchers to protect systems include data encryption, blockchain storage usage, and also device-level security measures (Gu et al., 2023). Nevertheless, the use of these methods becomes very problematic because medical data processing is very time-consuming requiring a higher computational load.

Malicious hackers may attempt to execute hidden movements such as deciphering the model or gaining knowledge about some patients' records (Joshi et al., 2022). Therefore, it is important to develop high-performing models while guaranteeing that the federated system remains secure from new threats.

Medical data-related challenges

Section 4 provides an overview of existing datasets used for implementing FL systems for heart disease detection. However, it becomes clear that none of those datasets were originally intended to train a FL system. Thus researchers were required to employ a combination of datasets (Misonne and Jodogne, 2022; Obeidi, 2023) while mitigating insufficient data, data noise, lack of standard evaluation criteria, and requirement of artificial splitting.

Handling non-IID data becomes highly challenging, especially in medical data. Even though FL is better at dealing with different types of data than traditional methods, having uneven data can reduce the net performance of the aggregated model. Further, the learning rate of the central model can be affected by the distribution patterns of the data that exist under different nodes of the federation network. Therefore, a clear requirement for a public dataset that can be used to benchmark the performance of FL-based heart disease detections can be identified.

Communication challenges

Communication between the participant nodes of a FL system holds high importance. With the possibility of nodes being spread across a vast geographical area, the connectivity can become unreliable throughout the federation process (Yu et al., 2020). As the communication over the network can fail midtime of the federation, attention needs to be given to failovers and restarts. Further, the communication protocol needs to distribute the model updates while keeping everything private and secure. Dealing with issues like slow networks, limited space for metadata, and making sure all the devices work together in synchronization receives high importance when using FL for heart disease detection. Thus, setting up a strong communication system that works well with different network conditions and keeping the data safe during transmission becomes challenging (Kaissis et al., 2020).

17.7 Conclusion

Heart disease detection plays a critical role in healthcare domain in smart city applications due to the high casualties involved. Hence, the field of early heart disease detection using artificial intelligence has received an abundance of research interest resulting in properly annotated heterogenous datasets and state-of-the-art ML models. From a theoretical point of view, these systems achieve good results but the practical implementation of them has been hindered due to privacy concerns and the lack of generalizability in the developed models. FL-based heart disease detection systems provide a workaround for the traditional ML infrastructure providing highly accurate and generalizable predictions. Though multiple researchers have utilized FL successfully in this domain, a lack of comprehensive surveys discussing the state-of-the-art techniques utilized in the domain can be identified. Hence, this paper explores the principles of federated heart disease detection, including standard architectures, communication protocols, and available datasets. The study pinpoints different ML techniques used specifically for structured and unstructured heart disease data as well. Apart from the standard techniques followed by the researchers, this paper has identified various challenges inherent to the field including the lack of a benchmark dataset, communication complexities, and security concerns. Further, the study provides recommendations for FL-based heart disease detection and future research directions, serving as a valuable asset for researchers and developers in smart city applications related to the healthcare domain.

REFERENCES

Ahsan, M. M., & Siddique, Z. (2022). Machine learning-based heart disease diagnosis: A systematic literature review. *Artificial Intelligence in Medicine, 128*, 102289.

Brisimi, T. S., Chen, R., Mela, T., Olshevsky, A., Paschalidis, I. C., & Shi, W. (2018). Federated learning of predictive models from federated electronic health records. *International Journal of Medical Informatics, 112*, 59–67.

Bharathi, S. K., Dhavamani, M., & Niranjan, K. (2022). A federated learning based approach for heart disease prediction. In *6th International Conference on Computing Methodologies and Communication (ICCMC)* (pp. 1117–1121). IEEE.

Fang, L., Liu, X., Su, X., Ye, J., Dobson, S., Hui, P., & Tarkoma, S. (2021). Bayesian inference federated learning for heart rate prediction. In *9th EAI International Conference on Wireless Mobile Communication and Healthcare (MobiHealth)* (pp. 116–130). Springer.

Goto, S., Solanki, D., John, J. E., Yagi, R., Homilius, M., Ichihara, G., & Deo, R. C. (2022). Multinational federated learning approach to train ECG and echocardiogram models for hypertrophic cardiomyopathy detection. *Circulation, 146*(10), 755–769.

Gu, X., Sabrina, F., Fan, Z., & Sohail, S. (2023). A review of privacy enhancement methods for federated learning in healthcare systems. *International Journal of Environmental Research and Public Health, 20*(15), 6539.

Guerra-Manzanares, A., Lopez, L. J. L., Maniatakos, M., & Shamout, F. E. (2023). Privacy-preserving machine learning for healthcare: open challenges and future perspectives. In *International Workshop on Trustworthy Machine Learning for Healthcare* (pp. 25–40). Cham: Springer Nature.

Hussain, M. W., & Roy, D. S. (2023). Performance Optimization Strategies for Big Data Applications in Distributed Framework. In *Intelligent Technologies: Concepts, Applications, and Future Directions*, Volume *2* (pp. 221–252). Singapore: Springer Nature Singapore.

Jafari, M., & Adibnia, F. (2023). HeartchainFL: Prediction of heart disease based on BigchainDB and federated learning. Available at SSRN 4409805.

Jalal, S. M., Hasan, M. R., Haque, M. A., & Alam, M. G. R. (2022). A horizontal federated random forest for heart disease detection from decentralized local data. In *10th Region 10 Humanitarian Technology Conference (R10-HTC)* (pp. 191–196). IEEE.

Joshi, M., Pal, A., & Sankarasubbu, M. (2022). Federated learning for healthcare domain pipeline, applications and challenges. *ACM Transactions on Computing for Healthcare*, *3*(4), 1–36.

Kaissis, G. A., Makowski, M. R., Rückert, D., & Braren, R. F. (2020). Secure, privacy-preserving and federated machine learning in medical imaging. *Nature Machine Intelligence*, *2*(6), 305–311.

Katarya, R., & Srinivas, P. (2020). Predicting heart disease at early stages using machine learning: A survey. In *International Conference on Electronics and Sustainable Communication Systems (ICESC)* (pp. 302–305). IEEE, Coimbatore, India.

Khan, M. A., Alsulami, M., Yaqoob, M. M., Alsadie, D., Saudagar, A. K. J., AlKhathami, M., & Farooq Khattak, U. (2023). Asynchronous federated learning for improved cardiovascular disease prediction using artificial intelligence. *Diagnostics*, *13*(14), 2340.

Li, J., Meng, Y., Ma, L., Du, S., Zhu, H., Pei, Q., & Shen, X. (2021). A federated learning based privacy-preserving smart healthcare system. *IEEE Transactions on Industrial Informatics*, *18*(3), (2021-2031).

Li, L., Fan, Y., Tse, M., & Lin, K. Y. (2020). A review of applications in federated learning. *Computers & Industrial Engineering*, *149*, 106854.

Linardos, A., Kushibar, K., Walsh, S., Gkontra, P., & Lekadir, K. (2022). Federated learning for multi-center imaging diagnostics: a simulation study in cardiovascular disease. *Scientific Reports*, *12*(1), 3551.

Meedeniya, D. (2023). *Deep Learning a Beginners' Guide*. CRC Press, www.routledge.com/9781032473246

Meedeniya, D., Kumarasinghe, H., Kolonne, S., Fernando, C., De la Torre Díez, I., & Marques, G. (2022). Chest X-ray analysis empowered with deep learning: A systematic review. *Applied Soft Computing*, *126*, 109319. https://doi.org/10.1016/j.asoc.2022.109319

Misonne, T., & Jodogne, S. (2022, June). Federated Learning for Heart Segmentation. In *14th Workshop on Image, Video, and Multidimensional Signal Processing (IVMSP)* (pp. 1–5). IEEE, Nafplio, Greece.

Nguyen, D. C., Pham, Q. V., Pathirana, P. N., Ding, M., Seneviratne, A., Lin, Z., & Hwang, W. J. (2022). Federated learning for smart healthcare: A survey. *ACM Computing Surveys (CSUR)*, *55*(3), 1–37.

Obeidi, Y. (2023). Global layers: Non-IID tabular federated learning. arXiv preprint arXiv:2305.19290.

Pradhan, B., Hussain, M. W., Srivastava, G., Debbarma, M. K., Barik, R. K., & Lin, J. C. W. (2022). *A Neuro-Evolutionary Approach for Software Defined Wireless Network Traffic Classification*. IET Communications.

Qiu, W., Qian, K., Wang, Z., Chang, Y., Bao, Z., Hu, B., & Yamamoto, Y. (2022). A federated learning paradigm for heart sound classification. In *44th Annual Interna-*

tional Conference of the IEEE Engineering in Medicine & Biology Society (EMBC) (pp. 1045–1048). IEEE.

Reddy, K. H. K., Roy, D. S., Mishra, T. K., & Hussain, M. W. (2023). *Handbook of Research on Network-Enabled IoT Applications for Smart City Services*. IGI Global.

Sakib, S., Fouda, M. M., Fadlullah, Z. M., Abualsaud, K., Yaacoub, E., & Guizani, M. (2021). Asynchronous federated learning-based ECG analysis for arrhythmia detection. In *IEEE International Mediterranean Conference on Communications and Networking (MeditCom)* (pp. 277–282). IEEE.

Salmeron, J. L., Arévalo, I., & Ruiz-Celma, A. (2023). Benchmarking federated strategies in Peer-to-Peer Federated learning for biomedical data. *Heliyon*. *9*(6), e16925.

Sohan, M. F., & Basalamah, A. (2023). A systematic review on federated learning in medical image analysis. *IEEE Access*, *11*, 28628–28644.

Wang, W., Li, X., Qiu, X., Zhang, X., Zhao, J., & Brusic, V. (2023). A privacy preserving framework for federated learning in smart healthcare systems. *Information Processing & Management*, *60*(1), 103167.

Wijethilake, N., Meedeniya, D., Chitraranjan, C., Perera, I., Islam, M., & Ren, H. (2021). Glioma survival analysis empowered with data engineering—A survey. *IEEE Access*, *9*, 43168–43191. https://doi.org/10.1109/ACCESS.2021.3065965

Witt, L., Heyer, M., Toyoda, K., Samek, W., & Li, D. (2023). Decentral and incentivized federated learning frameworks: A systematic literature review. *IEEE Internet of Things Journal* *10*(4), 3642–3663.

Yaqoob, M. M., Nazir, M., Khan, M. A., Qureshi, S., & Al-Rasheed, A. (2023). Hybrid classifier-based federated learning in health service providers for cardiovascular disease prediction. *Applied Sciences*, *13*(3), 1911.

Yaqoob, M. M., Nazir, M., Yousafzai, A., Khan, M. A., Shaikh, A. A., Algarni, A. D., & Elmannai, H. (2022). Modified artificial bee colony based feature optimized federated learning for heart disease diagnosis in healthcare. *Applied Sciences*, *12*(23), 12080.

Yoo, J. H., Jeong, H., Lee, J., & Chung, T. M. (2021a). Federated learning: Issues in medical application. In *8th International Conference Future Data and Security Engineering (FDSE)*. (pp. 3–22). Springer.

Yoo, J. H., Son, H. M., Jeong, H., Jang, E. H., Kim, A. Y., Yu, H. Y., & Chung, T. M. (2021b). Personalized federated learning with clustering: Non-IID heart rate variability data application. In *International Conference on Information and Communication Technology Convergence (ICTC)* (pp. 1046–1051). IEEE.

Yu, F., Zhang, W., Qin, Z., Xu, Z., Wang, D., Liu, C., & Chen, X. (2020). Heterogeneous federated learning. arXiv preprint arXiv:2008.06767

Zou, L., Huang, Z., Yu, X., Zheng, J., Liu, A., & Lei, M. (2022). Automatic detection of congestive heart failure based on multiscale residual UNet++: From centralized learning to federated learning. *IEEE Transactions on Instrumentation and Measurement*, *72*, 1–13.

18

Federated Learning for Heart Disease Detection Using a Grey Wolf Transfer Learning Model Based on Multi-perceptron Neural Networks

I. Janani
Sona College of Technology, Salem, India

G. Gokila Deepa
PPG Institute of Technology, Coimbatore, India

B. Dhiyanesh
SRM Institute of Science and Technology, Vadapalani Campus, Chennai, India

C. B. Selva Lakshmi
Velammal College of Engineering and Technology, Madurai, India

T. Yawanikha
Karpagam Institute of Technology, Seerapalayam, India

18.1 Introduction

Healthcare industries often make use of remote services through IoT sensing environments to monitor smart city patient conditions at the edge (Reddy et al., 2023). In a decentralized environment, using some form of machine learning (ML) technique to analyze data collaboratively with the help of the federated learning process (FLP), heart disease is the fatal result of a failure of heart function. Takayasu's arthritis (TA) is the most dangerous and rare cardiac vascular disease, characterized by a wide range of characteristics. So, predicting the disease's nature and effects with early treatment is difficult. During medical data analysis, the impact of disease rate is varied due to patient conditions and feature margins.

Technology that has been advanced globally for the use of the IoT in the medical field fully supports IoT because it monitors medical emergencies using them and assists patients in monitoring themselves. The World Health Organization will support

DOI: 10.1201/9781032631738-18

and help, and this technology will improve. Patient-level heart disease tracking for 24 hours and patient treatment-level information are easy to gather from doctors and hospitals. Large- and medium-sized arteries and their branches are damaged by the systemic inflammatory condition known as TA, also known as pulsatile disease. Young Asian women are the most affected. It typically affects the aorta and its major arteries, particularly the renal, carotid, and subclavian arteries. This can lead to stenosis, occlusions, or aneurysmal rupture of these essential arteries. Although cell-mediated immunity appears to be its primary pathophysiology, its exact reason is unknown. Suspicion and arterial symptoms are used to diagnose. Treatment is usually started with medical therapy with corticosteroids; however, lately, surgery has become more common due to the overall remission of the disease and the high relapse rates detected with medical treatment alone.

TA frequently has unexplained causes. It is an inflammatory condition, and cell-mediated autoimmune immunity is the cause. TRON mural fiber thickening in artery walls eventually causes ischemic alterations and pseudo-aneurysms-ML techniques to work. Google has constructed a secure and reliable cloud infrastructure to process this data and enhance our services.

Today, we're launching federated analytics, which uses data science techniques to examine unprocessed data kept locally on customers' devices. Similar to aggregate learning, it generates aggregate findings by doing local calculations on the data from each device. However, product engineers need more data. Associative analytics, unlike associative learning, strives to meet data science fundamentals (Hussain and Roy, 2023). This chapter explains the basic federated analysis techniques created in the quest for federated knowledge. It also explains how we applied those insights to brand-new domains and how current developments in data science technology offer higher accuracy and privacy for data science demands.

Research on consortium analysis methodologies is ongoing and has progressed beyond metrics and figures. Without letting raw data leave the devices, it is possible to train ML models with federated learning to gain aggregated insights into device data (Pradhan et al., 2022). For instance, the Gboard team wanted to find relevant phrases that users often type and add them to the dictionary for writing recommendations and spell-checking.

The association analysis approach is still in its infancy and requires more development to provide accurate answers to many typical data science questions. A thorough overview of federated research can be found. A combinatorial analysis technique for identifying everyday objects in data sets can be found in Discovering Federated Heavy Hitters with Differential Privacy. Through decentralized data aggregation and privacy protection, federated analytics enables us to rethink data science. We welcome additional input and advancements in this expanding subject.

In this section, we propose a multi-perceptron neural network (MPNN)-driven quantitative grey wolf optimized transfer learning (QGWOTL) model for detecting disease characteristics in smart city early and providing early treatment. First, we use Z-SVN for preprocessing to reduce the noise ratio. Additionally, CDIR helps calculate better clinical marginal disease rates by considering these factors. We can also develop a TADF method to marginalize feature weights. We compare the TADF and DFP result values based on actual edges to identify feature changes and create feature texture clusters. Furthermore, we select features using grey wolf optimized with SVM

(GWO-SVM) depending on edge clustering groups and classify them based on LSTMG-MPNN to predict risk type. In this way, we stratify patient status results by risk to increase priority, encouraging early diagnosis to save the patient's life (Abdellatif et al., 2022a).

This provides user interfaces for collaborative learning tasks using tensor flow-implemented ML models, such as training or testing sets. Our primary objective in creating these interfaces was to assess parallel learning algorithms used in various current models and data. This was not to examine how similar learning algorithm's function. It is highly recommended to support this website through donations. Improved weighted random forests (IWRF) methods for predicting cardiovascular diseases (CVDs) can be applied to identify significant features. Furthermore, the IWRF method can be implemented to generate new hyperparameters coupled with Bayesian optimization. The standard being proposed has better performance than other models. Its accuracy has improved by 2.4% and 4.6% on both datasets compared to previous studies. When the proposed methods were used for CVD detection, they achieved 99.2% and 98.52% accuracy. In addition, the Cleveland dataset model has a conversion rate of 95.73% (Abdellatif et al., 2022b) for extreme classification. Deep learning (DL) learns from time-domain signal representations, while traditional ML discovers expert features. With a score of 89.3, the suggested approach outperformed the baseline strategy by 9.1 in the challenge. Even though the experiment's results are not comparable, the method achieved 92.9% accuracy and a 7.1% error rate. This error rate is consistent with experts' 9.7% of "unknown" records (Gjoreski et al., 2020).

18.2 Related Works

The novel presents that a fast and efficient convolutional neural network (CNN) method can be invented to detect and classify electrocardiograms in real time. In addition, it has been indicated that a memory of 12 MB can process sample sizes of up to 90 kB within 9 ms of the estimated inference time. Moreover, the algorithm-based classifier achieves 99.1% classification accuracy and a 95% marginal F1 score. The developed classifier can be implemented in various peripheral devices for monitoring arrhythmias, thanks to the results obtained with it (Farag, 2022). The PCHF method provides key feature engineering techniques to improve performance and select the most significant features. We developed entirely redesigned features to obtain more accurate scores by strengthening the developed PCHF technique. The proposed decision tree (DT) method performs better than ML models and other advanced works, with 100% accuracy (Lakshmanarao et al., 2021). The proposed DL methods can be used to integrate with ML. Furthermore, expert features can learn from the spectro-photoscopy representation of the DL signal while testing standard ML techniques. The suggested approach outperformed the benchmark challenge method with a score of 89.3.9.1. However, the presented technique realized an overall accuracy of 92.9% and an error rate of 7.1%, but it isn't easy to compare it with experimental results directly. This error rate is very similar to the rate of records classified as "unknown" (9.7%) (Abubaker and Babayigit, 2023).

CVD classification accuracy can be improved to 98.23% by the proposed enhanced lightweight CNN method associated with the present advanced methods. In addition, electrocardiogram images can be processed on demand for CVD patients. Power limits in computers: the simple Bayes method produces 99.79% accuracy. As a result, this technique can be incorporated into the healthcare IoT ecosystem (Fitriyani et al., 2020). Stat lock and Cleveland dataset accuracy increased to 95.90% and 98.40%, respectively. Furthermore, it outperforms other models based on earlier studies. Furthermore, clinicians often use the CDSS heart disease model to diagnose a patient's health status depending on current symptoms. As a result, early treatment can prevent coronary heart disease deaths (Guo et al., 2020). References are required when using the platform for data mining based on the IoMT approach. It has been found that coronary artery disease mainly affects the elderly population, with atherosclerotic high blood pressure being the primary cause of this condition. The precision, agreement, and F-measure ratios for this cause are 96.6%, 96.8%, and 96.7%, respectively. Additionally, diabetes should also be considered as a factor when dealing with coronary artery disease, and preventive measures should be taken (Pathak et al., 2022).

The novel suggested that the MKL method can define the optimal core combination by maximizing similarity and avoiding overlap with significant objects. In the experiment, 960 PCG sessions were recorded in 40 CAD patients and 40 normal patients. With a KAPPA of 0.7850, the transformed additions achieve a maximum object precision of 89.25%. It is then combined with handcrafted features using the recommended MKL, which yields 91.19% accuracy and 0.8238 KAPPA. This work shows that it is possible to develop a highly accurate CAD diagnostic system by taking advantage of a PCG signal that is non-invasive and simple to acquire (Yang et al., 2023). The improved SMOTE using hyperband and extra trees (ET) outperformed recent CVD diagnosis advances by 99.2% and 98.52%, respectively, and provided better results than previous models. In addition, the sample from the generated Cleveland dataset was transformed into a 95.73% severity estimate. Doctors can assess heart disease using a prescribed model. As a result, starting treatment as early as possible can prevent CVD-related deaths (Padovano, et al., 2022).

The Focus Loss (FL) Framingham Heart Institute's data was used as the basis for the evaluation of the model to determine whether it could predict coronary heart disease. The FL model achieved an AUC value of 97.8%, surpassing comparable standards. These results suggest that using the FL model could improve coronary heart disease detection in the general population (Javeed et al., 2019). Regardless of the HRV-based features and ML classifiers selected, external validation findings were 20%–40% lower in accuracy, sensitivity, and specificity than cross-validation (CV). These findings propose that ML-based OSA detectors trained on public databases are currently insufficient for use in clinical settings, as well as a reliable assessment of these algorithms' true ability to predict (Mehrang et al., 2020).

The forecast method uses an RF model to predict HF and a Random Search Algorithm (RSA) to select features. The approach achieves 3.3% higher accuracy with only seven features than conventional RF models with more features. The offered method is more efficient and simpler than traditional RF models. In addition, the approach outperforms five other modern ML techniques. Improving the form's training accuracy achieves 93.33% classification accuracy. Ultimately, our process surpasses the 11 proposed HF detection approaches (Roy and Satija, 2023).

Candidate classifiers include extreme gradient regression, RFs, and logistic regression. The analysis findings indicated that the area under the curves for ICA and AFIB was 0.85 and 0.98, respectively. Positive and negative AFIB results were predicted with 91.9% and 100% accuracy, respectively. For ICAD, the highest ratios for multi-label and hierarchical classification were 56.9%, 88.4%, 69.9%, and 68.8%, individually (Procházka et al., 2018). Data preprocessing and enhancement, generating Mel spectrogram slice representations from lung sounds, and optimizing pre-trained YAMNet are all part of the framework. An experimental study on the TR dataset of respiratory databases reveals that the proposed framework surpasses existing single-proposal methods for binary Chronic obstructive pulmonary disease (COPD) severity classification and multiclass by 99.25% and 96.14%, respectively. Lung sounds are used to evaluate COPD severity (Wang et al., 2017).

The proposed technique integrates ML and adaptive image processing methods to identify the evolution of temperature ranges and measure respiration rates. Results from current cycling systems are consistent with an average 21-second delay in heart rate deceleration associated with activity level change. Other results indicated a mean transformation of 167 moments in respiratory temperature and 49 seconds in respiratory frequency (Abdar et al., 2019). CVD is the primary cause of death globally, but ML techniques can detect it early, potentially reducing mortality rates. However, ML faces challenges analyzing prognostic data due to category inequality and high-dimensionality problems, making diagnosing heart disease in real-world applications challenging. The suggested model demonstrated superior performance to other models, boosting accuracy rates by 2.4% and 4.6%, respectively, on both datasets (Jafari Tadi, et al., 2019). FROC examinations indicate that DL approaches can detect BAC at levels comparable to human professionals. A linear regression analysis between the two methods resulted in a coefficient of perseverance of 96.24%. Calcium mass spectrometry research indicates that the predicted calcium mass is precise. DL can be utilized in developing automated mammography schemes for BAC detection (Rizwan et al., 2021).

Resampling and class balancing methods were used to balance the data using a multilevel filtering strategy. As one of the most versatile algorithms of its kind, Nu-SVC supports four kernel functions: linear, polynomial, RBS, and sigmoid. Based on the data from the Z-Alizadeh Sani and Cleveland CAD datasets, the proposed NE-nu-SVC model is shown to be highly accurate at predicting CAD entities with 94.66% and 98.60% accuracy, respectively. The method can help doctors accurately identify coronary heart disease and modify more invasive diagnostic procedures (Ferdousi et al., 2021). A fully automated atrial fibrillation detection method incorporating multiple signal processing techniques and heterogeneous engineering features was developed and tested on a large CV database of 300 cardiovascular patients. Based on the test results, the CT test had 97% accuracy, 99% sensitivity, and 95% specificity. In contrast, the MRI test had 95% accuracy, 93% sensitivity, and 97% specificity. For CV and CD, the F1 scores were 97% and 96%, respectively (Wang et al., 2011). Briefly present the current wearable and implantable ECG sensor methods used to obtain AF data. Major difficulties in developing AF self-diagnosis methods are addressed in the conclusion. This review chapter is the first to systematically summarize all the issues surrounding AF self-diagnosis in one place. It has been emphasized that accurate, low-cost, and low-power self-diagnosis techniques are needed for effective AF treatment (Lai et al., 2019).

Sensor-generated synthetic data is used to train the dithering and test it. The Random Tree algorithm requires at least 0.01 seconds to create a sample and achieves 94%

accuracy in predicting diabetes probability; according to tests of several ML algorithms, it is the algorithm that produces the highest accuracy when implementing the proposed technique (X. Wen et al., 2020). The novel introduced a novel detection technique that utilizes the Likelihood Support Vector Machine (LSVM) model for absorption. The pump's flow pattern can be accurately characterized by combining it with the six suction indices. This helps determine whether the pump is at or near suction during suction. The proposed technique was evaluated based on two different pumps and in vivo experimental data (S. Kim et al., 2021). Using ML classifiers like K-Nearest Neighbors (KNN), DT, Naive Bayes (NB), Support Vector Machine (SVM), and Random Forest (RF), classical and SCD risk groups were automatically determined. A database of ECG measurement data from 28 ECG patients and 18 healthy subjects was utilized to evaluate the efficiency and significance of the proposed technique. An accurate prediction of SCD 30 minutes in advance can be made using a five-marker panel of arrhythmia risk, with KNN at 98.91%, SVM at 98.70%, DT at 98.99%, and RF at 99.49% in under 1 second. Automatic functions had an average accuracy of 97.46%.

All 16 features were retrieved after imputation for each partition of the four data sequences. Five statistically significant methods were applied to the classification. According to the examination findings, SVM achieved the highest sensitivity, precision, and accuracy among the five classifiers tested. This was done with scores of 0.968, 0.928, and 0.945. These findings suggest that the proposed feature extraction method classifies AF and RS. It can be the basis for designing a long-term home cardiac monitoring strategy and AF detection. The approach has shown superior performance to conventional methods in detecting and estimating PAD severity, especially when accounting for variations in patient height and arterial stiffness. CNNs trained in the process achieved over 90% success rates for specific patients. Further, accuracy is increased by 15% and over 40% in the R2 value for detection and severity estimation compared to traditional approaches without CPAR. EHR data has been pre-trained and can reveal connections between EHR codes, which can predict chronic diseases. The model showed the most significant improvement in predicting depression, as seen in the lower part of the precision recovery curve PRAUC, which increased from 0.70 to 0.76. This improvement was better than the most effective initial model. The model's interpretability was improved by adding self-focus weights within each row, which quantitatively showed the internal relationship between the different indices (W. Ning, et al., 2021).

The investigators created a hybrid DL model that uses CNN and LSTM to reconstruct ECG signals using Doppler sensors. This technique successfully recreates ECG signals even when the device is not connected. This is evidenced by a correlation coefficient of 0.86 between real and reconstructed ECG signals. The findings indicate that the Doppler sensor can remotely extract ECG signals for heart rate measurement (S. N. Ali, et al., 2023). A patient is diagnosed with arrhythmia and inadequate heart valves. A patient with a dysfunctional heart valve has abnormal temperature curves. This is despite experimental efforts to collect data on temperature curve variability from healthy participants. This subject's temperature range was 0.52°C lower than the others in all three experiment steps. The total temperature curve decreases during stasis and blood flow, although some curves show an increase (Karhade et al., 2022) (Table 18.1).

TABLE 18.1

Comparison of Different Methodologies at the Existing Level

References	Learning Type	Technique Used	Result Achieved
Gjoreski et al. (2020)	ML	Method for CHF detection	An accuracy of 93.2%
Abubaker and Babayigit (2023)	DL	Transfer learning approach	An accuracy of 94.2%
Ning et al. (2021)	DL	CNN	An accuracy of 99.85%
Hussain and Roy (2023)	DL	Framework	An accuracy of 38.93%
Karhade et al. (2022)	DL	Framework for the automated detection	Accuracy values of 99% and 99.48%,
Gupta et al. (2022)	DL	Filter-fusion technique	Accuracy of 98.80%
Li et al. (2019)	DL	Art U-Net model	Accuracy of 93.63%
Bhaskarpandit et al. (2023)	DL	FPGA	Achieved an accuracy value of 100%
Guo, et al. (2020)	ML	Recursion enhanced RF	96.6% accuracy
Abubaker and Babayigit (2023)	DL and ML	New lightweight CNN architecture	An accuracy of 99.79%

18.3 Materials and Methods

Most existing models fail to analyze the feature dimension related to the disease, leading to disease identification inaccuracy in smart cities. This is because property features have no mutual dependencies to predict. So, the federated learning model improves medical data detection accuracy. Increasing the non-feature relation doesn't create a mutual feature relation to take disease identification support margins into account. To resolve this problem, we propose a QGWOTL model based on MPNN to predict the disease's nature early for earlier treatment. The preprocessing uses Z-SVN to reduce the noise ratio.

With this attention, in Figure 18.1, the ideal medical margin disease rate is estimated using the CDIR. The TADF creates the disease feature pattern (DFP) to marginalize feature weights. When focusing on the actual margins, both TADF and DFP ideal values are compared to identify the feature variation needed to create clusters of features based on the actual margins. According to the marginalized cluster groups, the features are selected with GWO-SVM and classified to predict with LSTMG-MPNN by class and risk. The results are categorized by risk based on the patient's condition to emphasize earlier diagnoses to save patients.

18.3.1 Z-Score Vector Normalization (Z-SVN)

In this investigation, the Cleveland dataset was utilized. This dataset from the Cleveland Clinic Foundation contains 14 characteristics linked to patients' vital signs. This program uses 13 traits as forecasting variables, with one final feature as the target category. Prognostic indicators such as gender, age, chest discomfort, serum cholesterol, resting blood pressure, fasting blood glucose, maximal heart rate, and

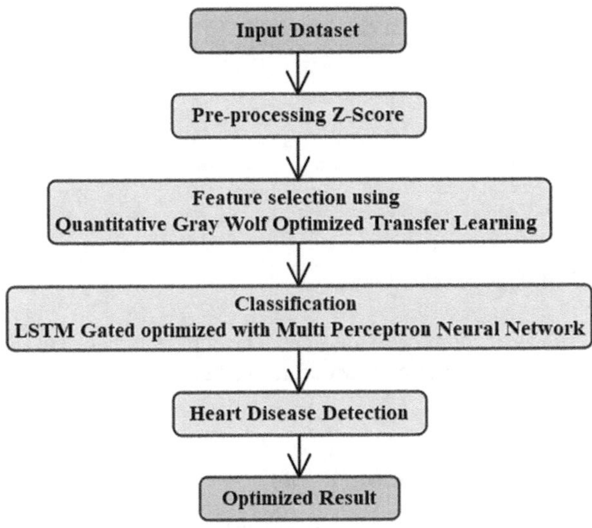

FIGURE 18.1 Architecture diagram LSTMG-MPNN.

electrocardiogram and ST-segment elevation can be used in this investigation. Exercise-induced angina, depression, sedation, thallium test findings, the number of injured blood vessels on fluoroscopy, and diagnosis are examples of anticipated symptoms. There are 303 values needed for data collection. There are six missing entries in the list, leaving 297 instead of 303.

To reduce feature dimensions, preprocessing based on bid filters is first done. The smart city information in the patient's record has been replaced. Verifies the sorted numeric index value against the equals, null, and null characteristics. It includes all the dimensions and features of the documents while normalizing them and removing any additional weights. A pre-processed dataset collected a variety of symptoms, including body temperature, immune level, phlegm, cough, erythrocyte sedimentation rate (ESR), C-reactive protein (CRP), and computed tomography (CT) transmission in Algorithm 1.

ALGORITHM 1: Z-Score Vector Normalization

Input: Initialize the data based on the heart dataset – c_{ds}
Output: Operate the processed dataset to filter – F_{ds}

Step 1: Archive identification of Discovery Panel= c_{ds}
Step 2: Compute for (c_{ds} → I during the initialization of the J feature.)
Step 3: NULL → Check if the exact secondary value is present.
Registration enables the elimination of empty properties and prevents progress.
Step 4: F_{ds} = Returns the efficient data record c_{ds}
Step 5: End for;
Step 6: R-F_{ds}

	age	sex	cp	trtbps	chol	fbs	restecg	thalachh	exng	oldpeak	slp	caa	
count	999.000000	999.000000	999.000000	999.000000	999.000000	999.000000	999.000000	999.000000	999.000000	999.000000	999.000000	999.000000	999.0(
mean	52.979980	0.637638	1.273273	129.630631	247.572573	0.167167	0.531532	156.737738	0.211211	0.786887	1.537538	0.433433	2.17
std	8.785098	0.480923	0.997189	15.991565	56.528643	0.373312	0.507219	20.106761	0.408372	0.923094	0.612448	0.854860	0.54
min	29.000000	0.000000	0.000000	94.000000	126.000000	0.000000	0.000000	71.000000	0.000000	0.000000	0.000000	0.000000	0.0(
25%	46.000000	0.000000	0.000000	120.000000	211.000000	0.000000	0.000000	147.000000	0.000000	0.000000	1.000000	0.000000	2.0(
50%	53.000000	1.000000	1.000000	130.000000	236.000000	0.000000	1.000000	160.000000	0.000000	0.500000	2.000000	0.000000	2.0(
75%	59.000000	1.000000	2.000000	140.000000	271.000000	0.000000	1.000000	172.000000	0.000000	1.400000	2.000000	1.000000	2.0(
max	77.000000	1.000000	3.000000	200.000000	564.000000	1.000000	2.000000	202.000000	1.000000	6.200000	2.000000	4.000000	3.0(

FIGURE 18.2 Normalization of the dataset.

Figure 18.2 shows the preprocessing steps. The approach represents dimensionality reduction based on filtering effects. Multiple attributes in each record denote patient information.

18.3.2 TA-Disease Prone Factor (TADF)

This method uses similarity of incidence based on infection rate, immunity-determined cardiac feature infected, spreading statistics, PHR immunity margins, and other pulmonary value measures measured according to the candidate feature section model, which has the most significant impact dependencies. By using Algorithm 2, it is determined by the mean rate that checks the spatial limits of cardiac feature limits. Candidate selection chooses the average marginal rate based on the occurrence of the continuous difference level, depending on the disease type. Also, the average rate is represented as an eigenvector for each event category, weighted depending on variance. Specific events are selected and created based on the values supported by the possibilities.

The pseudocode above was provided by an event predictor that computes event support for different event classes. Finally, an event is chosen as a possible event that generates a result.

ALGORITHM 2: TA-Disease Prone Factor

Input: preprocessed dataset $R - F_{ds}$
Output: Cardiac influence rate CIR→ F_{vs}

Step 1: Initialize data source from cardiac collective source $R - F_{ds}$
Step 2: Calculate the value of each source S.
For individual sequences, l
Step 3: Compute decision statements
For each Decision node
Step 4: Calculate recurrent comparisons based on distance vector approximation

$$Size_{(N)}$$

If F_v (frequent vector similarities)$\left(\mathbb{R}_{F\_ds}\right) \in s$, then

$$i = 1$$

Count = count +1.

Compute feature limits $F_{li} = \frac{\mathbb{F}_{\mathbb{V}}(\text{pi} + \text{AmR})}{\mathbb{F}_{\mathbb{V}}(\text{marginal weight})} \times \mathbb{F}_{\mathbb{V}}(F_{li})$ (18.1)

Compute spatial data forum Information data rate as IrPl.

$$\text{IrPl} = \frac{\mathbb{F}_{\mathbb{V}}(1-1)(\text{Lower}_{limit})}{\mathbb{F}_{\mathbb{V}}(1-1)(\text{marginal}_{\text{weight}})} \times \mathbb{F}_{\mathbb{V}}(1-1)(F_{li}) \quad (18.2)$$

Step 5: Compute mean cumulative index CI from an average mean rate of Event value

$$\text{Compute cardiac} - \text{I.R.} = \mathbb{C}_{\mathbb{I}} / \text{IrPl} \quad (18.3)$$

End

End

Step 6: Calculate the Cardiac Influence Rate (CIR).

$$\text{CIR} = \left(\frac{\text{Fv}(Upper_{limit})}{\text{Fv}(\text{marginal}_{\text{weight}})} \times \mathbb{F}_{\mathbb{V}}(F_{li}) \right) \times \text{Std}(\mathbb{I}_{\mathbb{R}}) \left(\frac{\text{Fv}(\text{Upper}_{\text{limit}})}{\text{Fv}(\text{marginal}_{\text{weight}})} \times \text{F}_{\text{V}}(\text{F}_{\text{li}}) \right) \times \text{Std}(\text{I}_{\text{R}}) \left(\frac{\text{Fv}(\text{Upper}_{\text{limit}})}{\text{Fv}(\text{marginal}_{\text{weight}})} \times \text{F}_{\text{V}}(\text{F}_{\text{li}}) \right) \times \text{Std}(\text{I}_{\text{R}}) \quad (18.4)$$

If CIR >Immunity margin, then

Add to Future vulnerable set Fv s $= \sum(\text{Sources} \in V_s) \cup s$

End

Stop

18.3.3 Disease Feature Pattern (DFP)

A DT is a tree-shaped model that when represented visually, uses decision rules to map data to its real target classes in a top-down manner. One prevalent supervised learning method appropriate for classification problems can accommodate constant and categorical-dependent variables. It concerns dividing the population into two or more equally sized sets based on the most significant liberated variable elements.

Entropy: It describes the amount of uncertainty in D.

Formula for two sections:

Information Gain: The information gain is calculated to determine the next split's attributes.

Gain=Entropy (D)-I (Attribute). Let assuming that, k_m logarithm process, $\mathcal{E}_i, z_i$ are the positive classes $(\text{i} = 1,2,3\ldots\text{n})$

Entropy level check

Level 1 entropy

$$\mathcal{E}_1 = \sum_{\mathcal{E}1=1} -(z_0) * k_m(z_1) + (z_1) * k_m(z_1) + \mathrm{F}_{\mathrm{vs}} \tag{18.5}$$

Level 2 entropy

$$\mathcal{E}_2 = \sum_{\mathcal{E}2=2} (z_0) * k_m(z_0) - (z_0) * k_m(z_0) + \mathrm{F}_{\mathrm{vs}} \tag{18.7}$$

Level 3 entropy

$$\mathcal{E}_3 = \sum_{\mathcal{E}3=3} \frac{-(z_0) * k_m(z_0)}{(z_1) * k_m(z_1)} + \mathrm{F}_{\mathrm{vs}} \tag{18.8}$$

Level 4 entropy

$$\mathcal{E}_4 = \sum_{\mathcal{E}4=4} (z_0) * k_m(z_0) + (z_1) * k_m(z_1)\mathrm{F}_{\mathrm{vs}} \tag{18.9}$$

Level 5 entropy

$$\mathcal{E}_5 = \sum_{\mathcal{E}5=5} -(z_0) * k_m(z_0) * (z_0) * k_m(z_0) + \mathrm{F}_{\mathrm{vs}} \tag{18.10}$$

Level 6 entropy

$$\mathcal{E}6 = \sum_{\mathcal{E}=6} (z_0) * k_m(z_0) * (z_0) + \mathrm{F}_{\mathrm{vs}} \tag{18.11}$$

Level 7 entropy

$$\mathcal{E}7 = \sum_{\mathcal{E}=7} (z_0) + k_m(z_0) * (z_0) * k_m(z_0) + \mathrm{F}_{\mathrm{vs}} \tag{18.12}$$

Here $\mathcal{E}_i, \mathcal{E}_j$ is gross entropy

$$\mathcal{E}_i = \sum_{\mathcal{E}=1\,to\,4} = k_m(\mathcal{E}_i^1) + k_m(\mathcal{E}_j^2) + k_m(\mathcal{E}_i^3) + k_m(\mathcal{E}_j^4) \tag{18.13}$$

$$\mathcal{E} = \sum_{\mathcal{E}=5\,to\,7} = k_m(\mathcal{E}_i^5) + k_m(\mathcal{E}_j^6) + k_m(\mathcal{E}_i^7) \tag{18.14}$$

Finally, entropy values are $\mathcal{E}_n$ heart disease prediction

$$\mathcal{E}_{n=} \int k_m(\mathcal{E}_i + \mathcal{E}_j) \tag{18.15}$$

DT Algorithm 3 implementation steps are provided.

ALGORITHM 3: Disease Feature Pattern

Step 1: Input dataset Entropy (S)
$S = \mathcal{E}_n$

Step 2: Feature select s Entropy (A)
Get feature selection output

Step 3: Pass the entropy values
$if_{entropy} = DT_{classifier}$

$$\left(\begin{array}{l}\text{Criterion} = \text{"entropy"} random_{state} = 1000, \max_{dep} th \\ = 5, \min_{samples\_leaf} = 3\end{array}\right)$$

$c_{if\_entropy fit}\left(x_{train} y_{train}\right)$

Step 4: Lastly, entropy with exactness
$y_{pred\_en} = C_{if_{entropy}\_predict}\left(x_{test}\right)$

Step 5: y_{pred_en}

Step 6: $\left(Print\ accuracy\ score\left(y_{test} y_{pred_{en}}\right)\right)$

Step 7: $e_m = accuracy\_score\left(y_{test} y_{pred_{en}}\right)$

e_m is a final result classification that categorizes data items into several target classes. Classification approaches assess how effectively the algorithm can assign target class labels to each incoming data set. In this situation, using a variety of risk indicators, classification algorithms are utilized to determine a person's propensity for heart failure. We use 200 of the 299 samples as training data and the other 99 as testing data before using these algorithms for classification.

18.3.4 Grey Wolf Optimized with SVM (GWO-SVM)

The GWO algorithm is a meta-heuristic search that mimics grey wolves' behavior as they explore, hunt, and encircle their prey. These wolves stalk their prey by surrounding them. The mathematical procedure for this behavior is as follows:

$$DS =\mid CD.XY_P - XY\left(temp\right) + Em \tag{18.16}$$

$$XY\left(temp+1\right) =\mid XY_p - XY\left(temp\right) - AB.DS \tag{18.17}$$

XY_P $\vec{X}$ signifies the prey's location, and Y denotes the grey wolf's position in numerous iterations. The coefficient vector is then formed.

$$\text{AB} = \left|2\,\text{ab.RND1} - \text{ab}\right| \tag{18.18}$$

$$\text{CD} = \left|2.\text{RND2}\right| \tag{18.19}$$

where *RND*1 *and RND*2 $\vec{2}$ are random vectors in (0 1). *aa* specifies movement, which is reducing linearly from the value two to 0 on diverse iterations:

$$a_a = 2 - temp * \frac{2}{\pi} \tag{18.20}$$

The ideal position of a grey wolf can be adjusted by altering its vector value.

$$A_B \; and \; C_D$$

These characters specify the solution, and the remaining wolves are transferred based on the three keys ($X\vec{X}$ 1, $X\vec{X}$ $\vec{2}$, 3). Furthermore, these are exposed in the form of the following equations.

$$XX(temp+1) = \frac{XX_1 + XX_2 + XX_3}{3} \tag{18.21}$$

$$XX_1 = XX_\alpha - AB_{1.}(DS_\alpha = |CD.XX_\alpha - XX| \tag{18.22}$$

$$XX_2 = XX_\beta - AB_{2.}(DS_\beta = |CD.XX_\beta - XX| \tag{18.23}$$

$$XX_3 = XX_\delta - AB_3(DS_\delta = |CD.XX_\alpha - XX| \tag{18.24}$$

The α and δ each wolf stays behind to hunt prey and provide protection in case of prey attack, AB1. The system can process any value that falls outside the range of -1 to 1.

$$Q(x_i x) = \varnothing(x_i)\varnothing(x) \tag{18.25}$$

In the near kernel function $Q(x_i x)$, the original data space is transformed into a higher-dimensional area using a dot product transformation function for easier data segmentation. Boost is a meta-algorithm that combines weak learners to enhance accuracy and ease data essentials. Momentum methods aim to improve prediction accuracy.

Step 1: Let p be positive and g be negative and then take a sample (S_i, y_i) and

$W_j = \frac{1}{2}$ is a sample input dataset, and T be the final iteration.

Step 2: The normalized $w_{i,j} \leftarrow w_{i,j}$ is the prospect of distribution, and *N* is the number of features.

$$\xi_t = \sum_r w_{i,j} |h_1(x_1) - y_1| 2 \tag{18.26}$$

Step 3: Least classification error is

$$W_1 = \frac{1}{2} \ln \left[\frac{1}{\xi_t^l} - 1 \right] \tag{18.27}$$

Step 4: Normalized weight calculated equation

$$w_{t+1,j} = w_{i,j}e^{-w}\,{}_{1}^{1}h\left(S^{1}\right) \tag{18.28}$$

Finalized fearer selection hypothesis

$$H\left(S\right) = \operatorname{sgn}\sum_{t-1}^{T} w_{1}e^{-w}\,{}_{1}^{1}h\left(S^{1}\right) \tag{18.29}$$

The following equations illustrate how the maximum distance between the hyperplane and the boundary becomes an optimization problem:

$$w^{T}x + k = 0$$

$$\min = \frac{1}{2}\left(w^{T}w\right) \tag{18.30}$$

$$y_{i}\left(w^{T}x_{i} + k\right) > 1 \tag{18.31}$$

Here $w^{T}x + k$ is the regularization parameter of the respective positive and negative support vectors.

The succeeding equation represents the contour:

$$\frac{w}{\|w\|}\left(x_{+}\right) - \left(x_{+}\right) = \frac{w^{t}\left(\left(x_{+}\right) - \left(x_{+}\right)\right)}{\|w\|} = \frac{2}{\|w\|} \tag{18.32}$$

The following formula expresses the classifier as a sum of support vectors

$$f\left(x\right) = \operatorname{sgn}\langle\sum_{i=1}^{N} y_{i}\alpha_{i}Q(+x) + b) \tag{18.33}$$

Here, x_i is the SVM data, N is the number ship class, and $Q\left(x_{i}, x\right)$ is the linear kernel equation.

18.3.5 LSTM-Gated Optimized with Multi-perceptron Neural Network (LSTMG-MPNN)

To effectively analyze sequence data at different time intervals using LSTM, introduce an adjusted LSTM unit thresholding system that detects temporal components. We suggest using the target regression prediction method in the hidden layer output at each time step. This will enable accurate performance measurements over a series of different periods. The model's output layer is activated with a sigmoid function, enabling multiple diagnostic label predictions for a patient. To classify the data, heart rate and cholesterol values were selected as significant risk factors for atherosclerosis.

The LSTM unit receives an input x_t and the previous output h_{t-1}, which results in a memory unit. The device also features input and output gates that act on it. Each LSTM cell has a forgetting gate f_t and a set of operations to perform represented by o_t.

1. Control which data to delete from the memory vector. Where b_f is a bias, and w_f is a set of weights.

$$\mathcal{C}_{T-1} using\ \mathcal{C}_{T-1}\ and h_{t-1} : f_t = f_{\left(w_f[h_{t-1x}]+b_f\right)}$$

2. Using x_t and h_{t-1}, create a matrix that allows updating specific information in $\left(\mathcal{C}_{T-1}\right)$.

$$i_t = fun^c{}_{\left(W_i \cdot \left(h_{t-1}x\right)+b_i\right)}.$$

3. Use *xt* and *ht*−1 to gather the information that should be included.

$$C_t = fun^c{}_{\left(W_i \cdot \left(h_{t-1}x+b_c\right)\right)}.$$

4. To translate, it is essential to integrate both new and extant data.

$$C_t = .C_{t-1} + i_t.C_t$$

5. Constant gradient decline can be implemented and trained to determine information that has been ignored, kept, or maintained.

It is necessary to process them before starting the forward propagation of the LSTM network to calculate the forgetting threshold. This threshold helps determine which input information should be forgotten and not impact future time steps. The 3D vector is smoothed between time steps t-1 and t to achieve this. Equation (18.34) is shown as the time vector is manipulated to become the input parameter of the output gate.

$$f_{(t)} = \left(w_{f[h_{t-1x}]+b_f}\right) + f_{(x)} \tag{18.34}$$

$$f_{(t)} = \left(w_{f[h_{t-1x}]+b_f} P_{\Delta t-1} \mathrm{t} + \mathrm{bf}\right) + f_{(x)} \tag{18.35}$$

The vector after smoothing the time interval between time slices is denoted as shown in Equation (18.35) using the smoothing formula.

$$P_{\Delta t-1} = \left(\frac{\Delta t-1}{60}, \left(\frac{\Delta t-1}{180}\right)^2, \left(\frac{\Delta t-1}{365}\right)^3\right) + f_{(x)} \tag{18.36}$$

In Equation (18.36), $\Delta t - 1$ represents the period interval in units of days. Use two-month, six-month, and one-year classes for infrequent patient withdrawals.

$$P_{\Delta t-1} \textit{within a reasonable range}$$

$$\widetilde{C}_t = \tanh_{f0}\left(w_c\left[h_{t-1}, x_t\right] + b_c\right) + f_{(x)} \tag{18.37}$$

$$C_t = f_t * C_{t-1} i_t * \widetilde{C}_t \; f_{(x)} \tag{18.38}$$

To update the transient state, we use the connection weights (w_c) and offsets (b_c) along with a temporary condition ($\tilde{c}_t$) that contains a new candidate value. The previous step's state information is stored in $\tilde{c}_{t-1}$, and c_t represents the updated time step.

The third forward propagation step determines the final network output, as shown in Equation (18.38).

$$h = \mathcal{O}_t * \tan h_{f_0} c_t \tag{18.39}$$

Where *ht* is the current hidden state and *ht*, and *Ct* will be used as input for the next step. The present study focuses on alternative methods for predicting heart disease in smart cities. It focuses on MLP, an artificial neural network (ANN) with three layers of nodes: input, hidden, and output. MLP employs a backpropagation algorithm and is trained using the backpropagation (BP) supervised learning method. The study also employed a technique for interpreting MLP in terms of BP.

The bias is represented by unit weights initialized with small random integers. The input data is passed directly to the network layer without changes. Each input is then linked to a hidden layer through weighted connections. An input unit provides the output that relates to it. To obtain the sum of the information, we multiply every input by the weight associated with it and add the consequences.

Here I_j is the multiple input and corresponding weight is to be calculated, O_j is the output, and each connection is connected to the related weight to be summarized.

$$\mathrm{I_j} = \sum_{\mathrm{i}} \mathrm{W_{ij}} \mathcal{O}_{\mathrm{i}} + \varnothing_{\mathrm{j+h}} \tag{18.40}$$

Here $W_{ij}\mathcal{O}_i$-weight and node-i and j, and $\mathcal{O}_i$-output of the bias nodes. Then logical functions are mapped with the smaller range of the process, and the function is usually 0 to 1.

Output node $\mathcal{O}_j$ is designed as,

$$\mathcal{O}_j = \frac{1}{1 + e^{-1} j} \tag{18.41}$$

Finally, apply the MLPNN algorithm to adjust the weights,

$$Err_j = \mathcal{O}_j\left(1 - \mathcal{O}_j\right)\left(T_j - 1\right) \tag{18.42}$$

Here $\mathcal{O}_j$ is the real output node j.

T_j is the target output node j.

The error can be estimated as a hidden layer

$$\mathrm{Err_j} = \mathcal{O}_\mathrm{j}\left(1-\mathcal{O}_\mathrm{j}\right)\sum_k Err_k \mathrm{W_{jk}} \tag{18.43}$$

Here W_{jk} is the connection node weight from node j to k. The consequence has been updated as follows:

$$\Delta \mathrm{W_{ij}} = (l)\,\mathrm{Err_j}\mathcal{O}_\mathrm{j} \tag{18.44}$$

$$\mathrm{W_{ij}} = \mathrm{W_{ij}} + \Delta \mathrm{W_{ij}} \tag{18.45}$$

Here l is the learning rate.

The bias adopted is as follows

$$\Delta \mathcal{O}_\mathrm{j} = (l)\,\mathrm{Err_j} \tag{18.46}$$

$$\mathcal{O}_\mathrm{j} = \mathcal{O}_\mathrm{j} + \Delta \mathcal{O}_\mathrm{j} \tag{18.47}$$

Finally, improving performance standards through standardization MLP with standardization technique accurately forecasts heart illness due to real-world heart disease data in smart cities. We present two approaches to address this problem and categorize cardiac diseases using MLP.

18.4 Results and Discussion

The results and discussion section discusses heart disease prediction for smart cities. Our comparison of the previous methods, DT, SVM, and RF, is used. Still, compared to the previous way of optimizing with LSTMG-MPNN, the proposed system has the most accurate results for accuracy, precision, and recall F score. We use Kaggle data. The dataset has been taken, and the dataset is called "heart.csv." The tools employed here are detailed in Table 18.2.

Based on all the information collected, the features of the dataset are described. Here, we discuss the confusion matrix solution for heart disease prediction and the following image for the confusion matrix of forecasts in Figure 18.3.

Figure 18.4 illustrates the precision calculated for heart disease prediction compared with various algorithms. The DT performance of the precision is 79%, the SVM performance of the precision is 89%, the RF performance of precision is 93%, and the proposed LSTMG-MPNN is 95.9%. The proposed system is the most effective result for precision.

$$\text{Precision} = \frac{\text{True positive}}{\text{True positive} + \text{False positive}}$$

TABLE 18.2

Simulation Parameters

Parameter	Method
Language	Python
Tools	Anaconda
Dataset	Heart.csv
Records size	30 kb
Total records	1000

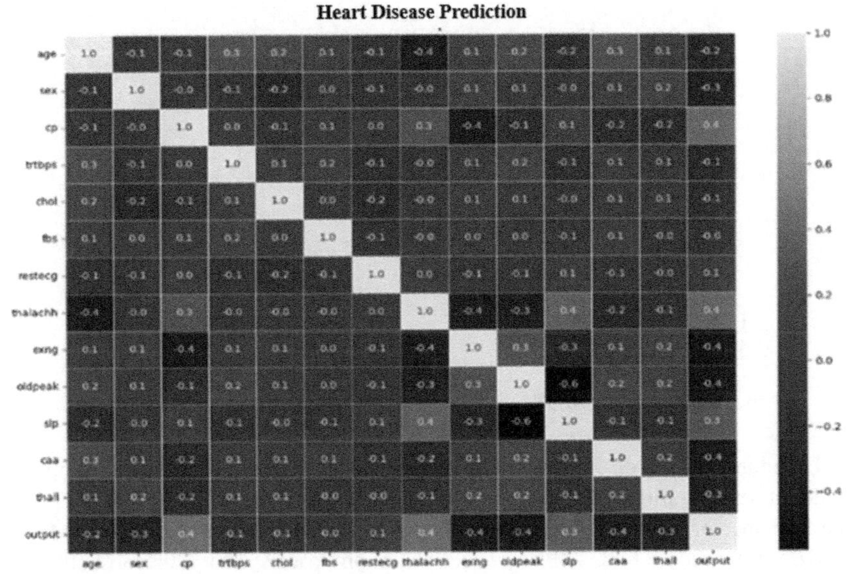

FIGURE 18.3 Confusion matrix.

The precision measurement value is precision = to 95.9%,

$$\text{Recall} = \frac{\text{True postive}}{\text{true postive} + \text{False negative}}$$

Recall measurement values are Recall = 96.1 %.

18.4.1 F1-Measure

The F1 measurement for heart disease prediction for ML and DP learning methods is based on calculation. Multiply the precision and recall values, then add the precision and recall values, then divide the upper and lower values. Finally, measure the F1-measure value for the percentage.

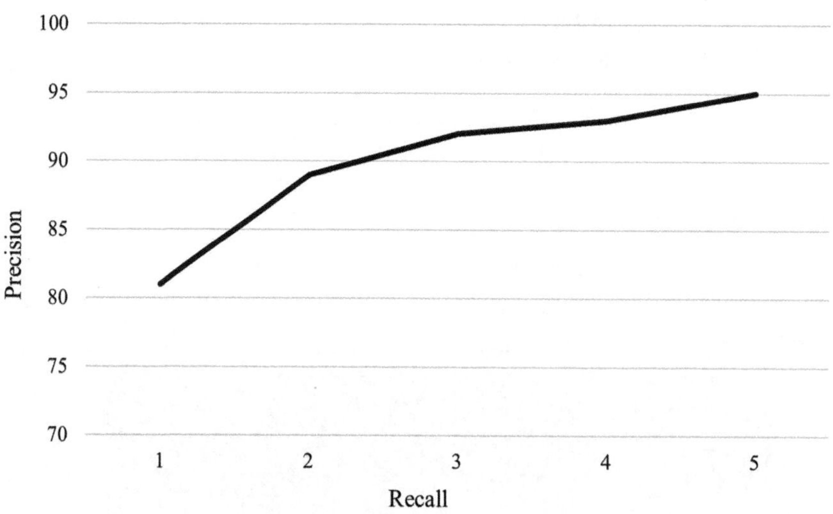

FIGURE 18.4 Precision and recall.

$$F1 = \frac{\text{precision X recall}}{\text{recall} + \text{precision}}$$

$$\text{F1 measure values} = 96.5\%$$

In Figure 18.5, the F-measure calculated for heart disease prediction is compared with various algorithms. The DT performance of the F-measure is 79%, the SVM performance of the F-measure is 89%, the RF performance of the F-measure is 92%, and the proposed LSTMG-MPNN is 96.5%. The proposed system is the most effective result for F-measure.

18.4.2 LSTMG-MPNN Algorithm

This category uses various methods to analyze the algorithm in the proposed system. The DT algorithm, SVM algorithm, and RF are compared with the developed system. Specifically, the LSTMG-MPNN proposed system is compared with RF. LSTMG-MPNN is the most significant achievement in heart disease prediction accuracy.

Table 18.3 and Figure 18.6 show algorithm accuracy: the DT accuracy is 93.5, the SVM accuracy is 94.5%, the RF accuracy is 95.1%, and the proposed LSTMG-MPNN accuracy is 96.5%. Finally, accuracy is given by the LSTMG-MPNN algorithm of the ML method.

Figure 18.7 shows performances based on precision, recall, and F1-measure, three-in-one compression. All the DT algorithms, SVMs, RF algorithms, and LSTMG-MPNN methods are compared, but the proposed LSTMG-MPNN system has the most excellent results and accuracy.

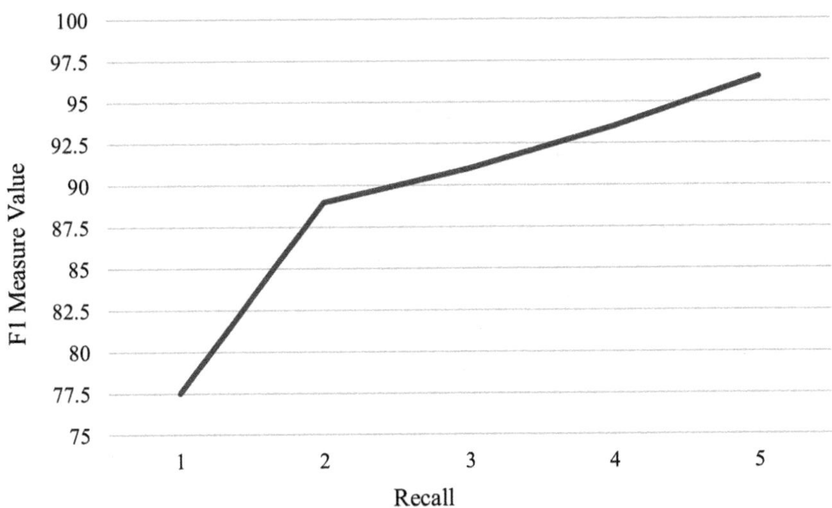

FIGURE 18.5 F-measure and recall.

TABLE 18.3
Proposed System Accuracy

Method	Accuracy (%)
DT	90.5
SVM	92.5
RF	94.1
LSTMG-MPNN	96.6

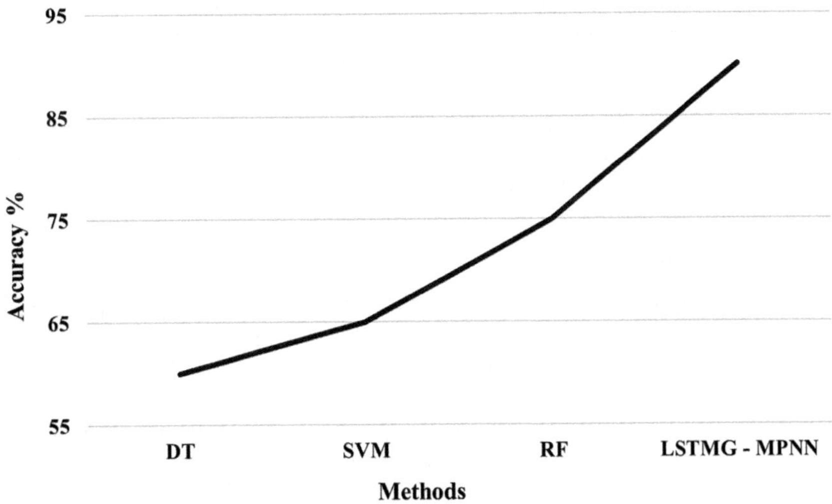

FIGURE 18.6 Proposed system-based accuracy.

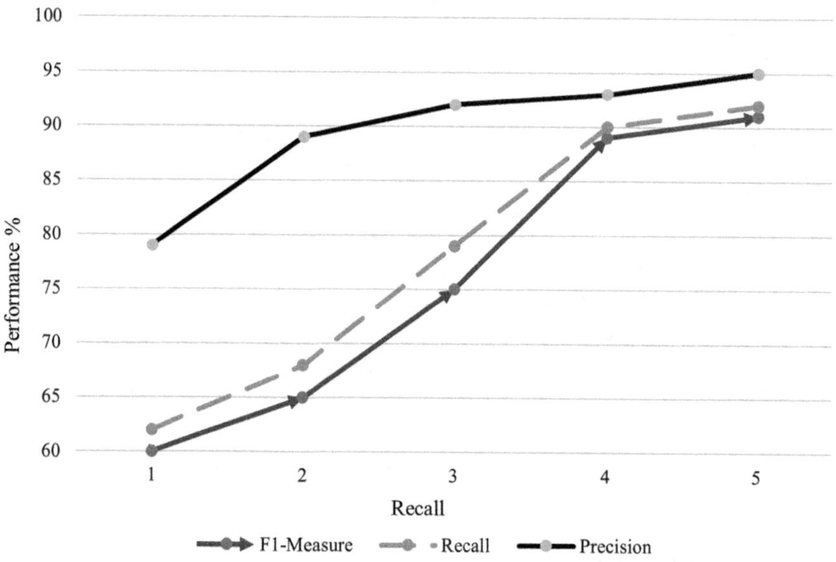

FIGURE 18.7 Performance algorithm based on precision and recall and F1-measure.

18.5 Conclusion

In this chapter, a method has been developed using LSTMG-MPNN to predict the development of heart disease in smart city. Before classification, the preprocessing stage uses Z-score normalization to get data from the dataset. After the feature section, with GWO-SVM optimizations, select the medical data feature. A classification method based on LSTMG-MPNN is used to classify feature selection data, and then feature selection is used to find and determine whether diseases have been found or not. Compared to other existing approaches, the proposed system achieves higher performance. The disease prediction accuracy is attained at up to 96.5%, as is the precision rate at up to 95.9%, recall at 96.1%, and F-measure at 96.5% with redundant time complexity. Identification supports early disease prediction for recommendations for diagnosis and treatment. In the future, further enhancements will be based on various methods for finding missing information or missing data.

REFERENCES

Abdar, M., U. R. Acharya, N. Sarrafzadegan and V. Makarenkov, "NE-nu-SVC: A New Nested Ensemble Clinical Decision Support System for Effective Diagnosis of Coronary Artery Disease," *IEEE Access*, vol. *7*, pp. 167605–167620, 2019, doi: 10.1109/ACCESS.2019.2953920.

Abdellatif, A., H. Abdellatef, J. Kanesan, C.-O. Chow, J. H. Chuah and H. M. Gheni, "Improving the Heart Disease Detection and Patients' Survival Using Supervised Infinite Feature Selection and Improved Weighted Random Forest," *IEEE Access*, vol. *10*, pp. 67363–67372, 2022a, doi: 10.1109/ACCESS.2022.3185129.

Abdellatif, A., H. Abdellatef, J. Kanesan, C.-O. Chow, J. H. Chuah and H. M. Gheni, "An Effective Heart Disease Detection and Severity Level Classification Model Using Machine Learning and Hyperparameter Optimization Methods," *IEEE Access*, vol. *10*, pp. 79974–79985, 2022b, doi: 10.1109/ACCESS.2022.3191669.

Abubaker, M. B. and B. Babayigit, "Detection of Cardiovascular Diseases in ECG Images Using Machine Learning and Deep Learning Methods," *IEEE Transactions on Artificial Intelligence*, vol. *4*, no. 2, pp. 373–382, 2023, doi: 10.1109/TAI.2022.3159505.

Ali, S. N., S. B. Shuvo, M. I. S. Al-Manzo, A. Hasan and T. Hasan, "An End-to-End Deep Learning Framework for Real-Time Denoising of Heart Sounds for Cardiac Disease Detection in Unseen Noise," *IEEE Access*, vol. *11*, pp. 87887–87901, 2023, doi: 10.1109/ACCESS.2023.3292551.

Bhaskarpandit, S., A. Gade, S. Dash, D. K. Dash, R. K. Tripathy and R. B. Pachori, "Detection of Myocardial Infarction From 12-Lead ECG Trace Images Using Eigendomain Deep Representation Learning," *IEEE Transactions on Instrumentation and Measurement*, vol. *72*, pp. 1–12, 2023, Art no. 4001812, doi: 10.1109/TIM.2023.3241986.

Farag, M. M., "A Self-Contained STFT CNN for ECG Classification and Arrhythmia Detection at the Edge," *IEEE Access*, vol. *10*, pp. 94469–94486, 2022, doi: 10.1109/ACCESS.2022.3204703.

Ferdousi, R., M. A. Hossain and A. E. Saddik, "Early-Stage Risk Prediction of Non-Communicable Disease Using Machine Learning in Health CPS," *IEEE Access*, vol. *9*, pp. 96823–96837, 2021, doi: 10.1109/ACCESS.2021.3094063.

Fitriyani, N. L., M. Syafrudin, G. Alfian and J. Rhee, "HDPM: An Effective Heart Disease Prediction Model for a Clinical Decision Support System," *IEEE Access*, vol. *8*, pp. 133034–133050, 2020, doi: 10.1109/ACCESS.2020.3010511.

Gjoreski, M., A. Gradisek, B. Budna, M. Gams and G. Poglajen, "Machine Learning and End-to-End Deep Learning for the Detection of Chronic Heart Failure From Heart Sounds," *IEEE Access*, vol. *8*, pp. 20313–20324, 2020, doi: 10.1109/ACCESS.2020.2968900.

Guo, C., J. Zhang, Y. Liu, Y. Xie, Z. Han and J. Yu, "Recursion Enhanced Random Forest With an Improved Linear Model (RERF-ILM) for Heart Disease Detection on the Internet of Medical Things Platform," *IEEE Access*, vol. *8*, pp. 59247–59256, 2020, doi: 10.1109/ACCESS.2020.2981159.

Gupta, K., V. Bajaj and I. A. Ansari, "An Improved Deep Learning Model for Automated Detection of BBB Using S-T Spectrograms of Smoothed VCG Signal," *IEEE Sensors Journal*, vol. *22*, no. 9, pp. 8830–8837, May 1, 2022, doi: 10.1109/JSEN.2022.3162022.

Hussain, M. W., & Roy, D. S. (2023). Performance Optimization Strategies for Big Data Applications in Distributed Framework. In *Intelligent Technologies: Concepts, Applications, and Future Directions, Volume 2* (pp. 221–252). Singapore: Springer Nature Singapore.

M. Jafari Tadi et al., "Comprehensive Analysis of Cardiogenic Vibrations for Automated Detection of Atrial Fibrillation Using Smartphone Mechanocardiograms," *IEEE Sensors Journal*, vol. *19*, no. 6, pp. 2230–2242, 2019, doi: 10.1109/JSEN.2018.2882874.

Javeed, A., S. Zhou, L. Yongjian, I. Qasim, A. Noor and R. Nour, "An Intelligent Learning System Based on Random Search Algorithm and Optimized Random Forest Model for Improved Heart Disease Detection," *IEEE Access*, vol. *7*, pp. 180235–180243, 2019, doi: 10.1109/ACCESS.2019.2952107.

Karhade, J., S. Dash, S. K. Ghosh, D. K. Dash and R. K. Tripathy, "Time–Frequency-Domain Deep Learning Framework for the Automated Detection of Heart Valve

Disorders Using PCG Signals," *IEEE Transactions on Instrumentation and Measurement*, vol. *71*, pp. 1–11, 2022, Art no. 2506311, doi: 10.1109/TIM.2022.3163156.

Kim, S., J.-O. Hahn and B. D. Youn, "Deep Learning-Based Diagnosis of Peripheral Artery Disease via Continuous Property-Adversarial Regularization: Preliminary in Silico Study," *IEEE Access*, vol. *9*, pp. 127433–127443, 2021, doi: 10.1109/ACCESS.2021.3112678.

Lai, D., Y. Zhang, X. Zhang, Y. Su and M. B. Bin Heyat, "An Automated Strategy for Early Risk Identification of Sudden Cardiac Death by Using Machine Learning Approach on Measurable Arrhythmic Risk Markers," *IEEE Access*, vol. *7*, pp. 94701–94716, 2019, doi: 10.1109/ACCESS.2019.292584.

Lakshmanarao, A., A. Srisaila and T. S. R. Kiran, "Heart Disease Prediction using Feature Selection and Ensemble Learning Techniques," *2021 Third International Conference on Intelligent Communication Technologies and Virtual Mobile Networks (ICICV)*, Tirunelveli, India, 2021, pp. 994–998, doi: 10.1109/ICICV50876.2021.9388482.

Li, H. et al., "Dual-Input Neural Network Integrating Feature Extraction and Deep Learning for Coronary Artery Disease Detection Using Electrocardiogram and Phonocardiogram," *IEEE Access*, vol. *7*, pp. 146457–146469, 2019, doi: 10.1109/ACCESS.2019.2943197.

Mehrang, S. et al., "Classification of Atrial Fibrillation and Acute Decompensated Heart Failure Using Smartphone Mechanocardiography: A Multilabel Learning Approach," *IEEE Sensors Journal*, vol. *20*, no. 14, pp. 7957–7968, 2020, doi: 10.1109/JSEN.2020.2981334.

Ning, W., S. Li, D. Wei, L. Z. Guo and H. Chen, "Automatic Detection of Congestive Heart Failure Based on a Hybrid Deep Learning Algorithm in the Internet of Medical Things," *IEEE Internet of Things Journal*, vol. *8*, no. 16, pp. 12550–12558, 2021, doi: 10.1109/JIOT.2020.3023105.

Padovano, D., A. Martinez-Rodrigo, J. M. Pastor, J. J. Rieta and R. Alcaraz, "On the Generalization of Sleep Apnea Detection Methods Based on Heart Rate Variability and Machine Learning," *IEEE Access*, vol. *10*, pp. 92710–92725, 2022, doi: 10.1109/ACCESS.2022.3201911.

Pathak, A., K. Mandana and G. Saha, "Ensembled Transfer Learning and Multiple Kernel Learning for Phonocardiogram Based Atherosclerotic Coronary Artery Disease Detection," *IEEE Journal of Biomedical and Health Informatics*, vol. *26*, no. 6, pp. 2804–2813, 2022, doi: 10.1109/JBHI.2022.3140277.

Pradhan, B., M. W. Hussain, G. Srivastava, M. K. Debbarma, R. K. Barik, and J. C. W. Lin (2022). *A Neuro-Evolutionary Approach for Software Defined Wireless Network Traffic Classification. IET Communications.*

Procházka, A., H. Charvátová, S. Vaseghi and O. Vyšata, "Machine Learning in Rehabilitation Assessment for Thermal and Heart Rate Data Processing," *IEEE Transactions on Neural Systems and Rehabilitation Engineering*, vol. *26*, no. 6, pp. 1209–1214, 2018, doi: 10.1109/TNSRE.2018.2831444.

Reddy, K. H. K., Roy, D. S., Mishra, T. K., & Hussain, M. W. (Eds.). (2023). *Handbook of Research on Network-Enabled IoT Applications for Smart City Services*. IGI Global.

A. Rizwan et al., "A Review on the State of the Art in Atrial Fibrillation Detection Enabled by Machine Learning," *IEEE Reviews in Biomedical Engineering*, vol. *14*, pp. 219–239, 2021, doi: 10.1109/RBME.2020.2976507.

Roy, A. and U. Satija, "A Novel Melspectrogram Snippet Representation Learning Framework for Severity Detection of Chronic Obstructive Pulmonary Diseases," *IEEE Transactions on Instrumentation and Measurement*, vol. *72*, pp. 1–11, 2023, Art no. 4003311, doi: 10.1109/TIM.2023.3256468.

Wang, Y., G. Faragallah, E. Divo and M. A. Simaan, "Detection of ventricular suction in an implantable rotary blood pump using support vector machines," *2011 Annual International Conference of the IEEE Engineering in Medicine and Biology Society*, Boston, MA, USA, 2011, pp. 3318–3321, doi: 10.1109/IEMBS.2011.6090900.

Wang, J. et al., "Detecting Cardiovascular Disease from Mammograms With Deep Learning," *IEEE Transactions on Medical Imaging*, vol. *36*, no. 5, pp. 1172–1181, 2017, doi: 10.1109/TMI.2017.2655486.

Wen, X., Y. Huang, X. Wu and B. Zhang, "A Feasible Feature Extraction Method for Atrial Fibrillation Detection From BCG," *IEEE Journal of Biomedical and Health Informatics*, vol. *24*, no. 4, pp. 1093–1103, April 2020, doi: 10.1109/JBHI.2019.2927165.

Yang, H., Z. Chen, H. Yang and M. Tian, "Predicting Coronary Heart Disease Using an Improved LightGBM Model: Performance Analysis and Comparison," *IEEE Access*, vol. *11*, pp. 23366–23380, 2023, doi: 10.1109/ACCESS.2023.3253885.

19

A Novel MistFog Federated Learning Model for Heart Disease Detection in Smart Healthcare

Mir Wajahat Hussain
Alliance University, Anekal, India

19.1 Introduction

A convergent network infrastructure that links real-world and digital items is what the term Internet-of-Things (IoT) refers. Incorporating cutting-edge technologies like wireless sensor networks, wireless body area networks, wearable, and implantable sensors and more, IoT demonstrates its potential to address the concerns in smart cities where health is of primary focus (Reddy et al., 2023b). The use of a plethora of IoT sensors generates huge data and needs immediate processing because of latency-sensitive data (Hussain et al., 2024). Further, the data from the traditional IoT-based systems must be delivered from the gateway to the source. The services provided by the IoT sensors are stringent in nature and the demand is continuously increasing for huge processing (Ashu et al., 2020; Hussain et al., 2021a, 2021b).

Cloud computing (CC) is an ideal platform for addressing higher computational requirements and follows a pay-per-use model. CC has immense computational and network resources and can address issues of scalability, data analysis, and reliability in a promising manner (Reddy et al., 2023b). Latency-sensitive applications are hampered by the geographical centralization of cloud data centers, which necessitates transmitting sensor data across multi-hop distances for processing. Fog computing (FC) may be defined as a virtual platform that extends the CC paradigm to the edge of the network and reduces cloud responsibilities (Tripathy et al., 2022) can help improve the quality of services (QoS). Fog can be used to facilitate the delivery of a wide variety of cutting-edge services, including those that require low latency, geographically dispersed, or mobile-friendly architecture. FC requires several hops for an application for processing which is prohibitive. Mist computing (MC) is a newer paradigm which is closer to the gadgets that emanate data and requires fewer hops. In MC, information is gathered and processed locally before being sent to a server. The MC environment has less storage than CC, FC, and transport power for long-term analytical data. MC environments, which operate near the edge and physical devices, have been

DOI: 10.1201/9781032631738-19

successfully applied to several systems for improved performance in multiple applications (Tripathy et al., 2022).

A critical issue in the healthcare sector is the prediction of heart diseases. Such disease might cause other issues like abnormal heart rhythms, heart attack, stroke, etc. can almost affect a considerable population worldwide. A patient's life might be in jeopardy if the detection is not done aptly, and hence real-time monitoring needs to be done (Tuli et al., 2020). Thus heart disease prediction includes constant health monitoring while decreasing medical expenditures and the need arise to push notifications to the doctors. Despite the huge data emanated from the sensors, machine learning (ML) algorithms might play a pivotal role in the detection of early diseases and their remedy.

Several works have profoundly discussed heart diseases; however, the focus has mostly been on improving the prediction accuracy while utilizing multiple ML algorithms. Despite several works, prediction accuracy continues to be low, and automatic detection of the disease is still a far dream. Another important issue that is overlooked in heart disease is how to reduce the execution time of the prediction in a real-time manner. Thus, automatic heart disease prediction is still an unaddressed problem based on the improvement of prediction accuracy and execution time.

This chapter discusses the prediction of heart disease while utilizing a Mist-Fog-layered architecture. The contributions of the chapter are enumerated as follows: (i) A novel model of MistFog utilizes IoT sensors, mist nodes, and fog nodes for automatic prediction of heart disease. (ii) Federated learning model is used which in turn utilizes an ensemble model for disease prediction. (iii) The proposed MistFog utilizes federated learning which aggregates the obtained predicted model from the worker nodes at the cloud for improved accuracy and lowering of execution time. (iv) Proof-of-concept for MistFog shows the proposed model is much better in terms of network consumption and thus intuitively shows improved performance.

This chapter is organized as follows: Section 19.2 discusses the existing state-of-the-art for heart disease prediction and captures several network, computing paradigms and learning models. Section 19.3 captures the proposed MistFog model for healthcare. Mathematical analysis/proof-of-concept is described in Section 19.4. The chapter concludes with Section 19.5 which further describes further avenues of this research.

19.2 Introduction to Related Work

The chapter's related work section will likely discuss previous research into healthcare-related applications of the computing paradigms, federated learning, and the works attempted. It also includes the core technologies and discusses briefly which the foundation for the proposed methodology.

19.2.1 Cloud Computing

CC usually refers to providing a service via the Internet. This service can be pretty much anything, from business software that is accessed via the web to off-site storage or computing resources (Hussain et al., 2022a, 2022b). CC can be described as the practice of using a network of remote servers hosted on the Internet to store, manage, and process data instead of a local server or a personal computer. Cloud is fast owing to the improvements in the network technologies which connect the user with the fast servers which host the actual application. The user accessing the service and the cloud platform spanned over several data centers uses the best-effort Internet for this communication.

19.2.2 Fog Computing

The above limitations of the centralized paradigm are effectively handled with the use of FC. FC as per the OpenFog Consortium is defined as "a system-level horizontal architecture that distributes resources and services of computing, storage, control and networking anywhere along the continuum from cloud to Things". It is a geographically distributed computing paradigm where a myriad of heterogeneous devices are connected at edge levels and offer flexible network, computing, and storage services. FC extends the CC near the edge of the network and is complementary to CC. FC is suitable for applications in which users require immediate services. FC is ideal for applications that require minimum data transmission rate and network latency with a throughput which is higher (Reddy et al., 2023b).

The issue with FC is that it takes several hops to reach the nearby fog server which is itself prohibitive for data which requires pre-processing. With the pre-processing only the relevant data will be moved to the next stage and hence can be a boon for resource-constrained devices. In the healthcare sector, where data is collected across various IoT-enabled devices, FC provides a critical paradigm for effectively processing information. Compared to cloud-based data centers, the latency, delay, or response time attained via FC-permitted devices to handle cardiac patients' data is considerably shorter due to the close placement of these gadgets to IoT-enabled devices.

19.2.3 Mist Computing

MC is much closer to the source of data and is ideally designed for time-centric applications. These time-centric applications will facilitate the improvement of higher throughput and low latency. With the help of MC only data emanating from multiple devices will be pre-processed which will enable only useful data to be moved further and thus help the processing time and bandwidth. MC offers multiple services for resource-constrained devices, namely, power, communication, bandwidth, and memory. It also ensures the usage of resources in an optimal manner. The advantages of MC include quicker response time, light-weighted computing, and promising for local decisions (Tripathy et al., 2022). Figure 19.1 describes the overall scenario of the computing paradigms in the context of IoT-based applications. The nascent topic of MC has shown significant promise for processing data at the network's edge, closer to where the data is created, reducing latency and bandwidth requirements, and enhancing privacy and security. Several articles have been published on applying deep learning to healthcare data management, a relatively new research area. Using an MC approach, it proposes a platform for deep learning strategies on massive healthcare data. To process data in a resource-constrained environment close to where the data is created, MC blends CC and edge computing.

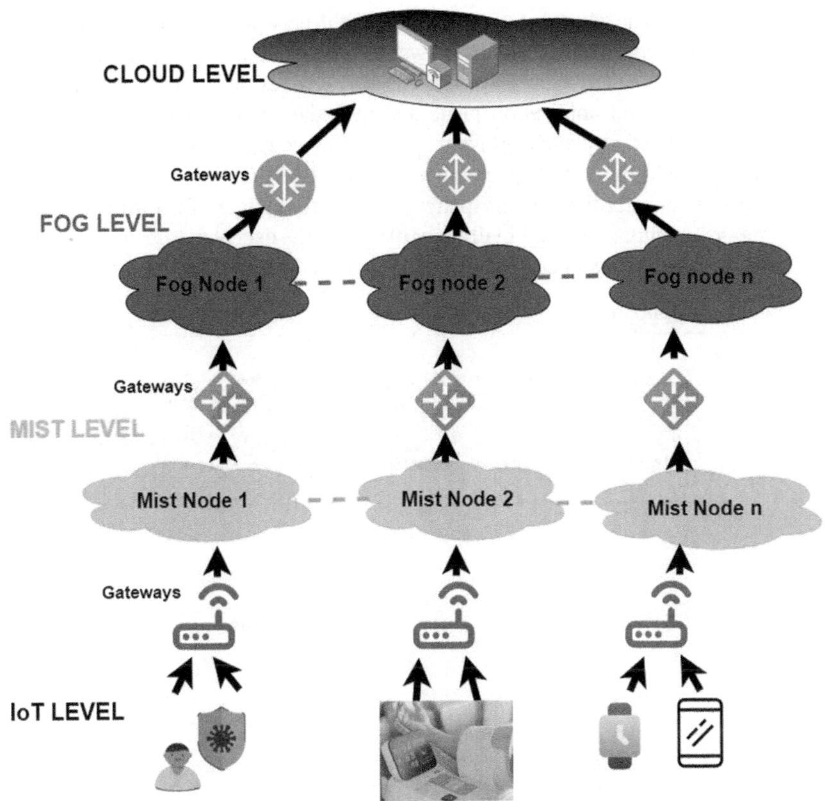

FIGURE 19.1 An overview of mist computing supported cloud computing framework.

19.2.4 Software-Defined Networking

In this world, the data generated continues to rise exponentially. This exponential rise of data is termed big data and requires an immense pool of computing resources which are met by a myriad of paradigms like CC, FC, and MC (Hussain et al., 2022b), (Hussain et al., 2020b). With this data generation, large data streams and data streams emanating from a large number of IoT devices connected to the Internet need to be pushed from to-fro which burdens the network (Hussain et al., 2021a). Erstwhile networks although handle several scenarios, there is a limit to the programmability. This paves the way to innovate the network to enable programmability and flexibility (Pradhan et al., 2022).

Software-defined networking (SDN) is regarded as the pioneer of the networking paradigm which has gained prominence in recent years (Hussain et al., 2020a, 2020b). The unique features of implementing customized policy make it more centric toward mass-scale deployment of complex systems. SDN's foundation is based on the separation of data and control plane (Hussain et al., 2021a, 2021b, 2021c). This separation is pertinent to application-aware networking and addressing the core requirements of today's network. The data plane enables forwarding of the data programmed entirely by the control plane. The control plane is the logic of the network and executes the required network-wide policy. The interaction between data and control plane is executed by a well-defined API called OpenFlow. OpenFlow enables the entire communication between the top-level application plane and the other two planes (control and data plane). The application plane deploys the network-wide policy. Application plane puts forth this policy to the control plane via northbound API (Hussain et al., 2022c). The control plane converts the network policy into rules which are forwarded to the data plane via the Southbound API. Finally, the rules from the data plane are clearly enforced and thus the data is forwarded. Figure 19.2 describes the overall planes of the SDN.

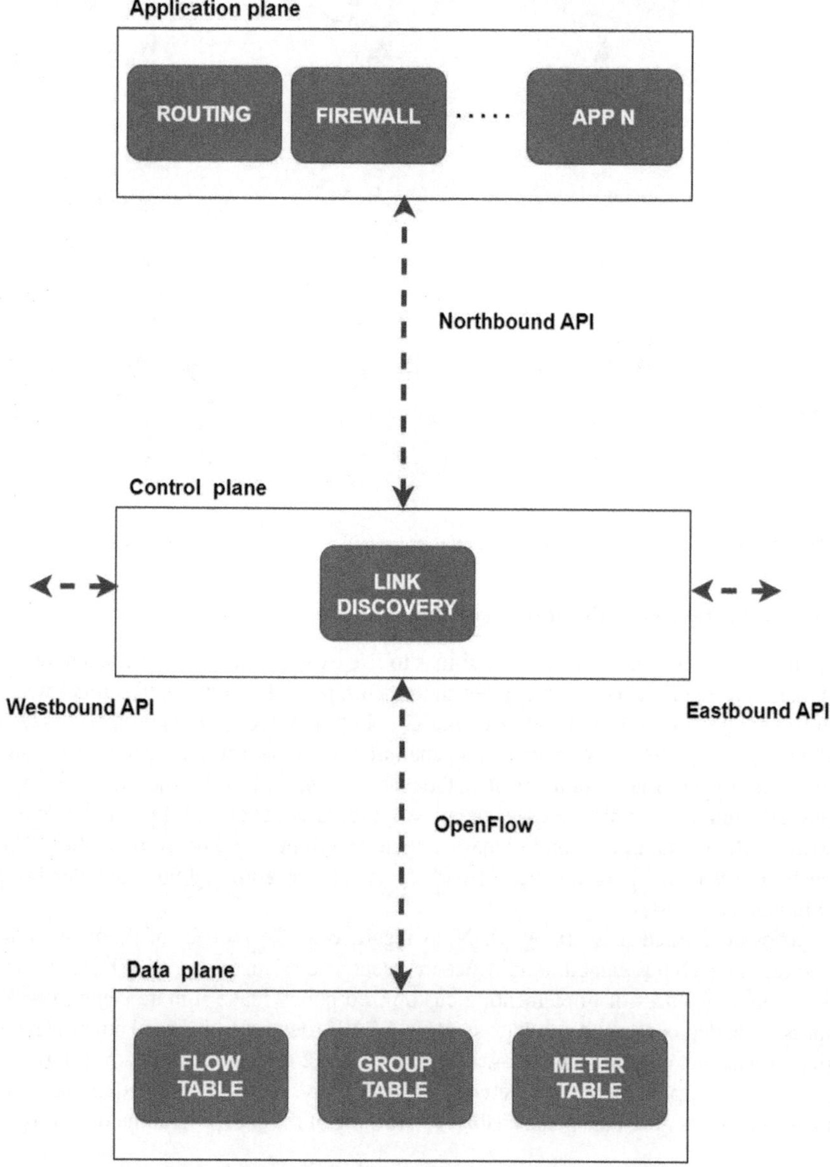

FIGURE 19.2 Overview of the SDN planar view.

19.2.5 Federated Learning

Federated learning is a type of novel machine learning technique which uses the distributed approach for creating the models (Li et al., 2020). Since FL uses the distributed approach of ML, so large number of distributed devices/servers can jointly form multiple models. FL is suitable where privacy and data diversity are of utmost concern, and when the datasets are available on an incremental basis (locally) rather than in a traditional centralized manner. The devices in FL learn locally and the global model is learnt by sending few pertinent parameters and this happens in a continuous manner. Further, the global model is initialized, created, and disseminated to all the devices which serves as a former step for the training process. The local model utilizes the local data for training the global data. The training model is further fine-tuned the global data by the knowledge updating of the specific characteristics and patterns (Zhang et al., 2021).

The local training is used for enhancing the model aggregation which is a sum of all the device insights. The central device/server for the FL captures the entire information available from all the devices. The entire process continues over multiple rounds which improves the global model entirely based on the information/intelligence over all the distributed devices participating.

19.2.6 Ensemble Model

Learning algorithms tend to operate in dynamic environments where the information is complex, and the data must be collected from a plethora of data streams. These data streams thus pose emerging challenges that traditional learning algorithms are incapable of efficiently like data changes over time, limited computational requirements. Ensemble methods have gained a lot of attraction to address diverse requirements and are promising. It is regarded as a powerful technique which combines several models to take an average model for higher accuracy and a stronger final prediction. Further ensembles not only help to improve accuracy, but a complex problem is also decomposed into simpler sub-problems. The main theme of the ensemble model is that individual models can have their own biases/weaknesses; however, the ensemble model integrates their strengths and addresses weaknesses, leading to improved performance. The focus of ensemble learning is not solely on a set of algorithms but how multiple algorithms are integrated to create a strong learner. Finally, the predictions of all the models are averaged for the final prediction (Krawczyk et al., 2017).

Healthcare has found multiple applications with the computing paradigms, namely, CC and FC. In the healthcare sector, where data is collected across various IoT-enabled devices, FC provides a critical paradigm for effectively processing information. Compared to cloud-based data centers, the latency, delay, or response time attained via FC permitted devices to handle cardiac patients' data is considerably shorter due to the close placement of these gadgets to IoT-enabled devices. Healthcare applications tend to generate immense data and to get valuable insights into various machine learning algorithms come into play. In addition to ML, deep learning is also in demand for analyzing large chunks of data obtained from electronic health records, medical pictures, and sensor data from wearable devices.

Several works have been attempted to address healthcare ailments, although heart diseases have also been profoundly discussed. Further among the works, IoT-based remote health monitoring has also been the prime focus. (Gia et al., 2017) put forth a lower cost solution for health monitoring model to obtain the health information of multiple patients having heart diseases. This solution utilizes and analyzes electrocardiography (ECG) for automatic diagnosis. In addition to the ECG, the solution also utilizes respiration rate and body temperature while considering fog layer and sensor nodes with a focus on energy minimization, getting automatic diagnosis of heart diseases. Gill et al. (2018) proposed a fog-based healthcare model for effectively managing heart diseases emanating from IoT devices. The proposed model includes resource management using fog nodes, data capture through IoT nodes acting as fog nodes, and using iFogSim toolkit to evaluate its performance. He et al. (2017) proposed a healthcare model which includes fog/cloud and sensor layer for complex event processing (CEP) for the personalized service for improvement in resources wastage and response time. Additionally, the model proposed is termed FogCepCare which includes optimizations for partitioning, clustering, and parallel processing to optimize the cloud/FC. Ali and Ghazal (2017) proposed an e-health IoT-based service utilizing SDN for real-time heart disease detection service through various controls of gesture and voice with the usage of smartwatches. The proposed real-time heart attack mobile detection service (RHAMDS) is intended to avoid vehicular collision through heart attack detection and was targeted to address road safety and traffic engineering. A framework Edge-of-Things Computation (EoTC) was proposed by Alam et al. (2019) to reduce the expenses pertaining to processing for services related to healthcare. The proposed methodology utilizes multiple virtual machines (VMs) and a distributed provisioning mechanism utilizing alternating direction method of multipliers (ADMMs) for suitable processing of healthcare data. With respect to results, EoTC framework outperforms the greedy method; however, it does take QoS criteria into account for evaluation. Another framework termed service level agreement (SLA) healthcare big data analytics (SLA-HBDA) was proposed by Sahoo et al. (2018) which utilizes integrated stream/batch data for healthcare predictive analysis. SLA-HBDA does not account for quality-of-service (QoS) delay; however, the proposed method performs better in terms of precision as compared to the Naive-Bayes (NB). Another promising model was proposed by Akrivopoulos et al. (2017), to lower storage, power consumption, and data transfer to-and-fro pertaining to ECG signal which enabled the detection of abnormal signals. Results of the proposed model show substantial improvements in key performance indicators like power consumed and abnormal event detection in ECG signals. Real-time heart disease detection was proposed by Azimi et al. (2018) having a hierarchical computing architecture (HiCH) leveraging convolutional neural networks (CNN) utilizing ECG signals. This HiCH model is utilized to outsource the decision-making process to the edge-based networks shifting the higher computing tasks to the cloud. Smart e-Health gateway was proposed by Rahmani et al. (2018) and utilized an intelligent layer between cloud and sensor nodes termed geo-distributed intermediary layer. Validation of the proposed model is done by IoT-enabled early warning score (EWS) application for healthcare. Consequently, the IoT-based application's availability is greatly enhanced by local decision-making in the event of poor Internet access or connection loss. Furthermore, both the learning algorithm's performance in a fully centralized CC core and its performance (e.g., accuracy) are maintained in this hierarchical architecture. Tuli et al. (2020) proposed a HealthFog-based model for real-time automatic heart disease analysis which combines ensemble deep learning at the edge level. The proposed model was delivered as a fog service which was evaluated in terms of bandwidth, latency, jitter, QoS, and accuracy and thus shows improvement as compared to the state-of-the-art.

Mostly the existing literature has focused on automatic detection leveraging IoT devices integrating Cloud-Fog paradigms. Although HealthFog is better in terms of several parameters but since heart disease imperatively requires detection at apt time, FC has a suitable latency that needs to be addressed. Additionally, since multiple paradigms are used for detection, a better use case of detection is federated model due to the convergence of multiple linear models to form a global model. Thus, this work presents a use-case on how to blend MC with FC and CC and leveraging federating learning with an ensemble model while also improving the network through several paradigms.

19.3 Components of the Integrated MistFog Model

The proposed integrated MistFog consists of the following: sensor-based devices, IoT sensors, gateway devices, mist broker nodes, and fog worker nodes. Figure 19.3 describes the following architecture of the MistFog architecture. The details of each of the following components are defined as follows:

1. **Sensor network**: In this architecture, multiple types of body sensors and wearable devices are used. The different types of sensors used are environmental, medical, activity, and smartwatches. They monitor a person's vital data such as blood pressure, heart rate, oxygen level, and glucose level.

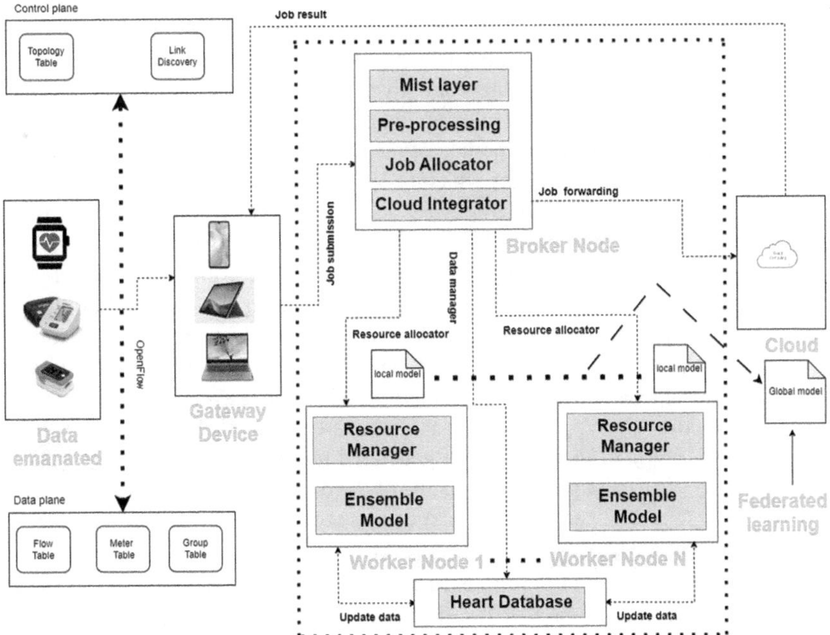

FIGURE 19.3 Architecture of the proposed MistFog model.

These components are utilized to retrieve and transfer data from the heart (data emanated) to the rest of the architecture's devices/module.

2. **Gateway devices**: Gateway devices are the recipients of the data from the sensor network. They act as the middleman for the sensors and the operational nodes. These serve as a data transmission bridge, allowing meaningful interpretation of the data. The gateway devices include laptops, smartphones, and tablets.
3. **Integrated MistFog model**: The integrated MistFog model comprises the following components:
   a) **Broker nodes**: This is the node that receives input data and the job requests supplied from the gateway device. This node includes several software components each with different functionality. The mist layer acts as the intermediate between where the data is generated and the data where it is processed (fog layer and cloud). This layer performs pertinent functionalities like data pre-processing and acts as a job allocator to the rest of the components. In data pre-processing, the heart dataset is fetched and all the sensor parameters are segregated to X coordinate and target variable to Y coordinate for fitting of the values in the machine learning algorithm. So, data pre-processing implies the segregation of data coordinates into X and Y. Further, the job is allocated by this module and is divided into a few tasks and is assigned to the number of worker nodes that use decentralized data and thus follows a federated learning approach to machine learning (Bonawitz et al., 2019). The data splitting is also handled by this module and hence this node acts as a fog orchestrator of the entire system. Since the healthcare data arrives in a streaming fashion, thus the model utilizes federated learning.
   b) **Worker nodes**: The job-allocated module divides the entire job into multiple tasks. These tasks are given as an input to the worker nodes. These tasks are allocated using the resources allocator and executed by the resource manager module of the worker nodes. These worker nodes also act as the fog nodes which execute the tasks. The worker nodes are either like the embedded devices like Raspberry Pi's or the nodes with less computing power. These resource modules might include storage for processing, sharing, and generating results for the data forwarded. The ensemble module is a part of the worker node and uses multiple machine learning algorithms (random forest, decision tree, and logistics regression) for the prediction of heart diseases. Further, this module is also capable of receiving results from other nodes and applies voting on whether the supplied data of the patient has a disease or not. After the processing of data, the result generated might be shared with the gateway devices to predict the results of the data. This approach of learning is a decentralized type and is known as the federated learning approach.
   c) **Cloud**: Sometimes the entire system is unable to process a large quantum of tasks and the infrastructure is unable to address such requirements. In such cases, CC can play a vital role in handling the higher

quantum of tasks. Although this module possesses a higher degree in terms of computing power, it comes at the expense of higher latency from the data emanated. This module will ensure the entire system to be made more robust and fault-tolerant and has added functionality of executing heavy tasks. Finally, the results are pushed to the cloud.

4. **Network paradigm**: As aforesaid, healthcare data has stringent network requirements. The use of multiple paradigms (cloud/fog/mist) requires a huge transfer of data from worker nodes for assimilating the global model obtained from the local model. The local model obtained from the worker nodes needs to be pushed towards the cloud. This huge transfer of data might become a bottleneck and might affect the execution time and the accuracy of the model. SDN is a promising model which addresses network requirements in an agile manner. SDN enables the decoupling of data and control planes. SDN executes a fine-grained policy based on the network global visibility from the controller (Hussain et al., 2021a, 2021b, 2021c). The controller enables huge transfer of data through and meets deadlines by creation of a special entry in the flow table and meter table.

19.4 Mathematical Analysis

Consider a network comprising gateway devices, fog nodes which act as a broker node and worker nodes. The various notations and the symbols are given in Table 19.1. In HealthFog (Tuli et al., 2020), the communication is the summation of moving the data from the gateway device to the broker node. From the broker node, multiple tasks are divided and sent to the multitude of worker nodes. The worker nodes obtain the data from the gateway devices. Thus, the communication cost is interpreted as

1. Communication cost of sending the data from the gateway device to the broker node

$$= T_x * F_c \tag{19.1}$$

2. Communication cost required to obtain the task data by the worker node from the gateway devices

$$= \left(F_c + 1\right)\frac{\sum_{i=1}^{n} W_i}{\sum_{i=1}^{x} T_i} \tag{19.2}$$

3. The total communication cost required to complete the job in HealthFog

$$= T_x * F_c + \left(F_c + 1\right)\frac{\sum_{i=1}^{n} W_i}{\sum_{i=1}^{x} T_i} \tag{19.3}$$

TABLE 19.1

Symbol Table Used.

S. No.	Symbol	Meaning
01	T_x	"x" number of tasks of the job
02	F_c	Communication cost required for moving data for each task to the fog broker node
03	M_c	Communication cost required for moving data for each task to the mist broker node
04	W_n	"n" number of worker nodes used in the network

In MistFog, the mist broker node obtains the data from the gateway device and acts as the forwarding device to the worker nodes. Thus, the communication cost is interpreted as

1. Communication cost required to obtain the job data by the mist node from the gateway device

$$-T_x * M_c \tag{19.4}$$

2. Communication cost required to obtain the task data by the worker node from the mist broker node

$$= F_c \frac{\sum_{i=1}^{n} W_i}{\sum_{i=1}^{x} T_i} \tag{19.5}$$

3. The total communication cost for the job completion in MistFog

$$= T_x * M_c + F_c \frac{\sum_{i=1}^{n} W_i}{\sum_{i=1}^{x} T_i} \tag{19.6}$$

Subtracting (19.6) from (19.3), we get

$$= T_x * F_c + (F_c + 1) \frac{\sum_{i=1}^{n} W_i}{\sum_{i=1}^{x} T_i} - \left(T_x * M_c + F_c \frac{\sum_{i=1}^{n} W_i}{\sum_{i=1}^{x} T_i} \right)$$

$$= T_x * F_c + (F_c + 1) \frac{\sum_{i=1}^{n} W_i}{\sum_{i=1}^{x} T_i} - T_x * M_c - F_c \frac{\sum_{i=1}^{n} W_i}{\sum_{i=1}^{x} T_i}$$

$$= T_x * F_c - T_x * M_c + (F_c + 1) \frac{\sum_{i=1}^{n} W_i}{\sum_{i=1}^{x} T_i} - F_c \frac{\sum_{i=1}^{n} W_i}{\sum_{i=1}^{x} T_i}$$

$$= T_x * \left(F_c - M_c\right) + F_c \frac{\sum_{i=1}^{n} W_i}{\sum_{i=1}^{x} T_i} + \frac{\sum_{i=1}^{n} W_i}{\sum_{i=1}^{x} T_i} - F_c \frac{\sum_{i=1}^{n} W_i}{\sum_{i=1}^{x} T_i}$$

$$= T_x * \left(F_c - M_c\right) + \frac{\sum_{i=1}^{n} W_i}{\sum_{i=1}^{x} T_i} \tag{19.7}$$

Since $F_c >> M_c$ and the other term, $\frac{\sum_{i=1}^{n} W_i}{\sum_{i=1}^{x} T_i}$ is positive, so it can be established that the communication cost is HealthFog which is much more than MistFog and hence the performance will be substantially improved.

19.5 Conclusion

This chapter addresses the pertinent issue of real-time heart disease detection utilizing novel paradigms of computing, network, and ML models. A novel MistFog model is proposed which aims to automatically predict heart diseases in real-time with better accuracy, improving execution time while capturing data through IoT/wearable devices. The worker nodes termed fog nodes locally predict the disease which are further integrated to form a global model at the cloud which in continuity improves the accuracy. Further a proof concept of MistFog model is proposed and is also compared with other models in terms of the network communication which shows its efficacy. Further, MistFog model needs to be analyzed experimentally with other prediction models and is treated as a future work.

Acknowledgment

The author acknowledges the support of Ms. Mahak Qayoom, Research Scholar, Amity Institute of English Studies and Research, Amity University, Noida, Uttar Pradesh, India, for eliminating typos and thoroughly proofreading several sections of this chapter.

REFERENCES

Akrivopoulos, O., Amaxilatis, D., Antoniou, A., & Chatzigiannakis, I. (2017). Design and Evaluation of a Person-Centric Heart Monitoring System over Fog Computing Infrastructure. *Proceedings of the First International Workshop on Human-Centered Sensing, Networking, and Systems*. https://doi.org/10.1145/3144730.3144736

Alam, Md. G. R., Munir, Md. S., Uddin, Md. Z., Alam, M. S., Dang, T. N., & Hong, C. S. (2019). Edge-of-things computing framework for cost-effective provisioning of healthcare data. *Journal of Parallel and Distributed Computing*, *123*, 54–60. https://doi.org/10.1016/j.jpdc.2018.08.011

Ali, S., & Ghazal, M. (2017, April 1). *Real-time Heart Attack Mobile Detection Service (RHAMDS): An IoT use case for Software Defined Networks*. IEEE Xplore. https://doi.org/10.1109/CCECE.2017.7946780.

Ashu, A., Hussain, M. W., Sinha Roy, D., & Reddy, H. K. (2020). Intelligent Data Compression Policy for Hadoop Performance Optimization. *Advances in Intelligent Systems and Computing, 80–89*. https://doi.org/10.1007/978-3-030-49345-5_9.

Azimi, I., Takalo-Mattila, J., Anzanpour, A., Rahmani, A. M., Soininen, J.-P., & Liljeberg, P. (2018). Empowering healthcare IoT systems with hierarchical edge-based deep learning. *Proceedings of the 2018 IEEE/ACM International Conference on Connected Health: Applications, Systems and Engineering Technologies*. https://doi.org/10.1145/3278576.3278597.

Bonawitz, K., Eichner, H., Grieskamp, W., Huba, D., Ingerman, A., Ivanov, V., … & Roselander, J. (2019). Towards federated learning at scale: System design. *Proceedings of Machine Learning and Systems*, *1*, 374–388.

Gill, S. S., Arya, R. C., Wander, G. S., & Buyya, R. (2018). Fog-Based Smart Healthcare as a Big Data and Cloud Service for Heart Patients Using IoT. *International Conference on Intelligent Data Communication Technologies and Internet of Things (ICICI) 2018*, 1376–1383. https://doi.org/10.1007/978-3-030-03146-6_161.

He, S., Cheng, B., Wang, H., Huang, Y., & Chen, J. (2017). Proactive personalized services through fog-cloud computing in large-scale IoT-based healthcare application. *China Communications*, *14*(11), 1–16. https://doi.org/10.1109/cc.2017.8233646.

Hussain, M. W., Pradhan, B., Gao, X. Z., Reddy, K. H. K., & Roy, D. S. (2020a). Clonal selection algorithm for energy minimization in software defined networks. *Applied Soft Computing*, *96*, 106617. https://doi.org/10.1016/j.asoc.2020.106617.

Hussain, M. W., Reddy, K. H. K., Rodrigues, J. J. P. C., & Roy, D. S. (2020b). An Indirect Controller-Legacy Switch Forwarding Scheme for Link Discovery in Hybrid SDN. *IEEE Systems Journal*, *15*(2), 3142–3149. https://doi.org/10.1109/jsyst.2020.3011902.

Hussain, M. W., Reddy, K. H., & Roy, D. S. (2020b). A counter-based approach for reducer placement with augmented Hadoop rack-awareness. *Turkish Journal of Electrical Engineering & Computer Sciences*, *29*(1). https://doi.org/10.3906/elk-2001-106.

Hussain, M. W., Reddy, K. H. K., & Roy, D. S. (2021a). Resource Aware Execution of Speculated Tasks in Hadoop with SDN. *International Journal of Advanced Science and Technology*, *28*(13), 72–84. http://sersc.org/journals/index.php/IJAST/article/view/1282.

Hussain, M. W., & Sinha Roy, D. (2021b). Enabling Indirect Link Discovery Between SDN Switches. *Proceedings of the International Conference on Computing and Communication Systems*, 471–481. https://doi.org/10.1007/978-981-33-4084-8_45.

Hussain, M. W., Moulik, S., & Roy, D. S. (2021c). *A Broadcast Based Link Discovery Scheme for Minimizing Messages in Software Defined Networks*. IEEE Xplore. https://doi.org/10.1109/GCWkshps52748.2021.9681933.

Hussain, M. W. & Roy, D. S. (2022a). Intelligent node placement for improving traffic engineering in hybrid SDN. *Lecture Notes in Electrical Engineering*, *776*, 287–296. https://doi.org/10.1007/978-981-16-2911-2_31.

Hussain, M. W. & Roy, D. S. (2022b). A counter-based profiling scheme for improving locality through data and reducer placement. *Intelligent Systems Reference Library*, 101–118. https://doi.org/10.1007/978-981-16-8930-7_4.

Hussain, M. W., Khan, M. S., Reddy, K. H. K., & Roy, D. S. (2022c). Extended indirect controller-legacy switch forwarding for link discovery in hybrid multi-controller

SDN. *Computer Communications*, *189*, 148–157. https://doi.org/10.1016/j.comcom.2022.03.017.

Hussain, M. W. & Roy, D. S. (2023). Performance optimization strategies for big data applications in distributed framework. *Studies in Computational Intelligence*, *2*, 221–252. https://doi.org/10.1007/978-981-99-1482-1_10.

Hussain, M. W. (2024). Centralized traffic engineering in SDN for 6G networks. *Towards Wireless Heterogeneity in 6G Networks in Taylor & Francis CRC Press.* https://doi.org/10.1201/9781003369028

Krawczyk, B., Minku, L. L., Gama, J., Stefanowski, J., & Woźniak, M. (2017). Ensemble learning for data stream analysis: A survey. *Information Fusion*, *37*, 132–156. https://doi.org/10.1016/j.inffus.2017.02.004.

Li, L., Fan, Y., Tse, M., & Lin, K.-Y. (2020). A review of applications in federated learning. *Computers & Industrial Engineering*, *149*, 106854. https://doi.org/10.1016/j.cie.2020.106854.

Nguyen Gia, T., Jiang, M., Sarker, V. K., Rahmani, A. M., Westerlund, T., Liljeberg, P., & Tenhunen, H. (2017, June 1). *Low-cost fog-assisted health-care IoT system with energy-efficient sensor nodes*. IEEE Xplore. https://doi.org/10.1109/IWCMC.2017.7986551.

Pradhan, B., Hussain, M. W., Srivastava, G., Debbarma, M. K., Barik, R. K., & Lin, J. C. (2022). *A Neuro-Evolutionary Approach for Software Defined Wireless Network Traffic Classification*. IET Communications. https://doi.org/10.1049/cmu2.12548.

Rahmani, A. M., Gia, T. N., Negash, B., Anzanpour, A., Azimi, I., Jiang, M., & Liljeberg, P. (2018). Exploiting smart e-Health gateways at the edge of healthcare Internet-of-Things: A fog computing approach. *Future Generation Computer Systems*, *78*, 641–658. https://doi.org/10.1016/j.future.2017.02.014.

Reddy, K. H., Srivastava, G., Goswami, R. S. & Roy, D. S. (2023a). A hybrid optimized intelligent resource-constrained service scheduling for unified IoT applications in smart cities. *IEEE Transactions on Network and Service Management*, 1–1. https://doi.org/10.1109/tnsm.2023.3341296.

Reddy, K. H. K., Roy, D. S., Mishra, T. K., & Hussain, M. W. (Eds.). (2023b). *Handbook of Research on Network-Enabled IoT Applications for Smart City Services*. IGI Global.

Sahoo, P. K., Mohapatra, S. K., & Wu, S.-L. (2018). SLA based healthcare big data analysis and computing in cloud network. *Journal of Parallel and Distributed Computing*, *119*, 121–135. https://doi.org/10.1016/j.jpdc.2018.04.006.

Tripathy, S. S., Mishra, K., Barik, R. K., & Roy, D. S. (2022). A novel task offloading and resource allocation scheme for mist-assisted cloud computing environment. *Lecture Notes in Networks and Systems*, *431*, 103–111. https://doi.org/10.1007/978-981-19-0901-6_10.

Tuli, S., Basumatary, N., Gill, S. S., Kahani, M., Arya, R. C., Wander, G. S., & Buyya, R. (2020). HealthFog: An ensemble deep learning based Smart Healthcare System for Automatic Diagnosis of Heart Diseases in integrated IoT and fog computing environments. *Future Generation Computer Systems*, *104*, 187–200. https://doi.org/10.1016/j.future.2019.10.043.

Zhang, C., Xie, Y., Bai, H., Yu, B., Li, W., & Gao, Y. (2021). A survey on federated learning. *Knowledge-Based Systems*, *216*, 106775. https://doi.org/10.1016/j.knosys.2021.106775.

20

Energy-Efficient and Delay Tolerant Prediction of Heart Disease in IoT-Enabled Mist Computing Platforms

Subhranshu Sekhar Tripathy
Kalinga Institute of Industrial Technology, Bhubaneshwar, India

Biswajit Tripathy and Sujit Bebortta
Ravenshaw University, Cuttack, India

Umar Muhammad Modibbo
Modibbo Adama University, Yola, Nigeria

20.1 Introduction

One of the most critical global health problems that need new approaches to early detection and prognosis is heart disease (Verma et al., 2022). As cloud computing and Internet of Things (IoT) rise, there is an immense opportunity to solve problems more productively (Talaat 2022). The approach for improving the prediction and prevention of heart diseases discussed in this work is a state-of-the-art technology based on the integration of deep reinforcement learning (DRL) algorithms with mist computing within an IoT-based smart city environment (Islam et al., 2015; Reddy et al., 2023).

The treatment cost of heart disease in the modern healthcare environment compels an accurate and early prediction (Rahmani et al., 2018). Early diagnosis allows timely treatment and better outcomes of the patients (Rahmani et al., 2018). However, IoT devices found in a healthcare environment usually produce live data that may be beyond the capacity of traditional prediction algorithms. This problem needs to change the paradigm toward de-centralized more efficient methods of processing.

A decentralized approach to data processing can also be considered a possible solution offered by mist computing that is located as an intersection point between IoT and cloud computing. Mist computing solves problems with latency and bandwidth constraints through the localization of computing resources close to where data is produced (Vermesan and Friess, 2022, Xu et al., 2014, Alam et al. (2019). This architecture, in particular, which requires prompt decision-making and real-time monitoring, is favored for the healthcare industry (Jiang et al., 2014, Rahmani et al., 2018, Faust et al., 2018).

DOI: 10.1201/9781032631738-20

In this chapter, we employ DRL algorithms known for their ability to identify complex patterns and learn from sequential information. This aims to enhance the accuracy of cardiac disease prediction, scalability and overall efficacy by seamless integration of DRL with mist computing in an IoT environment (Tuli et al., 2019a, 2019b, Dietterich 2000, Wang et al., 2021). First, we ran various tests and conducted a number of analyses to assess the feasibility of our strategy and compare it with other popular cloud technologies. Thus, our initial results indicate that the processing overhead has been substantially minimized while prediction accuracy has significantly improved. All these improvements lower the latency and energy which are very vital components of timely serviceable healthcare delivery (Ali and Ghazal, 2017, Rajasekaran et al., 2019).

The combination of DRL, mist computing, and IoT represents a change that healthcare practices may influence. This leading-edge technology can revolutionize the patient care and significantly improve health outcomes by providing early diagnosis and intervention in cases of cardiac mortality. We discuss the technical details and results of our study in chapters to come, focusing on the enormous capacity this approach provides for revolutionizing cardiovascular illnesses forecasting.

20.1.1 Motivations

In the healthcare industry, edge computing and artificial intelligence (AI) are fast becoming popular technologies, especially in dealing with heart disease prediction and management issues among individuals using IoT systems. We can be involved in machine learning studies that bring together integer linear programming techniques in order to classify vast healthcare IoT devices generated data to make quick decisions (Constant et al., 2017; Rajkomar et al. 2018; Hussain and Roy, 2023, Hussain, 2024).

The integer linear programming model has been successfully used as a mathematical optimization method to solve various problems in decision-making. It helps define the boundaries and determine how they should be balanced against the goals such as simulation costs or realism. Integer linear programming which is a practical tool to optimize some decisions and resource allocation in the IoT environment of healthcare and reinforcement learning refer to a framework for understanding the real world in interactive perception.

The edge processing of load-off removing is just a fraction of how integer linear programming is utilized in the health field of IoT (Moosavi et al., 2016, Azimi et al., 2018, Alam et al., 2019). This method is set towards well-elaborated peripheral computing technologies, which can be used from the network edge as efficiently as possible. Its implementation occurred because the edge computing systems should answer the latency issue. In edge computing, data is processed at the source or close to it, this results in a reduction of the response time dramatically compared to traditional methods which require the transmission of data to cloud-based centralized services to process it (Verma et al., 2022, Abdelmoneem et al., 2019, Preden et al., 2015).

Nevertheless, the edge devices of the network also frequently lack performance, so resource management is critically needed (Dogo et al., 2019). Applying previous examinations as a tool for improvement of resource management can be exercised better through edge computing optimization techniques (Preden et al., 2015). The system can dynamically tune performance and, when workloads and computer resources fluctuate constantly, it would balance the jobs. These efficiency gains also result in user experience improvement (Dogo et al., 2019; Ketu and Mishra, 2022; Fazel et al., 2023).

Integer linear programming is utilized for edge computing where heart disease monitoring and prediction are done with goals of optimizing resource utilization, decreasing latency, and improving the system performance (Quy et al., 2022; Pallewatta et al., 2022). In this investigation, we present a perception-computing architecture in which decision-making nodes at the edge of the network determine whether to deal with the job locally, send it to a neighboring fog node, distribute it to another node, or send to the cloud (Kumari et al., 2022).

First of all, we will introduce a mathematical foundation for the offloading problem and will also employ effective ILP optimization techniques. We put forward the steps for a tiered method that ensures objectivity in the situation of local information insufficiency (Firouzi et al., 2022; Kar et al., 2023). Fog devices in this system, sometimes, accept tasks from the higher-level agents with an enlarged view of the whole system and thus contributing to faster decision-making (Mahmud et al., 2020).

Along with other factors, such as latency, energy usage, and network bandwidth, the task allocation in the suggested framework, which is based on ILP optimization technique, is optimized by taking into account the input of these factors (Gupta et al., 2017). With reduced energy usage from mist nodes and superior average in-service delay for healthcare activities, this method unveils an easy solution to the expediency of task scheduling in dynamic healthcare settings (Mahmud and Buyya, 2019).

The following is a summary of the main contributions made by this study:

- It is raised the next issue which defines the coordination of healthcare shifting from mist–fog–cloud layer. We will not only apply modern offloading methods but also achieve them by altering the task offloading tactics in real-time environment.
- Depending on their needs for continuous data streams, diverse healthcare applications are divided into four main groups. A unique mechanism is developed to move task offloading from the fog layer to the cloud based on the condition of the fog layer, and each application type is given an appropriate delay.
- When compared to three current state-of-the-art solutions, i.e., deep neural network (DNN), Q-learning network, and proposed DRL model, simulation results show that the proposed healthcare IoT strategy significantly reduces latency delay and energy consumption for job offloading. In the age of IoT and edge computing, our discovery paves the path for more effective and responsive cardiac disease prediction and management.

20.1.2 Objectives and Contribution

- Create a deep learning ensemble technique that integrates with a large framework architecture to support the processing of collected data by mist and fog.
- The DRL framework was developed to expedite the calculation of cardiac patient diagnostics by using the deep learning ensemble approach over the mist computing layer. To mimic the processing of relevant data, a system is

utilized that combines the IoT, fog computing, fog computing environment, and the cloud.

- To assess the efficacy of the DRL-based mist deployment, many performance criteria are employed. These include recall, accuracy, precision, energy efficiency, and transmission latency.
- By shifting computationally demanding tasks to cloud computing devices, we can swiftly disseminate critical healthcare data while easing the pressure on resource-constrained IoT sensors.

20.1.3 Organization

The remaining chapters are structured as follows: Section 20.2 deals with the background studies with a brief emphasis on the fog computing layer, cloud platform, mist computing, IoT perception layer, and application layer along with their functionalities. Section 20.3 deals with the features of the proposed framework used for obtaining crucial measures of performance such as usage of network bandwidth, energy consumption, and delay. Section 20.4 deals with simulation outcomes and experimental setup. Section 20.5 deals with the challenges of the proposed approach in real-world deployment. Section 20.6 deals with the conclusions and finally Section 20.7 presents the future scope to the research.

20.2 Background Technology

Computing technologies are essential for managing a variety of data types in the healthcare industry, from tiny datasets to large ones, as well as for supporting complex IoT applications (Mahmud et al., 2022). These technologies cover a broad range of functions, such as computing, storage, and communication (Fan et al., 2020; Hengst 2000). As a result, healthcare computer solutions have a different architectural foundation than conventional or specialized models. Healthcare-focused computing technologies' main goal is to offer a range of services that are specifically catered to the demands of healthcare applications. These tools comprise Serverless Computing, Infrastructure as a Service, Software as a Service, Platform as a Service, Mobile Backend as a Service, and Function as a Service, in addition to other functionalities. Particularly, these services are designed for the specific needs of healthcare applications, thus functioning ideally in the existing workflows and processes. The computer technologies' deployment models in healthcare could be public, private, or hybrid prototypes that combine public and private infrastructures (Xu et al., 2014; Mahmud et al., 2022; Tuli et al. 2019a).

The study of computing technologies in healthcare is one of the most important areas of study which attracts a lot of attention (Shen et al., 2007; Bebortta et al., 2020; Hussain, 2024). Many different computer architectures have been designed and put forth in recent times specifically for healthcare IoT ideas.

The section "Cloud, Fog, and Mist computing in connection to healthcare IoT applications" tackles fundamental structures of core computing technologies with an emphasis on Healthcare. The five layers of the classic architectural framework of the healthcare IoT ecosystem are perception, mist, fog, cloud, and application layers

(Jiang et al., 2014; Rajkomar et al., 2018; Fan et al., 2020; Zhao et al., 1999; Pallewatta et al., 2022). The medical setting architectural approach is illustrated in Figure 20.1.

20.2.1 IoT Layer

In the hierarchy of computing technologies purposely created for healthcare IoT applications, the layer for healthcare IoT resides in the top tier (Tripathy et al., 2023; Bebortta and Singh, 2022). This fundamental level, which is placed close to the exact healthcare environment as well as the end users, plays a significant role in the detection of physical items and data collection using the different kinds of smart devices and sensors supported by the IoT network (Hengst 2000; Hussain and Roy (2023).

In general, a wide array of gadgets generates data and this needs thorough work with these sensors installed for fitting into specific healthcare practices. Data fetching and offering to the higher architectural levels are the responsibility of this tier (Bebortta et al., 2023a; Bebortta et al., 2023b). This layer enables real-time data streams due to the possibility of dispersing intelligent healthcare devices and sensors across geographical boundaries (Talaat 2022; Rahmani et al., 2018).

20.2.2 Mist Layer

In the architecture of computing technologies for healthcare IoT applications, the second layer is composed of healthcare mist (Tripathy et al., 2023; Bebortta et al., 2023b). In particular, this layer has attracted the most urgent need for time-sensitive data processing that is an essential necessity in the healthcare industry. Mist computing environment even extends further to the interaction between healthcare sensors and actuator controllers, which lies fully within this cloud-like network level. The latter layer is concentrated on the rule-based preprocessing performed by means of

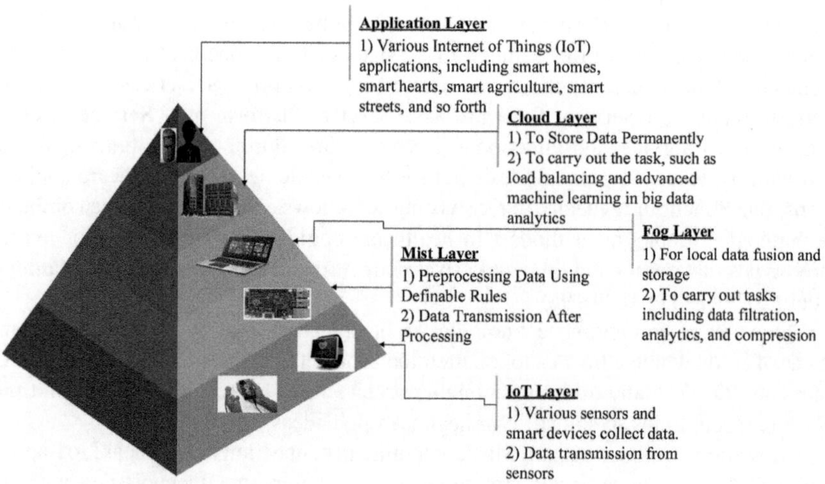

FIGURE 20.1 Layered architecture of computing technologies for IoT.

medical sensors. This preparation includes some important activities such as data filtering, aggregation of data, and fusion. While the bandwidth, memory, and power are modest, the healthcare layer can give a wide list of services. In the sphere of healthcare, this feature is a very important aspect of optimal usage and benefit from all the healthcare resources (Rajkomar et al., 2018; Shen et al., 2007; Tripathy et al. 2023c).

20.2.3 Fog Layer

The third essential layer inside the healthcare IoTs fabric of computer systems technology structure is the healthcare fog level. Critically, the responsibility of performing data processing from perception layer and pre-processed data from healthcare mist layer is underscored at this level. A healthcare fog network consists of several fog nodes situated at the network system boundary and provides functions at the healthcare fog level (Bebortta et al., 2023c; Tripathy et al., 2023a).

These fog nodes are distributed among different layers of the healthcare network infrastructure and comprise a wide variety of networking nodes such as routers, gateways, switches, access points, and servers dedicated only to this network type. The fog nodes can be of diverse dimensions including cloud-to-edge device connectivity which will facilitate the data traversal across the space. These fog nodes flawlessly unite with IoT healthcare smart devices on the edge network thus eliminating the need to transfer data to a centralized system. The healthcare fog can form a good interaction with the cloud layer which is a harmonious wave that will give the right storage and computing power when needed. In the healthcare sector, fog nodes contain the feature to offer a mix of services that are contractible and also have computational and storage support for static or dynamic working modes (Shen et al., 2007; Bebortta et al., 2020).

20.2.4 Cloud Layer

The fourth most vital segment in the meticulously designed layering of computing technologies for healthcare IoT applications is the healthcare cloud layer. It is well known for being a high-performance solution provider with hundreds of computing cores. An array of powerful computers which consist of considerable processing power, strong internet connection, extensive storage, and specialized data analytics tools are designed to be located in this layer.

The healthcare cloud layer is the base foundation for all major healthcare computing operations because of its ability to support a large storage capacity and execute resource-intensive calculations. It provides long durability as well as a variety of computation analyses which are selectively developed to satisfy the requirements of healthcare. The healthcare cloud layer constitutes an important element of the healthcare IoT architecture because it is the center of expertise for coordinating all interactions between the different levels easily. Moreover, the healthcare fog, mist, and application layers must be built on it as a key service provider. The healthcare cloud layer has been set up to immediately take on and execute computation-demanding operations when data processing power is higher than what the mist or fog layers can supply the same for a smooth data flow (Xu et al., 2014; Tripathy et al., 2023).

TABLE 20.1

A Comprehensive Tabulated of State-of-the-Art Studies

Articles	Study Domain	Issues	Problem Classification
Talaat (2022), Rahmani et al. (2018)	Application	Computational offloading in healthcare systems, performance evaluation	Waiting time, turnaround time, load balancing, early warning score, compression ratio
Rajkomar et al. (2018), Bebortta et al. (2020), Tripathy et al. (2023)	Management	Managing healthcare data, prediction using electronic health records	Area under receiver operating curve, precision, recall, F-measure, prediction accuracy
Bebortta and Singh (2022), Tripathy et al. (2023), Bebortta et al. (2023b)	Application	Offloading healthcare tasks in mist layer	Energy efficiency, latency, precision, recall, F-measure, accuracy, bandwidth utilization

20.2.5 Application Layer

The fifth and highest tier in the architectural arrangement of custom computing technologies for IoT applications in healthcare is the healthcare application layer. Social and economic benefits for the healthcare sector are achieved by this layer which works as a user interface between different healthcare stakeholders and the complexity of the computer system.

A vast range of services are provided to the healthcare IoT application and their associated members by the user-friendly user interfaces developed by the healthcare application layer. These healthcare-related apps embrace a broad-spectrum area, such as smart medical services, telemedicine, health monitoring, and also sophisticated medical services.

Healthcare application developers and end users may interact with the underlying healthcare fog and cloud layers without difficulty thanks to the crucial role the healthcare application layer plays in creating a direct line of communication. By ensuring that innovations and solutions in healthcare effectively reach their target audiences, this seamless connection helps improve healthcare services and results (Mahmud et al., 2022; Bebortta and Singh, 2022). In Table 20.1, a comprehensive account of the state-of-the-art work surveyed in this chapter along with their domain, issues, and problem classification is provided.

20.3 Features of Proposed Framework

20.3.1 Delay Model

As most jobs relating to a healthcare system are time-sensitive in nature and need on-time dispersion of the desired services, it is crucial to ascertain the delay of the system under consideration. Here, we treat the method for transferring control between the local computing network and the cloud computing node as a binary variable $\tau_j \forall j \in$ J which may be written as

$$\tau_j = \begin{cases} 0, \text{ locally compute} \\ 1, \text{ offload to mist node} \end{cases}$$

You may find out how long it takes to complete a job locally by using,

$$\tau_j^{\text{local}} = \frac{P_{tasks}}{f_j} \tag{20.2}$$

where $j \in$ J refers to the IoT device's CPU's processing frequency (f_j). However, if the job is delegated to the mist node, timing of the execution can be expressed as the ratio of the total duration of transmission τ_j^{Tx}, propagation lag τ_j^{prop}, waiting time τ_j^{q}, and task processing time τ_j^{exe} to the computational frequency of the mist nodes f_N, where

$$\tau_j^{mist} = \frac{\sum_{j \in J} \left(\tau_j^{Tx} + \tau_j^{prop} + \tau_j^{q} + \tau_j^{exe} \right)}{f_N} \tag{20.3}$$

20.3.2 Network Model

In the context of healthcare, we have proposed the concept of data transfer speed for fog node j as a critical metric in order to explain how communication flows within the healthcare IoT ecosystem. This rate signifies the speed at which healthcare data can be efficiently transmitted between fog node j and the healthcare cloud server, which holds paramount importance regarding the overall efficiency and productivity of the healthcare fog computing system.

$$T_j^{fog} = \text{Blog}_2 \left(1 + \frac{P_j^{tx} g_j^2}{N_0 B} \right) \tag{20.4}$$

The healthcare data transmission rate can be expressed as a function that considers various factors. Such factors like the connection factors such as the connection speed of healthcare fog node, the transmission power P_j^{tx}, and the wireless channel gain g_j for both the cloud server and the healthcare fog node as well as channel noise power spectral density indicated by N_0. With this trait, they together result in the transfer speed of data, for data exchange between the jth healthcare fog node and the central healthcare computer server, to be smooth while ensuring the optimum efficiency and reliability of healthcare information flow.

20.3.3 Energy Consumption Model

The energy requirement for the jobs that are passed on from the IoT device layer to the mist nodes changes with some crucial parameters such as the operation being performed and the frequency of the CPU. The local computing device energy utilization calculation can be done in the following manner (Bebortta et al., 2020):

$$\varepsilon_j^{loc} = \rho\left(f_j\right)^2_{\mathrm{p_{tasks}}} \quad (20.5)$$

The power coefficient of the chip's design is expressed by the symbol ρ in the equation above (20.5).

Furthermore, the amount of tasks that, n_{tasks}, would be offloaded may translated to the energy usage as the share of the tasks that will be transferred, i.e., s_{tasks}.

$$\varepsilon_i^{loc} = \rho\left(\mathrm{fj}\right)^2_{\mathrm{S_{tasks}}} \quad (20.6)$$

As a result, we ultimately determine the amount of energy used to offload jobs n_{tasks} as,

$$\varepsilon_j^{Tx} = \varepsilon_j^{loc} \times \tau_j^{Tx} \quad (20.7)$$

Figure 20.2 depicts the testbed setup for the proposed approach in a layered manner.

20.4 Simulation Results

20.4.1 Experimental Setup

We have presented a mist computing model for processing patients' data relevant to cardiac patients in the prior section of the study. In order to anticipate the development

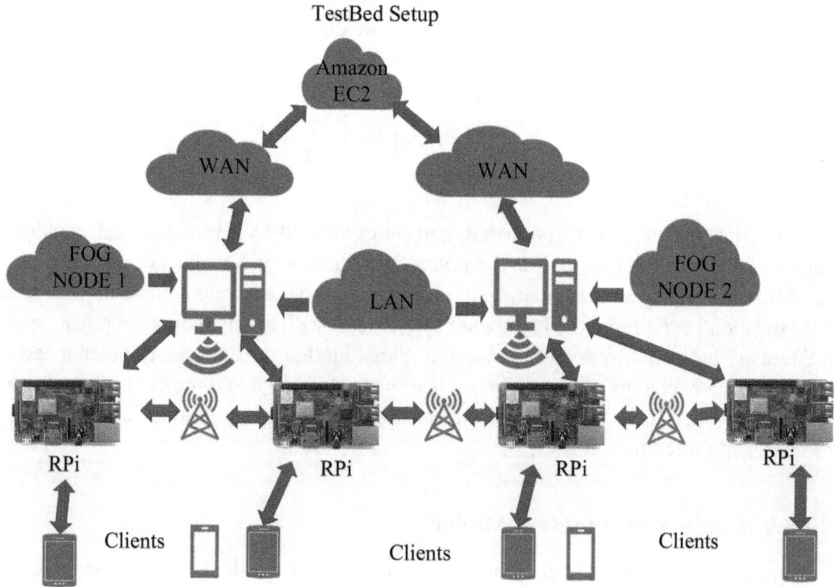

FIGURE 20.2 Testbed setup.

of cardiac disorders and evaluate the precision of these predictions, this model makes use of an intelligent DRL framework. The Cleveland heart disease dataset, which was extracted from 303 patient records, consists of 14 variables, to build on the framework established in reference (Alam et al. 2019). The 14 variables in this dataset include 13 different features as well as a goal attribute intended to show the frequency of heart illnesses in patient records. A result of "1" specifically indicates the existence of cardiac disease, while "0" indicates the absence of this ailment. The 13 elements include information gathered from non-invasive clinical investigations, as well as patient demographics like age and gender. The target attribute, which is essential to our inquiry, is derived from invasive coronary angiograms and encoded as "0" for the absence of heart disease and "1" for its existence. It is crucial to emphasize that Robert Detrano, a member of the Cleveland Clinic Foundation, put a lot of effort into gathering the data.

In this phase of our research, using DRL in an IoT environment powered by mist computing, we conduct a number of rigorous tests to assess the efficacy of our proposed algorithm for heart disease identification. Comparative analysis in the field of heart disease detection is the topic of our first project. We make use of the previously described Cleveland heart disease dataset to simplify the training and testing of our neural network. We classify cases in this dataset according to whether or not patients have cardiac disease, taking into account various age groups and gender. The information also includes four types of chest discomfort: non-anginal discomfort, atypical angina, classic angina, and people who are asymptomatic. Additionally, the results of the resting electrocardiogram (ECG) are divided into three categories: "0" for normal, "1" for an aberrant ST-T wave, and "2" for possible or certain enlarged left ventricle. The slope of the peak workout ST section is another categorization factor and is divided into three categories denoted by the numbers "1," "2," and "3." These numbers represent an upward, horizontal, or downward slope on the ST section graph, accordingly. The dependent variable, which is used to calculate the incidence of cardiovascular illness, is encoded as "0" when any major blood artery has a narrowing of less than 50% and "1" when the narrowing is greater than 50%.

Our method, which is specifically adapted for an IoT environment based on mist computing and supported by the capabilities of DRL, performs well in the domain of heart disease detection, and this full experimental approach allows us to thoroughly examine this performance.

In Figure 20.3, we present a thorough comparison of training accuracy when using the dataset of heart illness, taking into account various numbers of mist computing nodes for three different approaches: DNN, Q-learning, and our suggested DRL method. This work explains how the models' performance alternates with the number of mist nodes. Our findings support a recurring pattern: the accuracy rate goes up as the number of nodes exceeds the threshold. Every node actively learns from the heart disease data it receives for training, which accounts for this improvement. Additionally, as the network grows to include more mist nodes, each node has the chance to benefit from the combined learning experiences of its forerunners. Reason being, models have a tendency to adjust to the sample training data based on the cumulative knowledge supplied by earlier mist nodes, training performance of the models slowly improves across subsequent cycles over the training dataset. It is also noteworthy that across all occurrences of mist nodes in the network, our proposed DRL strategy consistently outperforms both the DNN and Q-learning methods. This improved performance highlights the effectiveness of our DRL technique for heart disease detection in an IoT environment powered by mist computing.

Our investigation is strengthened by Figure 20.4, which shows how testing accuracy changes as the quantity of mist computing nodes rises. It should be mentioned that every mist node only receives a small portion of the training information, which restricts its capacity to accurately replicate the suggested model. As a result of the limitations on individual node learning capacities, testing accuracy decreases as the number of nodes grows. However, compared to both the DNN and Q-learning approaches, our suggested DRL approach consistently outperforms them, displaying a significant advantage. This consistent improvement in performance highlights the

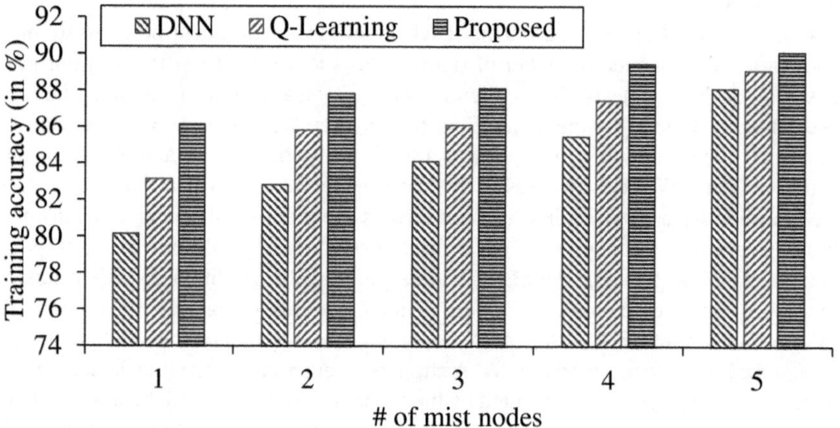

FIGURE 20.3 Evaluation of training accuracy in % for DNN, Q-learning, and proposed DRL framework over different numbers of mist computing nodes.

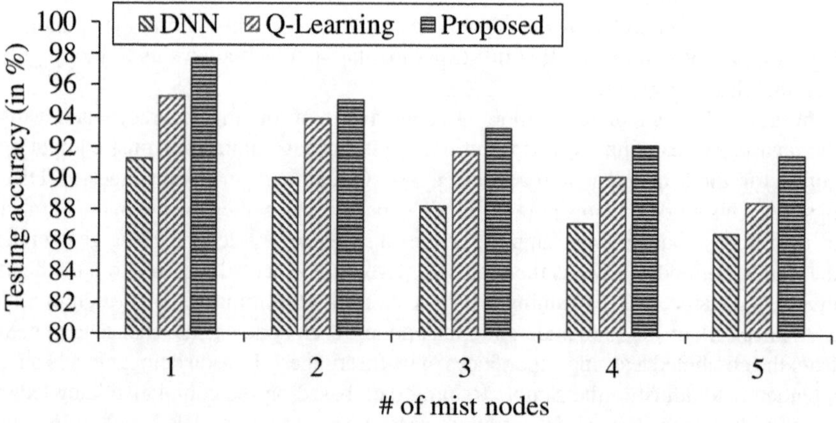

FIGURE 20.4 Comparison of testing accuracy in % for DNN, Q-learning, and proposed DRL framework over different numbers of mist computing nodes.

flexibility and efficacy of our suggested DRL strategy, even in circumstances where the dataset is dispersed among an increasing quantity of mist nodes within the network.

20.4.2 Evaluation of Different Computing Platforms

The extended interactions between components of multiple layers present in our mathematical model reflect the issue that has been widely discussed. In order to implement this conceptual framework, we took advantage of the iFogSim simulation platform that was built in detail using Netbeans IDE (Gupta et al., 2017; Mahmud and Buyya, 2019). The modular structure of our simulation lies in iFogSim since it relies on well-crafted classes written in the Java programming language for translating our ideal system into a computational model. This testbed on deep learning and Q-learning algorithms was also important in verifying the suitability of our proposed architecture. It was designed to perform as a testbed of the real world that was meticulously constructed about whether IoT apps work in an environment dominated by mist–fog–cloud.

The primary function of the experiment is that it allows different IoT gadgets to be connected effortlessly with gateway sensors, which means smooth transferring data from cloud servers through mist nodes and fog notes. In the scaling center of this system is the Broker layer, which governs resources and job start across multiple fog nodes. Significantly, the experimental testbed facilitates network teamwork rendering a suite of representational state transfer (REST) tasks enabled through HTTP RESTful APIs. A master node is necessary, via a local area network (LAN), to manage and control compute nodes as well as brokers through it. To make sure customer info is kept safe and private, each broker maintains a separate network. In the course of our research, we took advantage of iFogSim's capabilities to create a smart healthcare system. Different learning models were carefully applied to various brokers within this architecture. Within the IoT-mist network, these models were in charge of handling and processing shared data. It is important to highlight that interested readers are urged to study the thorough work written by authors in (Kumari et al., 2022), which gives a deeper exploration of the experimental setup and its possibilities, in order to gain a complete grasp of iFogSim and its delicate operational aspects.

Figure 20.5 provides a thorough investigation of the cloud, mist, and fog computing platforms' capabilities in the context of our suggested DRL model, with an emphasis on latency. This comparison accounts for the typical latency throughout a variety of communication rounds lying within. Notably, the outcomes show that the mist computing platform routinely outperforms its cloud and fog equivalents. In particular, mist computing achieves an impressive 4.5% average latency reduction when compared to fog, and an even more significant 14% reduction when compared to the cloud.

In Figure 20.6, the energy consumption is analyzed to compare the DRL architecture suggested by us in comparison with other possible approaches such as cloud computing layers. Based on the assessment, mist computing, involving a decentralized processing application shows superiority in terms of energy efficiency. Compared to fog computing, it shows a considerable decrease in average energy use of 3.85%. Compared to the cloud, it becomes obvious that significantly 17.45% of energy is saved when reducing the performance growth and therefore showing an imbalance between them.

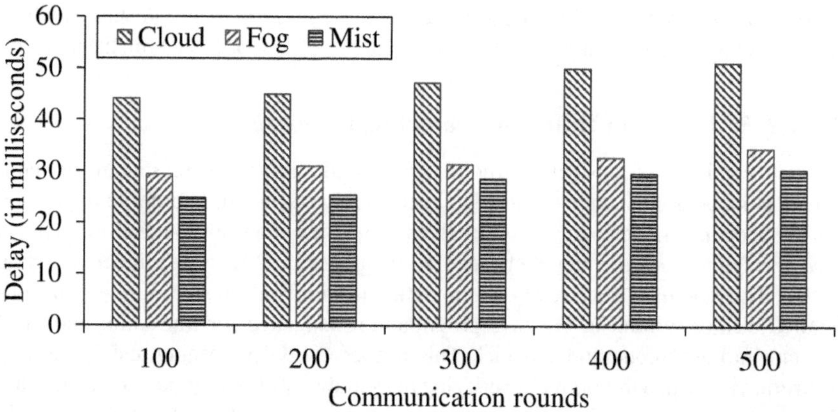

FIGURE 20.5 Comparison of delay in milliseconds for cloud, fog, and proposed mist framework over varying numbers of communication rounds.

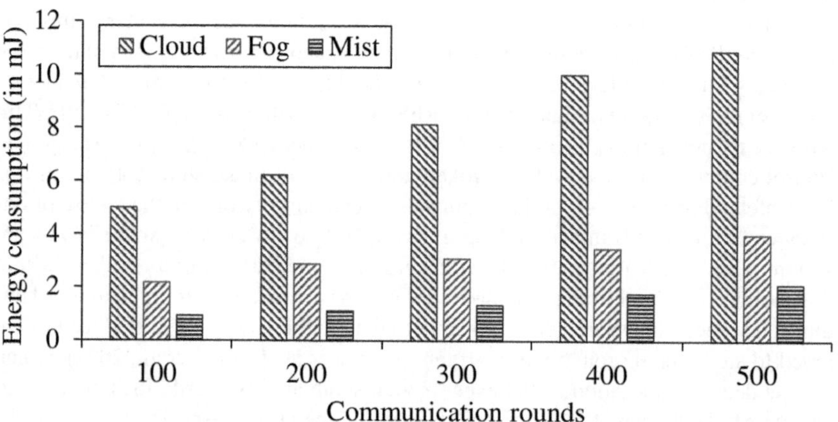

FIGURE 20.6 Comparison of energy consumption in milli-joules for cloud, fog, and proposed mist framework over varying numbers of communication rounds.

From Figure 20.7, we now shift our focus to network bandwidth where the functionality of cloud, fog, and mist computing platforms is evaluated in light of our proposed DRL architecture. The findings emphasize the greatest mists computing efficiency that persistently overcomes fog and cloud rivals. Compared to fog computing and cloud, the average network bandwidth deployed by the mist computing layer displays a noticeable decrease of 6.1% and an even more impressive decline at 10.5%, respectively, further increasing its lead over these two technologies

These performance assessments highlight the real advantages of the mist computing platform in our IoT ecosystem, which is especially designed for heart disease detection through DRL. Mist computing stands out as the best option because it excels in reducing latency, using less energy, and using network bandwidth prudently—all of

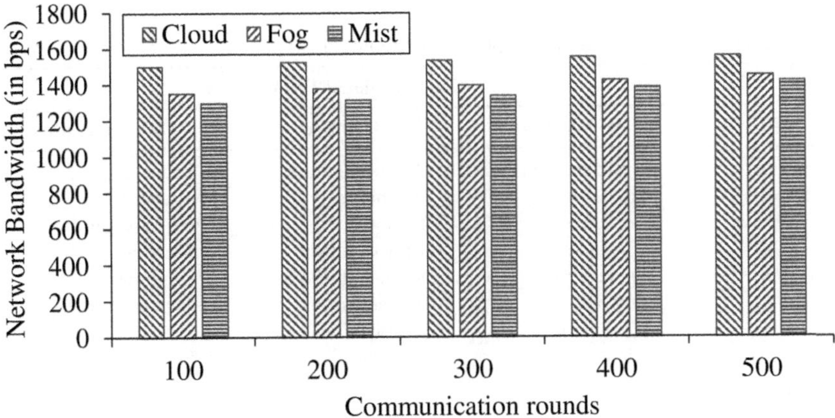

FIGURE 20.7 Comparison of network bandwidth in bits per second for cloud, fog, and proposed mist framework over varying numbers of communication rounds.

TABLE 20.2

Bandwidth and Latency Comparison

		Computing Frameworks		
		Cloud	**Fog**	**Mist**
Bandwidth (Mbps)	Up-link	1.91	81.42	90.15
	Down-link	2.07	100.39	109.42
RRT (milliseconds)		18.14	1.93	1.51

TABLE 20.3

Evaluation of the Computational Frameworks in the Context of a Healthcare Recognition Application

	Computational Frameworks		
	Cloud	**Fog**	**Mist**
Recognition time (in milliseconds)	3.58	3.57	3.55
Response time (Milliseconds)	743.54	163.13	143.89

which are crucial for assuring the effectiveness and efficiency of healthcare applications.

In Table 20.2, the bandwidth and latency comparison for the cloud, fog, and mist layer is presented. In Tables 20.3 and 20.4, the evaluation of the computational frameworks in the context of a health recognition application of the healthcare sector is presented. In Figure 20.4, an analytical comparison of different computing technologies is given. Finally, Table 20.5 provides a potential study of the computer systems based on the IoT.

TABLE 20.4

An Analytical Comparison of Computing Technologies

	Computational Technologies		
	Architecture	**Advantages**	**Disadvantages**
Cloud computing	• Utilizing central processing paradigms • Facilitating processing over the Internet • Built upon cloud agility	• Affordable storage capabilities • Simple to expand • Utilizes a global network driven by the Internet and robust TCP/IP protocol	• Reduced latency/ extended response time • Security vulnerabilities • High bandwidth expenses • Elevated power consumption • Concerns around data privacy and security on the Internet • Lack of offline support
Fog computing	• Based on the idea of decentralized computing • CISCO came up with it • Allow processing over the Internet • Brings the cloud to the edge of the network	• Allows for real-time data analysis • A faster response time • Keeps private information safe • Value for money • Natural to be scalable • It can be set up in private, public, or hybrid mode	• There are security issues • There are privacy and security issues with data over the internet • There are no offline supports
Mist Computing	• Allows light computing • Allows direct communication with the cloud • Stands in the middle of cloud and fog	• It can be used with both fog and mist computing platforms • It has a faster response time • Used to make local decisions • It's cost-effective in nature • It can be scaled up or down	• Problems with security • Problems with data privacy and security over the Internet • Only supports light computing

TABLE 20.5

A Potential Study of the Computer Systems Based on the Internet of Things

Requirements	Cloud Computing	Fog Computing	Mist Computing
Security	Chances are high	Not likely at all	Not likely at all
Communicating to each other (between the client and server)	A lot of hope	One hope	One hope

(*Continued*)

TABLE 20.5 (Continued)

Requirements	Cloud Computing	Fog Computing	Mist Computing
Cost of computing	Significant	Insignificant	Insignificant
Distribution by location	Located in one place	Located in multiple places	Located in multiple places
Delay for jitter	Significant	Insignificant	Insignificant
Waiting time	Significant	Insignificant	Insignificant
Awareness of location	No	Yes	Yes
Assistance with Mobility	Yes (but limited)	Yes	Yes
The number of service units	Insignificant	Significant	Significant
Area of service	Inside the Internet	At the network edge (local network)	At the network edge (local network)
How much power is used	Significant	Insignificant	Insignificant
Real-time support for communication	Yes	Yes	Yes
Protective measures	Can be defined	Can be explained	Can be explained

20.5 Challenges

1. Massive IoT data processing: Processing the enormous volumes of real-time data produced by IoT devices in healthcare settings is difficult because of its volume, velocity, and variety.
2. Latency and bandwidth constraints: When working with IoT-generated healthcare data, traditional prediction algorithms encounter latency and bandwidth issues that impede the timely transmission of crucial information.
3. Decentralized data processing: Logistical and technical issues arise from the requirement for decentralized processing to be moved closer to the data source, as suggested by mist computing.
4. Complex data patterns: Thus, predicting heart disease requires an understanding of complex patterns in the data because standard algorithms may find it difficult to deal with healthcare information due to their complicated nature.
5. DRL integration: By introducing DRL algorithms into the mist computing framework, issues related to training and fine-tuning these models for healthcare prediction applications are also presented.
6. Scalability: Some of the challenges associated with scalability include ensuring that there are capacities to scale up a system capable of handling an increasing amount of healthcare IoT data while preserving forecast accuracy.
7. Energy consumption: In order to prevent using more than the required energy, it is crucial to find a right harmony between the computational needs of DRL routines and IoT-dependent power-efficient processing.
8. Comparative evaluation: Also, there are problems with benchmarking and performance measurement in the case of testing or assessment for comparison between mist computing proposed DRL-based system versus other traditional methodologies based on cloud environment.

20.6 Conclusions

This study presented a deep mist framework to estimate the prevalence of heart disease for smart healthcare systems. The suggested framework was developed on top of the low latency, energy-efficient mist computing platform, and it made use of the DRL algorithm to aid prediction. The IoT device/application layer, mist layer, fog layer, and cloud layer were the four levels that made up the proposed architecture. With the highest prediction accuracy of 97.6714%, the proposed DRL algorithm quickly converges and exceeds the benchmark schemes addressed in this work, DNN and Q-learning, in terms of prediction accuracy, for training and testing sets over varying numbers of mist computing nodes. Further, the best performing algorithm suggested by the study, i.e., DRL was tested for different performance measures as discussed in this chapter like delay, energy consumption, and network bandwidth utilization over the cloud, fog, and mist computing layer. The simulations and data for making predictions conducted for this study make it clear that the suggested DRL algorithm fully satisfies the majority of QoS criteria for current healthcare systems.

20.7 Future Scopes

The potential for this research's future use is enormous:

- The integration of DRL with mist computing in healthcare IoT systems is anticipated to advance further as technology develops. Future research can concentrate on improving these systems' prediction capacities by creating more sophisticated DRL algorithms and maximizing their integration with mist computing. This might result in the very accurate and timely prediction of numerous health issues, including heart illnesses, allowing for proactive healthcare measures.
- Scaling the capacity of mist computing systems will be important for handling vast quantities of data in healthcare. The standardization of protocols and frameworks for interoperability between researchers and developers will bring together various IoT devices under the umbrella of cloud platforms. Therefore, healthcare professionals will have access to IoT and mist computing without compromising the clinical integrity of patient data.
- Possible apps in the future would focus on developing individualized health plans for each patient. What is more, AI and DRL algorithms can make personalized medicine possible. They would build systems that not only detect diseases but also recommend treatment plans tailored to a person's specific health information, genetics, and habits.
- With the help of advanced technology in healthcare setting, ethical considerations and moral issues will be more weighty. These issues should be looked into by future studies on data privacy, consumer consent, and the ethical implementation of AI in medicine. Apart from that safe data sharing frameworks are designed, measures to comply with healthcare regulations taken and the biases as well as fairness within algorithms of prediction are worked out.

REFERENCES

Abdelmoneem, R. M., Benslimane, A., Shaaban, E., Abdelhamid, S., & Ghoneim, S. (2019, May). A cloud-fog based architecture for IoT applications dedicated to healthcare. In *ICC 2019-2019 IEEE International Conference on Communications (ICC)* (pp. 1–6). IEEE, Washington, DC.

Alam, M. G. R., Munir, M. S., Uddin, M. Z., Alam, M. S., Dang, T. N., & Hong, C. S. (2019). Edge-of-things computing framework for cost-effective provisioning of healthcare data. *Journal of Parallel and Distributed Computing*, *123*, 54–60.

Ali, S., & Ghazal, M. (2017, April). Real-time heart attack mobile detection service (RHAMDS): An IoT use case for software defined networks. In *2017 IEEE 30th Canadian conference on electrical and computer engineering (CCECE)* (pp. 1–6). IEEE, Windsor, ON, Canada.

Azimi, I., Takalo-Mattila, J., Anzanpour, A., Rahmani, A. M., Soininen, J. P., & Liljeberg, P. (2018, September). Empowering healthcare IoT systems with hierarchical edge-based deep learning. In *Proceedings of the 2018 IEEE/ACM International Conference on Connected Health: Applications, Systems and Engineering Technologies* (pp. 63–68). Washington, DC.

Bebortta, S., Panda, M., & Panda, S. (2020, February). Classification of pathological disorders in children using random forest algorithm. In *2020 International Conference on Emerging Trends in Information Technology and Engineering (ic-ETITE)* (pp. 1–6). IEEE, Vellore, India.

Bebortta, S., & Singh, S. K. (2022). An intelligent framework towards managing big data in internet of healthcare things. In *Computational Intelligence in Pattern Recognition: Proceedings of CIPR 2022* (pp. 520–530). Singapore: Springer Nature Singapore.

Bebortta, S., Tripathy, S. S., Basheer, S., & Chowdhary, C. L. (2023b). DeepMist: Towards deep learning assisted mist computing framework for managing healthcare big data. *IEEE Access*.

Bebortta, S., Tripathy, S. S., Basheer, S., & Chowdhary, C. L. (2023c). FedEHR: A Federated Learning Approach towards the Prediction of Heart Diseases in IoT-Based Electronic Health Records. *Diagnostics*, *13*(20), 3166.

Bebortta, S., Tripathy, S. S., Modibbo, U. M., & Ali, I. (2023a). An optimal fog-cloud offloading framework for big data optimization in heterogeneous IoT networks. *Decision Analytics Journal*, *8*, 100295.

Constant, N., Borthakur, D., Abtahi, M., Dubey, H., & Mankodiya, K. (2017). Fog-assisted wiot: A smart fog gateway for end-to-end analytics in wearable internet of things. arXiv preprint arXiv:1701.08680.

Dietterich, T. G. (2000, June). Ensemble methods in machine learning. In *International Workshop on Multiple Classifier Systems* (pp. 1–15). Berlin, Heidelberg: Springer Berlin Heidelberg.

Dogo, E. M., Salami, A. F., Aigbavboa, C. O., & Nkonyana, T. (2019). Taking cloud computing to the extreme edge: A review of mist computing for smart cities and industry 4.0 in Africa. *Edge Computing: From Hype to Reality*, 107–132.

Fan, J., Wang, Z., Xie, Y., & Yang, Z. (2020, July). A theoretical analysis of deep Q-learning. In *Learning for Dynamics and Control* (pp. 486–489). PMLR.

Faust, O., Hagiwara, Y., Hong, T. J., Lih, O. S., & Acharya, U. R. (2018). Deep learning for healthcare applications based on physiological signals: A review. *Computer Methods and Programs in Biomedicine*, *161*, 1–13.

Fazel, E., Najafabadi, H. E., Rezaei, M., & Leung, H. (2023). Unlocking the power of mist computing through clustering techniques in IoT networks. *Internet of Things*, *22*, 100710.

Firouzi, F., Farahani, B., & Marinšek, A. (2022). The convergence and interplay of edge, fog, and cloud in the AI-driven Internet of Things (IoT). *Information Systems*, *107*, 101840.

Gupta, H., Vahid Dastjerdi, A., Ghosh, S. K., & Buyya, R. (2017). iFogSim: A toolkit for modeling and simulation of resource management techniques in the Internet of Things, Edge and Fog computing environments. *Software: Practice and Experience*, *47*(9), 1275–1296.

Hengst, B. (2000, August). Generating hierarchical structure in reinforcement learning from state variables. In *PRICAI* (pp. 533–543). Melbourne, Australia.

Hussain, M. W. (2024). Centralized traffic engineering. In *Towards Wireless Heterogeneity in 6G Networks* (pp. 180–193). CRC Press https://doi.org/10.1201/9781003369028

Hussain, M. W., & Roy, D. S. (2023). Performance optimization strategies for big data applications in distributed framework. In *Intelligent Technologies: Concepts, Applications, and Future Directions*, Volume *2* (pp. 221–252). Singapore: Springer Nature Singapore.

Islam, S. R., Kwak, D., Kabir, M. H., Hossain, M., & Kwak, K. S. (2015). The internet of things for health care: A comprehensive survey. *IEEE Access*, *3*, 678–708.

Jiang, L., Da Xu, L., Cai, H., Jiang, Z., Bu, F., & Xu, B. (2014). An IoT-oriented data storage framework in cloud computing platform. *IEEE Transactions on Industrial Informatics*, *10*(2), 1443–1451.

Kar, B., Yahya, W., Lin, Y. D., & Ali, A. (2023). Offloading using traditional optimization and machine learning in federated cloud-edge-fog systems: A survey. *IEEE Communications Surveys & Tutorials*, *25*(2), 1199–1226.

Ketu, S., & Mishra, P. K. (2022). Cloud, fog and mist computing in IoT: an indication of emerging opportunities. *IETE Technical Review*, *39*(3), 713–724.

Kumari, N., Yadav, A., & Jana, P. K. (2022). Task offloading in fog computing: A survey of algorithms and optimization techniques. *Computer Networks*, *214*, 109137.

Mahmud, R., & Buyya, R. (2019). Modelling and simulation of fog and edge computing environments using iFogSim toolkit. *Fog and edge computing: Principles and paradigms*, *1*.

Mahmud, R., Pallewatta, S., Goudarzi, M., & Buyya, R. (2022). Ifogsim2: An extended ifogsim simulator for mobility, clustering, and microservice management in edge and fog computing environments. *Journal of Systems and Software*, *190*, 111351.

Mahmud, R., Ramamohanarao, K., & Buyya, R. (2020). Application management in fog computing environments: A taxonomy, review and future directions. *ACM Computing Surveys (CSUR)*, *53*(4), 1–43.

Moosavi, S. R., Gia, T. N., Nigussie, E., Rahmani, A. M., Virtanen, S., Tenhunen, H., & Isoaho, J. (2016). End-to-end security scheme for mobility enabled healthcare Internet of Things. *Future Generation Computer Systems*, *64*, 108–124.

Pallewatta, S., Kostakos, V., & Buyya, R. (2022). QoS-aware placement of microservices-based IoT applications in Fog computing environments. *Future Generation Computer Systems*, *131*, 121–136.

Preden, J. S., Tammemäe, K., Jantsch, A., Leier, M., Riid, A., & Calis, E. (2015). The benefits of self-awareness and attention in fog and mist computing. *Computer*, *48*(7), 37–45.

Quy, V. K., Hau, N. V., Anh, D. V., & Ngoc, L. A. (2022). Smart healthcare IoT applications based on fog computing: Architecture, applications and challenges. *Complex & Intelligent Systems*, *8*(5), 3805–3815.

Rahmani, A. M., Gia, T. N., Negash, B., Anzanpour, A., Azimi, I., Jiang, M., & Liljeberg, P. (2018). Exploiting smart e-Health gateways at the edge of healthcare Internet-of-Things: A fog computing approach. *Future Generation Computer Systems*, *78*, 641–658.

Rajasekaran, M., Yassine, A., Hossain, M. S., Alhamid, M. F., & Guizani, M. (2019). Autonomous monitoring in healthcare environment: Reward-based energy charging mechanism for IoMT wireless sensing nodes. *Future Generation Computer Systems*, *98*, 565–576.

Rajkomar, A., Oren, E., Chen, K., Dai, A. M., Hajaj, N., Hardt, M., ... & Dean, J. (2018). Scalable and accurate deep learning with electronic health records. *NPJ Digital Medicine*, *1*(1), 18.

Reddy, K. H. K., Roy, D. S., Mishra, T. K., & Hussain, M. W. (Eds.). (2023). *Handbook of Research on Network-Enabled IoT Applications for Smart City Services*. IGI Global.

Shen, D., Chen, G., Cruz, J. B., Kwan, C., & Kruger, M. (2007, March). An adaptive Markov game model for threat intent inference. In *2007 IEEE Aerospace Conference* (pp. 1–13). IEEE, Bigh Monrana.

Talaat, F. M. (2022). Effective prediction and resource allocation method (EPRAM) in fog computing environment for smart healthcare system. *Multimedia Tools and Applications*, *81*(6), 8235–8258.

Tripathy, S. S., Bebortta, S., & Gadekallu, T. R. (2023c). Sustainable fog-assisted intelligent monitoring framework for consumer electronics in industry 5.0 applications. *IEEE Transactions on Consumer Electronics*.

Tripathy, S. S., Rath, M., Tripathy, N., Roy, D. S., Francis, J. S. A., & Bebortta, S. (2023a). An Intelligent Health Care System in Fog Platform with Optimized Performance. *Sustainability*, *15*(3), 1862.

Tuli, S., Basumatary, N., & Buyya, R. (2019a, November). Edgelens: Deep learning based object detection in integrated iot, fog and cloud computing environments. In *2019 4th International Conference on Information Systems and Computer Networks (ISCON)* (pp. 496–502). IEEE.

Tuli, S., Mahmud, R., Tuli, S., & Buyya, R. (2019b). Fogbus: A blockchain-based lightweight framework for edge and fog computing. *Journal of Systems and Software*, *154*, 22–36.

Verma, P., Tiwari, R., Hong, W. C., Upadhyay, S., & Yeh, Y. H. (2022). FETCH: a deep learning-based fog computing and IoT integrated environment for healthcare monitoring and diagnosis. *IEEE Access*, *10*, 12548–12563.

Vermesan, O., & Friess, P. (2022). European research cluster on the internet of things. In *Internet of Things-Global Technological and Societal Trends from Smart Environments and Spaces to Green ICT* (pp. 1–7). River Publishers.

Wang, Y., Nazir, S., & Shafiq, M. (2021). An overview on analyzing deep learning and transfer learning approaches for health monitoring. *Computational and Mathematical Methods in Medicine*, *2021*, 1–10.

Xu, B., Da Xu, L., Cai, H., Xie, C., Hu, J., & Bu, F. (2014). Ubiquitous data accessing method in IoT-based information system for emergency medical services. *IEEE Transactions on Industrial Informatics, 10*(2), 1578–1586.

Zhao, G., Tatsumi, S., & Sun, R. (1999). RTP-Q: a reinforcement learning system with time constraints exploration planning for accelerating the learning rate. *IEICE Transactions on Fundamentals of Electronics, Communications and Computer Sciences, 82*(10), 2266–2273.

Index

Pages in *italics* refer to figures and pages in **bold** refer to tables.

For Product Safety Concerns and Information please contact our EU representative GPSR@taylorandfrancis.com Taylor & Francis Verlag GmbH, Kaufingerstraße 24, 80331 München, Germany

Batch number: 10397790

Printed by Printforce, the Netherlands